Health Technology
Assessments by the
National Institute for Health
and Clinical Excellence

Innovation and Valuation in Health Care

Series Editor: **Michael Schlander**, University of Applied Economic Sciences; Institute for Innovation and Valuation in Health Care, Ludwigshafen and Eschborn, Germany

Health Technology Assessments by the National Institute for Health and Clinical Excellence: A Qualitative Study
Michael Schlander

Michael Schlander

Health Technology Assessments by the National Institute for Health and Clinical Excellence

A Qualitative Study

Forewords by Peter S. Jensen and Panos G. Kanavos

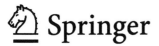 Springer

Michael Schlander
Institute for Innovation
and Valuation in Health Care
University for Applied Economic Sciences
Eschborn 65760
Ludwigshafen 67059
Germany

ISBN: 978-0-387-71995-5   e-ISBN: 978-0-387-71996-2

Library of Congress Control Number: 2007926599

Foreword I

The last decade has witnessed remarkable advances in children's mental health treatments, with evidence clearly demonstrating the efficacy of a number of treatments for conditions such as attention-deficit/hyperactivity disorder (ADHD), autism, anxiety disorders, and major depression (MTA Cooperative Group, 1999a; McCracken et al., 2002; Walkup et al., 2001; March et al., 2004). Unfortunately, even though a number of efficacious treatments have now been established, available evidence also suggests that most children with these conditions are not diagnosed (Leaf et al., 1996; Zuckerbrot and Jensen 2006). Even among the fraction (about one-third) who are diagnosed, most of these do not receive the high quality, effective forms of treatment demonstrated in research studies (MTA Cooperative Group, 1999b; Jensen et al., 2001b). "Usual care" is often minimally intense.

For these treatment research advances to be relevant in policy contexts, where various health needs essentially compete against one another for scarce dollars, they need to demonstrate "value for money." Thus, treatments must not only be shown to be efficacious, but also to be sufficiently effective in terms of dollars spent, so that policy-makers can justify this expense from the perspective of other benefits that could have been purchased with the same monies.

In the area of ADHD, the National Institute for Health and Clinical Excellence (NICE) recently completed a technology appraisal of ADHD, examining and comparing the major ADHD treatment options using cost-effectiveness analysis (NICE, 2006b).

While such efforts on the part of health care decision-makers are not just laudatory but increasingly essential, this relatively new area of health policy research, particularly in a relatively young field like child psychiatry, is rife with critical decision points, many of which could substantially change policy recommendations and, ultimately, children's health.

This monograph by Michael Schlander carefully dissects each of the steps of the NICE ADHD appraisal process, and notes a number of potential problems both within and outside the appraisal process itself, such as the small number of studies meeting inclusion criteria; chosen studies' heterogeneity in design (i.e., inclusion of efficacy and effectiveness studies without considering differences in such studies) and endpoints (clinical global ratings vs. narrow-band symptom scales); not adhering to originally agreed-upon search criteria; and critical omissions of specific studies and recently published or presented reports.

As Michael points out in this incisive critique, cost-effectiveness analyses almost always involve "implicit assumptions." This invariably means that thorny choices must be made by the study team. Such thorny choices, if not explicitly discussed and reviewed on their strengths and limitations by persons with a range of expertise – clinical, statistical, economic, and policy-relevant – will almost certainly generate substantial controversy. Some controversy is always likely, even when all necessary expertise is involved in the appraisal process, since economic decisions may be based on the final recommendations. But if this range of expertise is not present throughout, controversy seems inevitable. While the focus of this monograph is the NICE ADHD analysis and appraisal process, the careful step-by-step critique might be used as a guide for future appraisal processes, not just for NICE, but for all health care policy analysts as well.

PETER S. JENSEN
Ruane Professor of Child Psychiatry
Center for the Advancement of Children's Mental Health
Columbia University, New York, NY

Foreword II

In recent years there has been a proliferation of health technology assessment (HTA) initiatives internationally aimed at introducing rationality in the decision-making process and informing reimbursement decisions for the inclusion of new technologies in national reimbursement lists. The National Institute for Health and Clinical Excellence (NICE) in England and Wales stands prominently among these initiatives.

While efforts have been made for health technology assessments, and the resulting guidance to policy-makers, to adhere to an agreed upon process ensuring transparency, robustness and inclusiveness, in addition to scientific and analytical rigor, it may be the case that, occasionally, this process is less than optimal. The current study on Attention Deficit Hyperactivity Disorder (ADHD) in children and adolescents reviews the NICE appraisal process, confirms the transparent, inclusive and participatory nature of the appraisal, but identifies a number of inconsistencies in the assessment itself and problems in the way the evidence was presented. Having identified these shortcomings, the study at hand offers significant lessons for policy-makers, not only in England and Wales, but, given NICE's international standing, in other settings as well.

The first lesson is that processes are not infallible and continuous efforts are required to ensure not only procedural consistency, but also analytical rigor. Second, however well existing processes may work, there may be a need to define and have consensus on the precise parameters of technology assessments with all stakeholders in light of the available evidence base for a particular disease or therapy area. And third, the transferability of the results to other settings may also transfer the unintended inconsistencies of the original assessment.

While generalizations about the NICE appraisal model cannot be made simply by examining the process and evidence based on ADHD, the present study highlights certain shortcomings that should be addressed in order to improve even further HTA and its use in decision-making.

Professor PANOS G. KANAVOS
Senior Lecturer in International Health Policy
Head, Medical Technology Research Unit LSE Health
London School of Economics
London, UK

Preface

The present volume introduces a new series on "Innovation and Valuation in Health Care." This series of publications will scrutinize relevant health care issues and their implications for rational policy making. The series will primarily focus on themes related to public health issues and the economics of health care delivery.

The series starts with a critique of a recent National Institute for Health and Clinical Excellence (NICE) technology appraisal, evaluating therapeutic options for attention-deficit/hyperactivity disorder (ADHD) in children and adolescents and providing guidance on the use of medication.

During the past decades ADHD has emerged as one of the most common diagnoses in children and adolescents. ADHD is of particular public health interest, as many of the consequences of ADHD are of a social and economic nature, for example affecting academic and professional achievement of patients. In this respect, ADHD manifests as a behavioral disorder associated with substantial long-term sequelae. The principal evidence-based treatment options for ADHD are pharmacotherapy and psychosocial interventions. While these have been shown to be clinically effective, their impact on long-term outcomes remains to be established. Not surprisingly, the NICE assessment team faced a daunting task during this review, involving innumerable choices at various decision nodes.

Informed health care policy recommendations hinge on the availability of high-quality systematic reviews summarizing the available evidence. Great efforts towards transparency, reliability, and scientific rigor have been implemented by NICE to arrive at sound and economically valid health technology assessments. Using the example of the NICE appraisal of ADHD treatment strategies, the present monograph illustrates how an economic evaluation may nevertheless fall short of delivering relevant answers.

It is hoped that the exploration of issues potentially underlying the problems associated with this technology assessment may stimulate debate about the further improvement of appraisal processes. This should be of interest not only to professionals including physicians and other providers of health care, as well as policymakers beyond the United Kingdom, but also to patients (and their parents, in the case of children with ADHD).

Institutions commissioning and analysts authoring such technology reports are vested with particular responsibility for future health care delivery. At NICE, technology assessment reports greatly influence the outcome of the subsequent appraisal process. Many policy-makers and health care providers will digest only the guidance ultimately issued by NICE and the abstracts of systematic reviews, like those from the Cochrane Library. Hence, a balanced presentation of conclusions, highlighting limitations and future research needs, is of paramount importance.

Health technology assessments (HTAs) may contribute to improvements of health care delivery. In order to provide valid input to prioritization problems, the methods of HTAs should enable using the best currently available evidence, and their economic component needs to reflect social values. We hope that this series will stimulate the debate about appropriate public health and health care policy recommendations, notably including their economic underpinnings.

February 2007   MICHAEL SCHLANDER
                                   Professor of (Health Care & Innovation) Management
                                   Institute for Innovation & Valuation in Health Care;
                                   University of Applied Economic Sciences
                                   Eschborn and Ludwigshafen
                                   Germany

Acknowledgments

Perhaps, first of all the National Institute for Health and Clinical Excellence (NICE) should be recognized as an institution that has created sufficient transparency as to enable the present case study. In this respect, NICE clearly has set a new standard for organizations engaged in health technology assessments.

Then, I would like to thank numerous fellow health economists who discussed key findings of this case analysis when I first presented it at the Annual Meeting of the International Society for Pharmacoeconomics and Outcomes Research (ISPOR) in Philadelphia, May 2006. I am also indebted to three anonymous peer reviewers of *Current Medical Research and Opinion* who provided many constructive suggestions. The manuscript further benefited greatly from suggestions by Stuart Donovan, Ikeston, Derbyshire, and Andrew Terris, Heidelberg, Germany, who helped to eliminate some of those idiosyncrasies that German natives tend to produce when they use the English language to communicate. I am also grateful to the editors of *Current Medical Research and Opinion* who kindly gave their permission to use material that was published earlier in their journal.

The tranquility of Josef Schrott's secluded hideaway in Kohlern, high above Bozen, South Tyrol (Italy, also known as "Colle" above Bolzano, Sudtirolo/Alto Adige), provided an ideal environment to work on key components of the present text. I would like to thank Cornelia, as well as Hendrik and Matthias, for their extraordinary patience with their husband and father while I enjoyed my time reading and writing on shady places under the lime trees of Kohlern.

Summary

Results of Health Technology Assessments (HTAs) have become increasingly relevant to health care policy-makers worldwide. The National Institute for Health and Clinical Excellence (NICE) in England is widely regarded as a role model for the implementation of HTAs incorporating economic evaluation based on the logic of cost-effectiveness.

Beyond guidance on medical technologies to the National Health Service of England and Wales based on technology appraisals, NICE also issues clinical guidelines which are distinct from the HTAs in that their scope is usually broader, and in that development of the former is led by clinical experts, and the latter by economists.

The focus of this present report is the NICE appraisal process underlying its guidance concerning treatments for attention-deficit/hyperactivity disorder (ADHD) in children and adolescents, issued in March 2006.

ADHD is of particular interest as a test of the robustness of the NICE approach because it is associated with a number of descriptors that characterize a complex clinical decision problem.

Specifically:

- Prevalence estimates of ADHD vary depending on the population studied and diagnostic criteria used.
- ADHD is commonly associated with co-existing conditions, which include psychiatric comorbidities (such as "externalizing" symptomatology related to oppositional defiant disorder and conduct disorder, and "internalizing" symptomatology related to anxiety and depression) as well as a range of other psychiatric, neurological, and somatic disorders.
- International differences arise when different diagnostic criteria are used (e.g., DSM-IV in North America, and ICD-10 criteria in Europe) or when different standards of care and therapeutic preferences influence study designs, and this potentially confounds the interpretation of the results of studies across geographic boundaries.
- The diagnosis prevalence of ADHD appears to be increasing coincidently with increased awareness of this condition and the increased use of psychostimulants in many countries, which in turn has led to controversy about the putative overuse of these interventions in this population.

- The variety of assessment instruments used to measure clinical outcomes in ADHD, the inherent variability in calculating health-related quality of life (HRQoL) outcomes, alongside the emergence of new treatment options, many of which are associated with higher unit costs than earlier options, collectively exacerbate the difficulties of conducting HTAs of interventions in this condition.

The objective of the present report is to explore how NICE appraisal processes can accommodate these clinical complexities. To this end, a qualitative study was done of NICE Technology Appraisal No. 98, "Methylphenidate, atomoxetine and dexamfetamine for attention deficit hyperactivity disorder (ADHD) in children and adolescents (Review of Technology Appraisal 13)," published in March 2006. The data for this study consisted of all relevant technical documents produced by NICE (including meeting minutes and announcements) that were made publicly available (www.nice.org.uk). All key steps of the appraisal process were identified. In addition, a comprehensive review of the literature on ADHD treatment strategies was conducted.

The NICE appraisal process consists of three stages – "scoping," "assessment," and "appraisal," each of them offering defined opportunities for stakeholders to provide input into the evaluation process. A fourth component of the appraisal process is "appeal" by consultees when there are pre-defined grounds for doing so.

NICE had reported a first appraisal of the use of interventions for hyperkinetic disorder (ADHD per ICD-10) in October 2000. It recommended the use of methylphenidate as part of a comprehensive treatment program for severe ADHD.

NICE subsequently reviewed the evidence and in 2005 concluded that:

- Where drug treatment is considered appropriate, methylphenidate, atomoxetine, and dexamphetamine are recommended within their licensed indications.
- There are no significant differences between individual drugs in terms of efficacy or side effects – a conclusion derived as a consequence of paucity of evidence used for assessment.
- Given the limited data used to inform response and withdrawal rates, it is not possible to distinguish between the different strategies on the grounds of cost-effectiveness.
- If there is a choice of more than one appropriate drug, the product with the lowest cost should be prescribed.

In the underlying assessment, the economic model was, in the absence of identified effectiveness differences, driven by drug acquisition costs, and a treatment strategy had been recommended as "clearly optimal" that consisted of 1st line dexamphetamine sulphate, 2nd line methylphenidate hydrochloride (immediate-release formulations), and 3rd line atomoxetine hydrochloride.

The Final Appraisal Determination further stated that the decision about choice of intervention should be based on:

- The presence of comorbid conditions (e.g., tic disorders, Tourette's syndrome, epilepsy).

- The adverse event profile.
- Compliance issues (e.g., the need to administer a midday dose at school, and its associated implications).
- The individual preferences of the patient and/or parent/guardian.

Final guidance was published in March 2006, after an appeal had been dismissed, and reflected the Final Appraisal Determination. Clinical guidelines are in preparation.

Key aspects of the critique include the following:

Critique 1: Scoping

- Despite the documented importance of psychosocial interventions in ADHD, this remained beyond the scope of the NICE appraisal. This omission, therefore, precludes the evaluation of such interventions alongside drug therapy. Existing evidence was not used to its full potential. In contrast, the scope for clinical guideline development does encompass psychosocial treatment.
- Although part of the scope, the assessment failed to address the potential impact of diagnostic criteria and co-existing conditions on the clinical and cost-effectiveness of treatment strategies assessed.

Critique 2: Data selection by the Assessment Group

- The effectiveness review of the HTA focused on hyperactivity measures at the expense of other ADHD-defining core symptoms of inattention and impulsivity.
- One third of the studies selected for effectiveness review were <3 weeks treatment duration, in violation of inclusion criteria defined via the assessment protocol, which were introduced to ensure sufficient time to evaluate the impact of treatment on indicators of social adjustment.
- A number of high-quality, double-blind trials were either discounted or overlooked by the Assessment Group because they did not fit alongside a predetermined model.
- For the economic model, in order to enable QALY calculation based on clinical response rates, the most widely used ADHD-specific outcomes instrument – the group of Conners' scales – was not used by the Assessment Group. Instead, responders were defined by improvement of Clinical Global Impression (CGI) subscale scores, which are – besides their problematic psychometric properties – not exactly appropriate to provide normative information independent from baseline.
- The choice of the CGI-I (improvement) subscale as the primary outcome measure for cost-effectiveness evaluations by the Assessment Group substantially reduced the number of studies included in the economic analysis. Therefore, for one treatment modality (which was subsequently recommended for first-line treatment) a small-scale short-term study had to be added that had been excluded before for quality concerns.
- As ADHD is a chronic disorder, long-term treatment- and cost-effectiveness considerations are important. Yet, the Assessment Group evaluated studies of three to

eight weeks treatment duration, despite the availability of at least 15 randomized trials of ≥ 12 week treatment duration (although not all of these contained all of the elements selected for extraction by the Assessment Group, such as CGI-I data).

Critique 3: Efficacy, effectiveness, and the role of treatment compliance

- The Assessment Group did not address the wide-ranging issues surrounding the importance of the distinction between clinical efficacy and effectiveness.
- The assumptions made by the Assessment Group about the measurement and impact of non-compliance in ADHD remained a major issue throughout the appraisal. In effect, any clinical benefit potentially resulting from improved compliance was "assumed away" by the Assessment Group, without reference to the extensive literature on the subject.
- Artificially enhanced compliance in randomized clinical trials (RCTs) is an important confounder to their external validity in a "real world" setting. Reduced or non-compliance to stimulants in ADHD would likely manifest as a rapid return to symptoms. However, the potential implications of this were not considered in the NICE appraisal.
- This is important because data indicate that the majority of children with ADHD miss doses and/or do not refill prescriptions. Moreover, due to its PK/PD properties, methylphenidate is "unforgiving" of missed doses, and multiple dosing of immediate-release formulations throughout the day is required to maintain effectiveness. In addition, midday dosing may have social as well as compliance implications.
- Real-world evidence indicates that modified-release formulations of methylphenidate are associated with high response rates – perhaps as a result of reducing the non-compliance risk – a factor that was not adequately considered in the NICE appraisal.

Critique 4: Data synthesis across endpoints and studies

- Evidence remaining after selection of data for the primary economic analysis was insufficient to assess the relative value of alternative treatment approaches.
- In an attempt to overcome this shortcoming, the Assessment Group synthesized response rates across different effectiveness measures, and used the statistical mixed treatment comparison (MTC) technique to facilitate the integration of both direct and indirect evidence.
- To broaden the dataset available for analysis, the Assessment Group imported data from additional trials that reported different outcome measures (derived from clinical global impressions and narrow-band symptom scales). This raises important questions about the potential for the use of heterogeneous outcome measures to confound the conclusions.
- Although the use of meta-analyses is a well-accepted approach, the validity of this approach is a function of the internal validity and similarity of the trials to be included and assumes that relative treatment effects will be the same across trials. In the present ADHD assessment, this approach necessarily concealed effects of enhanced compliance associated with long-acting medications, including but

not limited to modified-release formulations of methylphenidate, in real-world settings, thus introducing a bias against this group of medications.

- In the NICE appraisal, there were multiple sources of potential bias relating to the small number of studies selected, wide variations in patient numbers between selected studies, short observation periods, heterogeneity of studies (including heterogeneous populations, study designs and endpoints), and compliance issues.

Critique 5: Economic model

- Symptom scales used for the assessment of ADHD do not usually qualify as instruments to measure HRQoL outcomes, contrary to their interpretation in the NICE Assessment Report.
- Deviating from the search strategy defined in the assessment protocol, several key publications were omitted, which may have impacted the overall outcome of the appraisal.
- The structure of the model resulted in double-counting of non-responders, which affected treatment options differently and was a source of distortion and bias.
- Compliance issues were effectively excluded from consideration in the economic model; three to eight (or twelve) weeks treatment duration in controlled trials were assumed to capture long-term treatment persistence.
- Although the economic model was extended to a time horizon of 12 years, clinically relevant long-term sequelae associated with ADHD were not addressed.

Critique 6: Appraisal and appeal process

- The Appraisal Consultation Document noted the ADHD core signs of inattention, hyperactivity, and impulsiveness, the difference between ICD-10 and DSM-IV definitions, and the potential influence of comorbidity on therapeutic outcomes in ADHD, although the Assessment Report had failed to adequately address those.
- The Appraisal Committee found that methodological flaws in some studies limited their persuasive value. However, the "flaw" of being open-label was an essential design component of a pragmatic real world study considered, increasing its external validity.
- An appeal was lodged on the basis of the omission of a key study from the assessment process, which might have influenced the Final Appraisal Determination. However, the appeal was dismissed.

Against the background of these observations, the conclusions of NICE are contrasted with insights from clinical long-term studies, from disease-specific effectiveness measures, and from other HTAs concerned with ADHD treatment strategies.

Specifically:

A number of long-term trials in ADHD have become available that may enable differentiation between treatment approaches, also by diagnostic criteria, by comorbidity, and by intensity of treatment. Retrospective database analyses lend support to the importance of treatment persistence in ADHD and indicate a differential impact of the products assessed. Furthermore, evidence is growing that non-stimulant interventions (e.g., atomoxetine), which are more expensive, are not more (or less) effective than stimulant drugs (e.g., methylphenidate). This might have implications for NICE guidance as well. These conclusions receive further support from concordant results of HTAs of ADHD treatment strategies in other jurisdictions.

It is therefore concluded that the NICE appraisal and guidance does not adequately reflect current knowledge of ADHD and its treatment. This however is more than an academic issue because it may have potentially for-reaching clinical practice implications.

With reference to the case analysis, four distinct domains of problems underlying the anomalies observed are suggested.

- Separation of clinical and economic perspectives.
  The appraisal was driven by economists without sufficient integration of clinical perspectives and expertise. This may have contributed, *inter alia*, to not taking into account the impact on the appraisal of different measurement instruments for ADHD, the role of treatment compliance in the clinical effectiveness of ADHD treatments, and the importance of adequate treatment duration.
- High level of standardization.
  The drive to establish consistency and transparency across the technology appraisal process reduced the rich clinical evidence base to a few short-term studies reporting clinical global improvements on a subscale that might be less than optimal, potentially resulting in bias and misleading results. An alternative approach – that is, to seek a solution specific to the condition and the available data, rather than define a problem to fit a common framework – may be a more pragmatic approach.
- Technical quality of assessment.
  Multiple shortcomings of a technical nature – such as a departure from search criteria specified in the assessment protocol, deviations from NICE reference case guidance, and a range of further anomalies and inconsistencies – may highlight an apparent shortfall in expected quality assurance systems for the technology assessment process, in addition to insufficient integration of clinical perspectives.
- Process-related issues.
  Within the highly structured NICE process, transparency is limited when commercial-in-confidence data are used. This may impede effective stakeholder participation. Transparency is also limited with regard to uninformative appraisal committee meeting minutes and to economic models used by assessment groups. This is a potentially serious constraint since technology appraisals rely heavily on assessment reports, and transparency is broadly considered a key feature of model quality.
  This notwithstanding, the predictability, inclusiveness, and overall publicity of the NICE appraisal process should be acknowledged.
  Referring to the "accountability for reasonableness" (A4R) framework proposed by Daniels and Sabin, however, NICE falls short of expectations despite an official commitment to adhere to the framework. Transparency is incomplete, appeals are restricted and do not allow to reopen debate, and the extent that the conditions of relevance and enforcement are met is subject to debate.

Suggested implications for international policy-makers include consideration of:

- *The objectives of health care provision*, since the underlying social value judgments made by NICE are not universally shared.
- *The extent of reliance on QALYs as an outcome measure*, as the narrow analytical focus of NICE was identified as a prime reason for the selective use of the clinical evidence, which simultaneously caused exclusion of a wider evidence base that was inconsistent with QALY-based outcomes measurement.
- *Flexibility in use of analytic approaches*, as greater flexibility compared with the NICE reference case might drive alternative evaluation techniques and provide increasingly robust guidelines.
- *The technology appraisal process.* Although relatively transparent, the NICE approach does not fully meet A4R criteria. Also NICE transparency is impeded by commercial-in-confidence data (submitted by manufacturers of technologies assessed) and intellectual property rights (concerning models developed by review teams) that restrict third-party participation in technology appraisals.
- *The timing of technology appraisals.* A fundamental paradox of cost-effectiveness evaluations is that early data are needed for policy impact, while reliable data require practical experience. This has been cited as a reason why modeling in economic evaluation is "an unavoidable fact of life." At the same time, this should encourage to strive for more consistent use of information from studies not yet published in peer-reviewed journals, such as abstracts and conference presentations.
- *The use of multidisciplinary assessment teams.* The present case study of NICE's ADHD appraisal highlights some of the constraints that may arise when economists and clinicians work independently. The case supports the conception that greater integration of these disciplines at all stages of the appraisal process would more likely achieve the goals of each.
- *Quality assurance.* Standardization is not synonymous with quality consistency of HTAs. Apparently, additional precautions are warranted to achieve greater transparency in the quality assurance of the NICE process. Specific processes should be implemented to ensure high quality of evidence synthesis and economic models.
- *Implementation*, which may be achieved best when guidance is concordant with clinical needs and expectations, instead of defining separate clinical and decision-making perspectives, as was the case in the ADHD assessment.

Based upon the case analysis, possible ways forward are discussed, highlighting different international starting points, key ethical aspects related to the objectives of health care provision, institutional context, and a research agenda to take matters further.

In conclusion, international health care policy-makers contemplating whether to adopt NICE-like approaches appear well advised to consider both strengths and limitations of the NICE approach, in addition to the specific value judgments underlying NICE technology appraisals, which they may or may not share.

Contents

List of Tables

List of Figures

List of Boxes

Introduction

National Institute for Health and Clinical Excellence (NICE)
Attention-Deficit/Hyperactivity Disorder (ADHD)

Chapter 1
Introduction

If collectively financed health care cannot afford to fund all effective clinical interventions in the face of limited resources, choices are inevitable, and the need arises to determine which services are most worthwhile. International health care policy-makers have increasingly turned to cost-effectiveness analysis (CEA), which promises to inform about the trade-offs involved in prioritization decisions in an explicit, quantitative, and systematic way.

In the context of Health Technology Assessments (HTAs), cost-effectiveness analysis typically relies on best estimates of clinical efficacy and effectiveness. These estimates are produced by systematic reviews, which thus form an important component of a meaningful economic evaluation (Gilbody and Pettigrew, 1999).

1.1 National Institute for Health and Clinical Excellence (NICE)

Following the early examples of Australia and Canada, many jurisdictions have mandated the use of such evaluation in the context of reimbursement decisions, often related to pharmaceuticals (Morgan et al., 2006; Ontario Ministery of Health, 1994; Commonwealth of Australia, 1992). The National Institute of Health and Clinical Excellence (NICE), which was established as a Special Health Authority within the United Kingdom National Health Service (NHS), features prominently among these initiatives (see Buxton, 2006; Hutton et al., 2006; McMahon et al., 2006; Morgan et al., 2006; Henry et al., 2005; García-Altés et al., 2004; Stevens and Milne, 2004; Kanavos et al., 2000).

Since its inception as the "National Institute for Clinical Excellence" in April 1999, technology appraisals by the National Institute for Health and Clinical Excellence (NICE) have attracted international attention. Their high visibility has served to extend their influence beyond the Institute's primary remit, notably (though not limited to) providing guidance to the National Health Service (NHS) of England and Wales (cf. Figure 1.1). NICE is frequently being perceived as a role model

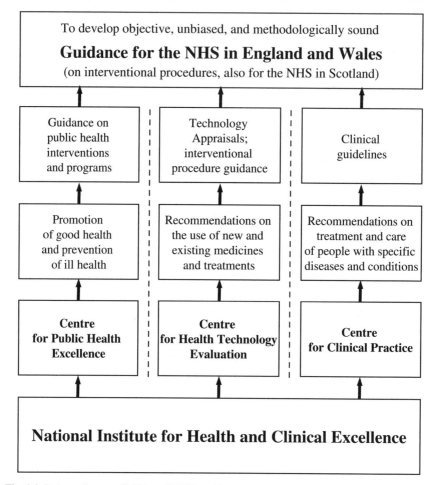

Fig. 1.1 Roles and responsibilities of NICE and its parts
NICE was established as a Special Health Authority for England and Wales in 1999 as part of the National Health Service (NHS) to promote clinical excellence and the effective (and cost-effective) use of resources. NICE comprises three distinct "Centres of Excellence" with separate, though related roles (NICE, 2005j). The present report is concerned with the Technology Appraisal role of NICE and its Centre for Health Technology Evaluation

for the implementation of cost-effectiveness analysis (CEA)[1] as an integral part of health technology assessments (HTAs), to support informed decisions about

---

[1] More precisely, NICE has adopted a specific variant of CEA often referred to as cost-utility analysis (CUA), using quality-adjusted life years (QALYs) as a comprehensive and universal measure of health outcomes. From here on, the term CUA will be applied to describe this approach, in contrast to CEA using *any* measure of health outcome (or "clinical effectiveness," which may include QALYs) that may be deemed appropriate in a particular decision-making context. Also, in the United States (and consequently some quotes of US literature in this paper) "cost-effectiveness analysis" is being used as an umbrella term comprising both CEA (as defined here) and CUA.

the rational allocation of health care resources in an environment of economic limitations.

While leading health economists have expressed concern that economic evaluation may not be used to its full potential (Drummond, 2004; Neumann, 2004), NICE has been acclaimed for representing "the closest anyone has yet come to fulfilling the economist's dream of how priority-setting in health care should be conducted" (Williams, 2004). It has been further suggested that "NICE tends to concentrate on the difficult choices, where there are usually trade-offs between increased benefit and increased costs," representing "these situations where economic analysis is likely to have the greatest added value, including the quantification of the uncertainty surrounding the decision" (Drummond, 2004).

In the most general terms, the expected role of technology appraisals is to provide the basis for NICE to issue guidance about the optimal use of a health technology (NICE, 2004c). NICE claims that its guidance "ends the uncertainty" over the value of a technology (NICE, 2006f) and "helps to standardise access ... across the country" (NICE, 2006f).

Implementation of NICE guidance is mandatory for the NHS in England and Wales, although its actual implementation has been subject to debate (e.g., Freemantle, 2004; Sheldon et al., 2004; Burke, 2002). Within the context of NICE this guidance is also expected to inform the development of clinical guidelines by National Collaborating Centres and Guideline Developers (NICE, 2006g,h, 2004a). NICE guidance should be reproduced unchanged within clinical guidelines and should be given the highest ranking for strength of evidence (NICE, 2004a), implying the assumption that highest quality standards will be attained consistently.

A review team of the World Health Organization (WHO) commissioned by NICE to appraise the methods and processes of its technology appraisal program "was impressed by the commitment to using rigorous methodology throughout the process of technology assessment" (WHO, 2003). A number of "particularly valuable achievements" were noted including transparency of the process, intensive participation of stakeholders, responsiveness to change, commitment to using the best available evidence, and use of academic centers of excellence for independent technology appraisal.

The review team confirmed that "published technology appraisals are already being used as international benchmarks" (WHO, 2003). The WHO team also made a number of recommendations to further enhance the operations of NICE and, explicitly, to "assist organizations with similar responsibilities in other countries to deal with their difficulties and meet their expectations" (WHO, 2003). Although limited to "consideration of the methods and scientific robustness" of technology appraisals, the WHO report was interpreted by observers as largely affirming NICE as "a leading organization internationally in the use of evidence about clinical and cost-effectiveness to inform decisions in the health sector" (Devlin et al., 2003).

This has led to a call by some health economists to internationally expand the NICE approach (for example, Quam and Smith, 2005; Neumann et al., 2005a; WHO, 2003; Maynard, 2001b). The European High-Level Group on Innovation and Provision of Medicines (G-10) engaged in debate about creating a "Euro-NICE"

(European Commission, 2002), although it recognized that pricing and reimbursement structures for medicines fall within the competence of the member states. Only in July 2006, the German grand coalition government agreed on the outline of a new health care reform, expanding the mission of the German Institute for Quality and Efficiency in Health Care ("Institut für Qualität und Wirtschaftlichkeit im Gesundheitswesen", IQWiG) to include "cost-benefit evaluations" of pharmaceutical products (Bundesministerium für Gesundheit, 2006a,b). These evaluations should adhere to "international standards" with explicit reference to NICE[2].

Current debate in North America also includes consideration of the experiences in the United Kingdom (McMahon et al., 2006; Wilensky, 2006). In the United States the troubled start of the new Medicare drug benefit, Medicare part D, has contributed to renewed interest in alternative approaches in order "to make drug choices ... on the basis of evidence about efficacy, safety, and economic value" (Avorn, 2006). The development of an independent information infrastructure has been proposed to disseminate data on pharmaceutical cost-effectiveness (Reinhardt, 2001, 2004), and the creation of one or more new institutes has been suggested to provide advice to Medicare on cost-effectiveness when determining the coverage of new medical interventions (Neumann et al., 2005a; Reinhardt, 2004). Leading NICE representatives have claimed that "the conditions ... seem ripe for a NICE in the United States" (Pearson and Rawlins, 2005).

The approach to economic evaluation adopted by NICE has not been without controversy (cf. Dolan et al., 2005; Maynard et al., 2004; Rawlins and Culyer, 2004; Gafni and Birch, 2003a; Dent and Sadler, 2002; Cookson et al., 2001; Lipman, 2001; Parfit, 2000; Smith, 2000; and many others). This is perhaps not very surprising in a field as ideologically charged and as generously subsidized as health care. In addition, guidance on the appropriate use of technologies does affect strong financial interests. Agencies like NICE are likely to draw fire from interested parties when their recommendations imply restrictions of use or denial of reimbursement (e.g., Ferner and McDowell, 2006; O'Brien, 2006; Iliffe, 2005; Burke, 2002; Ellis, 2001; Powell, 2001).

Nonetheless, the processes and transparency utilized by NICE have been widely regarded as exemplary (e.g., Schlander, 2007a; WHO, 2003; Towse and Pritchard, 2002; Buxton, 2001) and it has been asserted that "NICE demonstrates the potential of a new organization with a specific mandate to consider cost-effectiveness" (Neumann et al., 2005a). Furthermore, NICE recently updated its methods guidance for technology assessment, (among other aspects) endorsing probabilistic sensitivity analyses[3], thus assuming a leadership role in this important area (Buxton, 2006;

---

[2] Apparently there is still some confusion among German politicians with regard to terminology, such as the important differentiation between "cost-benefit" and "cost-effectiveness" / "cost-utility" evaluations.

[3] For a long time, the conventional approach to assessing parameter uncertainty in cost-effectiveness analyses has been by one-way or multi-way sensitivity analyses (Briggs, 2000, 2001; Petitti, 2000; Briggs et al., 1994), which indicate the range of possible results if key model parameters change. Probabilistic sensitivity analyses additionally convey information about the probability of each possible result. Such analyses may be based on Monte Carlo simulations (Briggs and Gray,

Claxton et al., 2005; NICE, 2004c). Indeed, the traditionally cautious and, for that matter (Smith, 2000), initially skeptical editors of the British Medical Journal have endorsed NICE as a "triumph" (Smith, 2004). They even suggested that "NICE is conquering the world" and "may prove to be one of Britain's greatest cultural exports, along with Shakespeare, Newtonian physics, the Beatles, Harry Potter, and the Teletubbies" (Smith, 2004).

However, little is known about the real-life robustness of the NICE approach. It remains to be established how well the highly standardized processes of NICE for health technology assessments and appraisals (see Chapter 3, *NICE Appraisal Process*) can accommodate complex clinical decision problems. One such example is the choice of optimal treatment for children and adolescents with attention-deficit/hyperactivity disorder (ADHD). The recent technology appraisal by NICE concerning treatments for ADHD (NICE, 2006b) may serve as an appropriate case study to explore the performance of NICE technology appraisals in practice.

Accordingly the focus of the present report will be a qualitative study of NICE Technology Appraisal No. 98, "Methylphenidate, atomoxetine and dexamfetamine for attention–deficit/hyperactivity disorder (ADHD) in children and adolescents (Review of Technology Appraisal 13)" (NICE, 2006b). The decision to analyze this particular case was motivated by the convergence of a personal scientific interest of this author in the areas of pharmaceutical market regulation and ADHD, and by an early observation that the scope published in August 2003 (NICE, 2003) excluded psychosocial interventions, which represent a therapeutic mainstay in most European countries (Taylor et al., 1998, 2004). The aim of the "appraisal of an appraisal" (cf. Blades et al., 1987) presented here will be to elucidate some of the challenges faced by decision-makers when addressing particularly difficult clinical problems. This study cannot – and is not intended to – invalidate the NICE technology appraisal process *per se*, or its results to date. Qualitative research is not a substitute for, but a complement to, quantitative work and, as such, it may enable the reader to "reach the parts other methods cannot reach" (Pope and Mays, 1995). Case study research has been recognized to be especially useful to explore contemporary phenomena not amenable to quantitative analysis, for instance where complex inter-related issues are involved (Pope and Mays, 1995), in particular in the field of health service organization and policy (Pollitt et al., 1990). Furthermore, such in-depth qualitative studies are unlikely to be repeated on a large scale as they are demanding and require thorough examination of a broad range of data (cf. Hill et al., 2000); in the present case, the technology assessment report alone was a 605-page document (King et al., 2004b; cf. Chapter 4, below). Indeed such independent in-depth analyses of technology appraisals have been rare (cf. Redwood, 2006; WHO, 2003; Hill et al., 2000; Blades et al., 1987).

Hence, the present study may provide insights on strengths (which would be reassuring) and weaknesses (which might cause concern) of the NICE technology

---

1999) using statistical or empirical (e.g., patient-level data on observed costs and effects from randomized clinical trials) distributions and may reflect parameter correlations (Ades et al., 2006; Claxton et al., 2005; Ades and Lu, 2003; Briggs et al., 2002; O'Brien and Briggs, 2002).

appraisal process under conditions of stress caused by complex analytical challenges, and identify potential areas for further improvement. Therefore, even if it turned out that the case analysis dealt with an exceptional outlier, its findings were still relevant, as one should expect that technology assessments by NICE consistently meet the highest quality standards, and provide robust information for stakeholders and decision-makers. This is an important requirement since economic evaluation is intended to enable meaningful comparisons across a wide range of morbidities and because resulting NICE guidance is specifically issued to influence the adoption of technologies and the practice of many physicians, thus affecting large numbers of patients. Given the high profile of NICE and its international standing as a presumed role model, these observations should be of interest to health care policy-makers not only in the United Kingdom.

1.2 Attention-Deficit/Hyperactivity Disorder (ADHD)

Broadly, ADHD is characterized by a "persistent pattern of inattention and/or hyperactivity/impulsivity that is more frequent and severe than is typically observed in individuals at a comparable level of development" (American Psychiatric Association, 1994). Although economic studies of ADHD are still in their infancy (Romeo et al., 2005) – and thus far have been published predominantly in the United States – it is already clear that this disorder is associated with a substantial economic burden (Matza et al., 2005a; Leibson and Long, 2003).

The case of the appraisal of ADHD interventions by NICE may be of particular interest for a number of reasons, all of which illustrate its relevance as well as its complexity:

First, even though DSM-IV-based (American Psychiatric Association, 1994) prevalence estimates vary widely (in 8- to 10-year-old children from 3.9% up to 19.8% in one study) and depend on the population studied and diagnostic criteria used (Faraone et al., 2003a), ADHD is believed to represent the most common psychiatric disorder in children and adolescents (Figure 1.2).

Second, ADHD is associated with high rates of co-existing (comorbid) conditions. Externalizing signs such as oppositional defiant disorder and conduct disorder occur in 50–60% of all children with ADHD, and internalizing mental health problems, notably, anxiety and depression, in 12–26% (Faraone et al., 2003a; Green et al., 1999). A wide range of other psychiatric, neurological and somatic disorders may be associated with or superimposed on signs and symptoms of ADHD[4] (Steinhausen et al., 2006; Schlander et al., 2005b; Gillberg et al., 2004; cf. Table 1.1).

---

[4] Green et al., in their systematic review (1999), provide the following estimates of psychiatric comorbidities: oppositional defiant and conduct disorders, 30%; conduct disorder, 28%; anxiety, 26%; depression, 18%; learning disabilities, 12% (Green et al., 1999). Based on a European sample of N=1,478 patients with ADHD or hyperkinetic disorder (Preuss et al., 2006), Steinhausen et al. (2006) reported the following rates of co-existing symptoms "of any degree:" oppositional-defiant

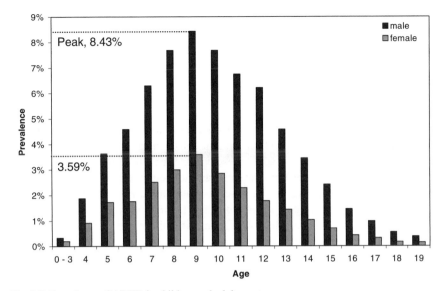

Fig. 1.2 Prevalence of ADHD in children and adolescents
Age and gender specific prevalence rates of ADHD based on administrative data from Nordbaden,
Germany, year 2003 (Schlander and Schwarz, 2005a, Schlander et al., 2007). For characteristics of
the comprehensive Nordbaden claims data base, cf. Box 1

Table 1.1 Prevalence of co-existing conditions in children and adolescents with ADHD

Co-existing disorders	ADHD patients	Control group	Relative Risk (CI[1])
Conduct and personality disorders	48.5%	5.2%	9.29(8.57–10.07)
Mood and affective disorders	38.0%	8.9%	4.29(4.02–4.57)
Specific development disorders	37.4%	13.4%	2.81(2.66–2.96)
Specific development disorders of scholastic skills	23.0%	2.8%	8.27(7.38–9.28)
Adjustment disorders	8.3%	1.6%	5.26(4.49–6.17)
Sleep disorders	4.5%	1.3%	3.19(2.67–3.80)
Incontinence (and polyuria)	4.4%	2.3%	1,95(1.68–2.26)
Mental retardation	3.8%	0.8%	4.85(3.86–6.10)
Tic disorders	2.4%	0.7%	3.26(2.55–4.16)
Disorders due to brain damage	1.8%	0.4%	4.95(3.54–6.92)
Pervasive development disorders	1.6%	0.5%	3.47(2.54–4.73)
Disorders associated with sexual development	0.7%	0.2%	3.43(2.16–5.46)
Disorders due to substance abuse	0.6%	0.2%	3.65(2.13–6.23)
Habit and impulse disorders	0.4%	0.0%	11.25(4.04–31.27)

Analyses of administrative data from Nordbaden, Germany, confirming high rates of psychiatric and developmental comorbidity among patients with ADHD in a large European sample (cf. Box 1). Differences between groups were all statistically highly significant (p<0.001).
Extended analyses also indicate higher rates of a broad range of somatic diagnoses among children
and adolescents with ADHD in Nordbaden. [1]CI, 95 % confidence intervals for relative risks.
Schlander et al., 2005b.

Third, the complexity of the situation is exacerbated by international differences in commonly accepted diagnostic criteria, notably DSM-IV in North America, and the more restrictive ICD-10 criteria (World Health Organization, 1992) that are preferred in Europe, giving a 1.7% prevalence for "hyperkinetic disorder" (HKD) in boys in the United Kingdom (cf. Taylor et al., 1991, 2004).

Both DSM-IV and ICD-10 use essentially similar lists of 18 symptoms of inattention (9), hyperactivity (5) and impulsivity (4), and both systems require that symptoms cause impairment (maladaptive behaviors inconsistent with age and developmental level), must have been present before the age of seven, persisted for at least six months, be pervasive, i.e., present in at least two settings (e.g., at school, at home, at work, during leisure time), and are not better accounted for by another mental disorder. Depending on the type of symptoms present, three subtypes of ADHD are differentiated, i.e., a predominantly inattentive type (about 10 to 15% of patients), a predominantly hyperactive and impulsive type (about 5%), and a combined type (about 80%).

Despite substantial overlap, ICD-10 criteria for hyperkinetic disorder (code F90.0; or F90.1 if additional symptoms of conduct disorder are present) are stricter as they require the presence of abnormal levels of *both* inattention and overactivity (corresponding to the combined category of DSM-IV), which should cause *impairment* in at least two settings. Thus the requirement for pervasiveness is more stringent under ICD-10. In addition, ICD-10 specifies that the *co-existent presence* of anxiety disorders, mood disorders, pervasive developmental disorders, and schizophrenia should pre-empt a diagnosis of hyperkinetic disorder. In general, the symptoms of children fulfilling the ICD-10 criteria correspond best to a more severely impaired combined subtype of ADHD according to DSM-IV (cf. Tripp et al., 1999; Wolraich et al., 1998; American Psychiatric Association, 1994; World Health Organization, 1992). The ICD system is used worldwide for recording morbidity statistics.

There also exist differences of standards of care (as exemplified, for instance, by lower prescription rates of psychostimulants in Europe compared to the United States; cf. below). Despite international convergence of standards of care, this raises issues related to the portability of the results of US studies to a European context (cf. Drummond and Pang, 2001).

Fourth, accrued data on ADHD is suggestive of an apparent increasing prevalence. However, this needs to be viewed in the context of raised awareness among parents, educators and health professionals of the adverse effects of behavioral and learning problems in children. This raised awareness is, perhaps, reflected by a striking increase in the number of prescriptions for psychostimulants in younger people in the US during the 1990s (Shatin and Drinkard, 2002; Robison et al., 1999, 2002; Kelleher et al., 2001), Canada (Miller et al., 2001; Hollander et al., 1996), and Australia (Valentine et al., 1995), and, with some time lag compared to the US, in a number of European countries (Schwabe and Paffrath, 2006; Köster et al., 2004;

---

disorder, 67%; conduct disorder, 46%; anxiety, 44%; depression, 32%; tics, 8%. No control group was assessed in this observational study.

Box 1 The Nordbaden project The Nordbaden project was initiated to build an integrated claims database within the context of the fragmented German health care system. The database enables physician, patient and diagnosis centered analyses of administrative prevalence, co-existing conditions, resource utilization and direct medical costs from the perspective of the German Statutory Health Insurance (SHI). Nordbaden is a region in the Southwest of Germany with a population of 2.7 million, 82 percent (or 2.2 million) of which are insured by SHI. Key sociodemographic population characteristics (Bundesministerium für Gesundheit, 2005; Statistical Office of the European Communities, 2005; Statistisches Landesamt Baden-Württemberg, 2005) in 2003 did not substantially deviate from Germany as a whole (with a population of 82.5m, of which 70.4m, or 85.7%, are insured by SHI).

The database covered all persons insured by SHI in the region of Nordbaden. An individual monthly gross income exceeding 3,825 Euro was required for parents in 2003 to be allowed to opt out of the SHI system; within the SHI system, children were co-insured with their parents at no extra premiums. The SHI system provided comprehensive coverage of medical services, without co-payments by children and adolescents below the age of 18 years, and with only moderate out-of-pocket payments required from adults. Within the SHI system, physicians were reimbursed on a fee-for-service basis, making underreporting unlikely and hence justifying the expectation that patient visits were indeed well captured within the claims database.

In accordance with established policies and principles for protection of privacy and confidentiality (Meier, 2003; Wichmann et al., 1998), the datasets from the Nordbaden region for all four quarters of 2003 were integrated, with personal identifiers (of patients and service providers) replaced by pseudonyms by the Regional Association of the Statutory Health Insurance Physicians (Kassenärztliche Vereinigung, KV) Nordbaden (now KV Baden-Württemberg). A data analysis plan and data transfer protocol had been established and approved by the data protection officer of the KV Nordbaden.

11,245 children and adolescents (age 19 years or less) with a diagnosis of hyperkinetic disorder (HKD) or hyperkinetic conduct disorder (HKCD) were identified in Nordbaden in 2003. For children age 6 years or less, 12-month prevalence rates were 1.26% in total, 1.72% for boys and 0.77% for girls; for children age 7-12 years, 4.97% (boys, 7.16%; girls, 2.65%), age 13-19 years, 1.31% (males, 1.99%; females, 0.60%). Prevalence was highest at age 9 (peak; overall: 6.1%; boys, 8.4%; girls, 3.6%; cf. Figure 1.2).

The ADHD group was matched with a non-ADHD cohort ("control group") on a 1:1 ratio based on age, gender, and type of health insurance (within the German SHI system), and the rate of co-existing conditions was compared between both groups (Schlander, 2005b) - see Table 1.1.

A key strength of claims databases is that they allow examining medical care utilization as it occurs in routine clinical care (Motheral et al., 2003). As for retrospective claims data analyses in general, an important limitation of the data is the lack of verifiable information about the quality of diagnosis and coding. The observed administrative prevalence of "HKD" and "HKCD" of 4.97% in children age 7 to 12 years in Nordbaden in 2003 appears consistent with a continuing trend toward increasing awareness and detection of ADHD in children and adolescents (Buitelaar and Rothenberger, 2004; Köster et al., 2004). Coded according to ICD-10, it appears extraordinarily high in light of high-quality epidemiological studies indicating a "true prevalence" of hyper-kinetic disorder (HKD and HKCD) in the range of 1.5% to 2.9% in school age children (Taylor et al., 2004; Brühl et al., 2000; Wolraich et al., 1998). A number of possible explanations seem conceivable, an obvious one being that many physicians might indeed prefer the broader DSM-IV criteria to establish a diagnosis of ADHD - whereas the reporting system enforces ICD-10 based coding. This hypothesis was supported by an *ad hoc* survey we conducted with a convenience sample of six German pediatricians, who indeed without exception confirmed that they adhered to DSM-IV diagnostic criteria but were required by the administrative system to code according to ICD-10. Source: Schlander et al., 2007.

Lohse et al., 2004; Criado Álvarez and Romo Barrientos, 2003; Schirm et al., 2001; Ekman and Gustafsson, 2000) including the United Kingdom (Wong et al., 2004) during the last decade (Figure 1.3).

Fifth, this has aroused much controversy and emotive debate both among professionals as well as in the general public about the possibility of overuse of psychotropic medications in children (Timimi, 2003; Rey and Sawyer, 2003; Breggin, 2002; Ekman and Gustafsson, 2000; Llana and Crismon, 1999; Jensen et al., 1999). In Europe, recent analyses of methylphenidate prescriptions in Germany did not provide evidence for overuse of stimulants (for a regional sample from the late 1990s, cf. von Ferber et al., 2003, and Schubert et al., 2001, 2002; for Nordbaden in year 2003, cf. Schlander et al., 2006d – see also Box 1), although over the last decade methylphenidate use in Germany has been growing faster compared to the United Kingdom, both in relative as well as in absolute terms (cf. Schlander, 2006b).

In the United States, the amalgam of scientific debate and opinionated dispute was illuminated by a sharp controversy which emerged between Steven Nissen (2006), a specialist for cardiovascular medicine from Cleveland, and a group of child and adolescent psychiatrists from the Massachusetts General Hospital at Harvard (Biederman et al., 2006a) and others after the Drug Safety and Risk Management Advisory Committee of the Food and Drug Administration (FDA) had recommended – on the basis of an 8 to 7 vote – a so-called "black box" warning about cardiovascular risks potentially associated with the use of psycho-stimulants. One month later, none of the members of the FDA's Pediatric Advisory Committee concluded that a black box warning was warranted, and meeting participants reported that they had been "impressed that the process … allowed

Rx Items Dispensed 1998-2005

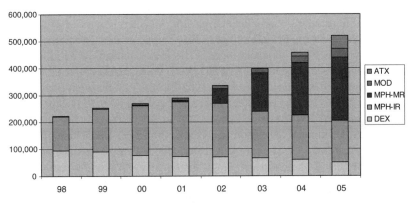

Fig. 1.3 ADHD-related prescriptions in England, 1998–2005
In England, data from the Prescription Pricing Authority (Department of Health, 1999–2006) show an increase in the number of prescription items of methylphenidate hydrochloride from 126,600 in 1998 to 389,200 in 2005. In 2005, methylphenidate hydrochloride modified-release formulations accounted for 60% (Concerta[R] XL, "MPH-MR12", 56%), and methylphenidate hydrochloride immediate-release formulations ("MPH-IR", Ritalin[R], Equasym[R], and generics) accounted for 40% (7%, 4%, and 29%, respectively).
The figure shows prescription items dispensed in the community in England, 1998–2005; DEX: dexamphetamine (Dexedrine[R] and others); MPH: methylphenidate; IR: immediate-release formulations (Ritalin[R] and generics); MR: modified-release formulations (Concerta[R] XL, Equasym[R] XL; Ritalin[R] SR imports); MOD: modafinil (Provigil[R], licensed for daytime sleepiness); ATX: atomoxetine (Strattera[R]); PEM: pemoline (Volital[R], available before 2002 only, not shown due to small volume).

for the airing of highly disparate and often passionate views regarding these issues" (Rappley et al., 2006).

The issue has been complicated by disagreement about the validity of ADHD as a distinct disease entity (Timimi, 2002; Breggin, 2002; DeGrandpre, 2000). Critics point to the lack of specific cognitive, metabolic or neurological markers and the absence of medical tests for ADHD and argue that the disorder may be best understood as a cultural construct (Timimi, 2004), whereas child and adolescent psychiatrists have maintained that the diagnostic status of ADHD merely "is a reflection of the state of affairs within psychiatry" (Buitelaar and Rothenberger, 2004). Important arguments include the existence of genetic risk factors for ADHD, supported by twin, adoption and family-genetic studies, the existence of physical counterparts in brain structure and function and DNA composition, and the strong predictive value of hyperactivity for poor psychosocial adjustment (cf. Young et al., 2005; Buitelaar and Rothenberger, 2004; Sergeant, 2004; Asherson et al., 2004; Taylor, 2004; Schachar and Tannock, 2002; Taylor et al., 1996; see also below, "long-term sequelae").

In addition, sixth, the substantial variety of instruments to measure clinical outcomes, symptom relief, and health-related quality of life across clinical studies aggravates existing difficulties in determining utility values to calculate quality-adjusted life years (QALYs) in patients with a diagnosis of ADHD (De Civita et al., 2005; Griebsch et al., 2005; Collett et al., 2003).

Seventh, the therapeutic armamentarium for ADHD, comprising two principal options – behavioral treatment and medication management – has been expanded by the emergence of new treatment options, notably extended- or modified-release preparations of methylphenidate (MPH-MR08, MPH-MR12) that eliminate the need for a midday dose, and atomoxetine (ATX), a non-stimulant compound, both of which have the potential to profoundly change the therapeutic landscape (Rappley, 2005; Patakis et al., 2004; Arnold, 2001).

Eighth, the resultant expectation of changes in service provision derived from the combined influences of increased awareness and more frequent diagnoses, growing acceptance of pharmacotherapy in the light of new clinical studies (in particular, MTA Cooperative Group, 1999a,b), and the availability of novel medication options that command higher unit costs compared to previously available options (Schlander, 2004a, 2006b), are likely to have important budgetary impacts (cf. Table 1.2 and Figure 1.4).

Finally, ADHD is associated with a substantial cost of illness. Health care costs for individuals with ADHD have been reported at twice those for individuals without the disorder (Leibson and Long, 2003). Parents and other family members of patients have also been found to have about 60% more medical claims than matched controls, and data strongly suggest that a child's ADHD places a substantial economic burden on parents and other family members (Swensen et al., 2003), including a negative impact on parents' absenteeism from work and productivity (Matza et al., 2005a).

The economic impact of ADHD is further exacerbated by its frequent persistence into adulthood (Wolraich et al., 2005; Wilens and Dodson, 2004; Mannuzza et al., 2003), thus constituting a chronic condition, and by serious long-term sequelae that have been linked to the disorder (Mannuzza and Klein, 2000). These sequelae include poor driving abilities (Barkley, 2004), higher risks of accidents and injuries (Swensen et al., 2004; Hoare and Beattie, 2003; Lam, 2002), increased rates of tobacco, alcohol and other substance use disorders (Wilens and Biederman, 2006), more frequent antisocial behaviors (Thapar et al., 2006; Mannuzza et al., 2004; Rasmussen and Gillberg, 2000) and encounters with the criminal justice system (Sourander et al., 2006; Johansson et al., 2005; Rösler et al., 2004; Siponmaa et al., 2001) across the lifespan, as well as relatively poor educational outcomes and lower-ranking occupational positions than controls (Murphy et al., 2002; Barkley, 2002; Mannuzza et al., 1997, 2004).

In light of these complexities, it has been suggested from a clinical perspective that a key feature of good practice is the involvement of specialists in the initial assessment of patients (Taylor, 2006). Once a diagnosis of ADHD has been established, which should have included a thorough differential diagnosis and a search for co-existent problems, it is a key feature of the decision-making context to select the appropriate course of treatment. Besides counseling and education, aiming to build up a treatment alliance with patients and their parents or guardians, and consulting with teachers, a critical choice is whether to begin with medication or

Table 1.2 Treatment options for ADHD in children and adolescents in the United Kingdom: product availability and acquisition cost

Trade name	Manufacturer	Active ingredient[1]	Formulation	Abbreviation	Cost/daily dose[2]	Assumed total daily dose[3]	Daily dosage schedule	Authorization[4]
Dexedrine	UCB Pharma Ltd., Slough	Dexamphetamine sulphate	Tablets (5mg)	DEX	£ 0.43	20mg/d	2 (–3) times	≤ 2000
Ritalin	Cephalon UK Ltd., Guildford, Surrey	Methylphenidate hydrochloride	Immediate-release tablets (10mg)	MPH-IR	£ 0.56	30mg/d	3 (2–4) times	≤ 2000
Equasym	UCB Pharma Ltd., Slough	Methylphenidate hydrochloride	Immediate-release tablets (5, 10, 20mg)	MPH-IR	£ 0.53	30mg/d	3 (2–4) times	≤ 2000
Concerta XL	Janssen-Cilag Ltd., High Wycombe, Bucks	Methylphenidate hydrochloride	Modified-release tablets (18, 36mg)	MPH-MR12	£ 1.23	36mg/d	1 time	2002 (Feb., 19)
Strattera	Eli Lilly & Co Ltd., Basingstoke, Hampshire	Atomoxetine-hydrochloride	Hard capsules (10, 18, 25, 40, 60mg)	ATX	£ 1.95[5]	Irrelevant (flat pricing)	1 (–2) times	2004 (May, 27)
Equasym XL	UCB Pharma Ltd., Slough	Methylphenidate hydrochloride	Modified-release capsules (10, 20, 30mg)	MPH-MR08	£ 1.17	30mg/d	1 time	2005 (Feb., 11)

[1] Note that exact licensed indications and ages differ between products.
[2] NHS acquisition costs (net prices, excluding VAT and not accounting for negotiated procurement discounts in some settings), taken from British National Formulary 51, March 2006; note that individual doses and thus costs may vary.
[3] Average assumptions underlying "cost per daily dose", not to be confused with treatment recommendations; doses need to be optimally titrated for each individual patient; see for instance Wilens and Dodson (2004).
[4] First authorization in UK, from electronic Medicines Compendium, available online at http://emc.medicines.org.uk, last accessed August 12, 2005.
[5] Due to its flat pricing policy, the cost per daily dose of ATX increases to £3.80 when administered twice daily.

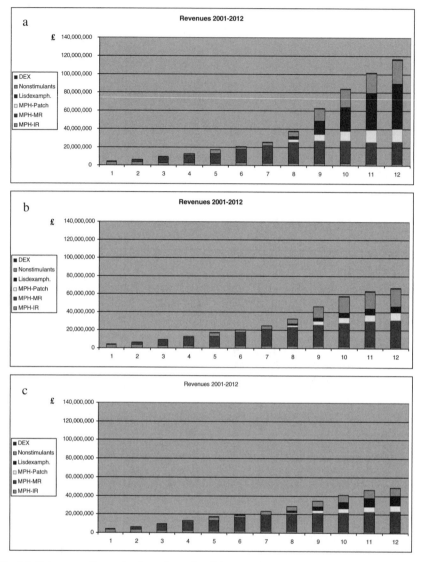

Fig. 1.4 Future spending projections: three plausible scenarios
Expenditures for pharmacotherapy for children and adolescents with ADHD in England (scenarios
for 2001–2012), from the perspective of the NHS.
a: "High Case"; b: "Base Case"; c: "Low Case". MPH: methylphenidate; IR: immediate-release
formulations (Ritalin[R], branded generics [Equasym[R], Medikinet[R]], generics; Focalin[R]); MR:
modified-release formulations (Concerta[R] XL, Equasym[R] XL, Medikinet[R] retard, Focalin[R] XR;
MPH-Patch: transdermal system (Daytrana[R]); LisDEX: lisdexamphetamine (NRP104); Nonstim-
ulants: atomoxetine (Strattera[R]), modafinil (Sparlon[R]) and armodafinil; DEX: dexamphetamine.
For further detail, see Box 2.
Data source: Schlander, 2006b.

Box 2 Budgetary impact analysis The growth of pediatric psychotropic prescriptions has become an international phenomenon (Wong et al., 2004). Beyond clinical implications, in an era of limited available resources, the economic dimension associated with increased health care utilization can no longer be ignored. In economic terms, the opportunity cost of medical interventions will be approximated by their budgetary impact - in particular, if a payer's perspective is adopted. Conventional cost-effectiveness analyses however do not provide information about the financial consequences of the adoption of health care programs, since incremental cost effectiveness ratios (ICERs) and derived measures do not indicate the size of numerator and denominator.

Consequently, budgetary impact analyses are requested by a growing number of health care policy-makers as an input into the decision-making process about health care resource allocation (Trueman et al., 2001). Therefore a forecasting model was developed (Schlander, 2006b) to project future pharmaceutical expenditures for children and adolescents (age 6–18 years) with a diagnosis of ADHD in England through 2012, specifying assumptions and assumed relationships between variables in a transparent manner. Key uncertainties were addressed using scenario analysis, combining objective information with specific assumptions about future events (Makridakis et al., 1998).

The model was restricted to pharmaceutical spending. It combined, in a hierarchical structure, (1) epidemiological information (demographic and prevalence data) with assumptions on (2) recognition rates (diagnosis prevalence), (3) rate of patients receiving drug therapy (treatment prevalence), (4) availability and adoption of new products (assumed to include a transdermal system of methylphenidate, which was approved as Daytrana[R] in the United States in April 2006, dexmethylphenidate, lisdexamphetamine mesylate, and armodafinil), incorporating information on therapeutic profiles, (5) diffusion and market shares for alternative preparations, by category and by product, including generic substitution, (6) treatment intensity (expressed as average number of days times defined daily doses), (7) acquisition cost per defined daily dose for each product, from the perspective of the NHS in England. For validation of the model, available data on the variables above were used to compare model outcomes with the historic evolution of drug spending in England.

On this basis, a number of scenarios were developed indicating a plausible range of future NHS spending on medication for ADHD in children and adolescents (Figure 1.4).

In strategic management, scenario analysis is a well-established tool to deal with environmental uncertainty (Goodwin and Wright, 2004). The practice of scenario planning implicitly acknowledges that "best guesses" of future events may be wrong. Therefore, any scenario should not be confused with a forecast of the future. Multiple scenarios are pen-pictures of a range of plausible futures. Though each individual scenario has an infinitesimal probability of actual occurrence, combined a range of scenarios can shed light on possible future outcomes.

Some important limitations of this study warrant discussion.

First, this analysis did not purport to convey value judgments. It had little to nothing to say about the clinical appropriateness of the prescriptions analyzed; its mere focus was their budgetary impact.

Second, there is substantial uncertainty around future events. Compounds in development may be discontinued, marketed drugs may be withdrawn because of serious adverse events, safety concerns may slow down diffusion of new products, and so on. The dynamic health policy environment is yet another factor.

Finally it should also be emphasized that this study was limited to ADHD in children and adolescents.

Source: Schlander, 2006b.

Table 1.3 Clinical choice of most appropriate ADHD treatment
The clinical choice between the two principal treatment options for ADHD in children adolescents, i.e., medication management and behavior therapy, including their most appropriate sequence, will be influenced by a number of criteria. Economic analyses have the potential to add important insights

Criteria (examples)	Complexity (examples)	Analytic approaches (examples)
Clinical effectiveness	Impact of diagnostic criteria, subtypes; co-existing conditions; therapeutic objectives (i.e., outcomes criteria and clinical endpoints)?	Systematic review of clinical evidence
Cost-effectiveness	Relies on clinical effectiveness synthesis	Cost-utility analysis (CUA)?
	Broader impact of ADHD on caregivers and on society as a whole?	
	Clinical margin (impact of severity of condition)?	Cost-effectiveness analysis (CEA)
	Intensity margin (impact of intensity – e.g., dose – of intervention chosen)?	
Affordability	True opportunity cost?	Budgetary impact analysis
	Appropriateness of level of analysis and of budget constraint?	Cost-benefit analysis (CBA)?
Preferences	Whose preferences (patients, parents; population sample) should count?	Cost-benefit analysis (CBA)
	Appropriate level of analysis?	Cost-utility analysis (CUA) for health state preferences?

behavior therapy, or the combination of both. In practice, the appropriate choice between alternative evidence-based treatment strategies will be influenced by the attitudes and preferences of stakeholders involved, including parents and schools, in addition to clinical guidelines informed by the results of systematic reviews on their effectiveness and economic implications. In principle, there are multiple conceivable ways in which economic evaluations might provide relevant insights (Table 1.3).

Each and all of the foregoing issues raises questions about how the application of the (conceptually) relatively simple logic of cost-effectiveness[5], as epitomized in real life by NICE, can accommodate these clinical complexities. In this regard, a critical appraisal will be of international interest given the high profile of NICE, and stimulate debate about the adoption of the NICE approach in other jurisdictional settings.

---

[5] Excellent introductions are offered by Drummond et al. (2005) and Gold et al. (1996). For a more critical account, see Ubel (2000) and Nord (1999).

A Note on Objectives and Methods

Objectives
Accountability for Reasonableness
Methods
Limitations

Chapter 2
A Note on Objectives and Methods

2.1 Objectives

The primary objective of the present report is to analyze the real-life performance and robustness of the process for technology appraisals and the methods for health technology assessments adopted by the National Institute for Health and Clinical Excellence (NICE). This report is focused on the application of these processes and methods, as put to practical use in a particularly challenging field of economic analysis, the evaluation of treatment strategies for attention-deficit/hyperactivity disorder (ADHD).

Thus the empirical part of this report will provide a critique of an application of economic evaluation methods on behalf of NICE, i.e., it will "appraise the appraisers" (Blades et al., 1987). This will lay the foundation for a broader discussion of implications for international health care policy-makers looking at NICE as a potential role model.

Occasionally, examples of the author's own work in this field will be used to illustrate context and relevance (e.g., European data on the administrative prevalence of ADHD and budgetary impact projections; cf. Chapter 1, *Introduction*), as well as to present recent cost-effectiveness evaluations directly related to the NICE appraisal (e.g., European adaptation of an economic model developed on behalf of the Canadian Coordinating Office for Health Technology Assessments, CCOHTA, and European cost-effectiveness analyses based on the landmark NIMH MTA Study, cf. Chapter 6, *Discussion*), and the methods underlying these data will be briefly delineated in *Boxes* (see pages 11, 17, 127, 133, and 176).

2.2 Accountability for Reasonableness

The analysis of the NICE processes will be guided by a framework developed by Norman Daniels and James Sabin who have argued that the legitimacy of controversial limit-setting decisions in public health care systems hinges on a fair institutional decision process (Daniels and Sabin, 1997, 1998, 2002). In order to narrow the scope of controversy, they have proposed principles of "accountability for reasonableness"

(A4R), which "fair-minded people" should accept based on the idea that there exists a core set of reasons – that all center on fairness – on which there will be no disagreement.

A key element of fair process under A4R (Table 2.1) involves transparency about the decision making, including the grounds for decisions (the *publicity* condition, opening decisions and their rationales for scrutiny by all affected, not just the members of the decision-making group). Second, the *relevance* condition imposes an important constraint on arguments, because arguments are required to rest on scientific evidence – though not necessarily a specific kind of evidence – and to appeal to the notion of "fair equality of opportunity." Although Daniels and Sabin acknowledge that stakeholder participation may improve deliberation about complicated matters, they believe it is neither a necessary nor a sufficient condition of A4R. However, they advocate an *appeals* component as an institutional mechanism to engage a broader segment of society in the process. This appeals process should provide those affected by a decision an opportunity to reopen deliberation, and offer decision-makers an option to revise funding decisions in light of further arguments. Fourth, *enforcement* entails voluntary or statutory regulation to make sure the first three conditions are met. It has been argued that proper enforcement of the decisions will also ensure that reasoning is decisive in priority-setting and not merely a theoretical exercise (Hasman and Holm, 2005).

Using A4R as a benchmark guiding the review of NICE processes turns out to be a timely endeavor: it was, to the knowledge of this author, not before August 2005 that Sir Michael Rawlins, Chairman of the Board of NICE, and Andrew

Table 2.1 Accountability for reasonableness framework
Conditions for fair priority-setting processes according to the "Accountability for Reasonableness" (A4R) framework developed by Daniels and Sabin (1997, 1998, 2002): Descriptors taken from Daniels (2001) and Mitton and Donaldson (2004)

Condition	Description
Publicity	Decisions regarding coverage of new technologies (and other limit-setting decisions) and their rationales must be publicly accessible.
Relevance	These rationales must rest on evidence, reasons and principles that fair-mined parties (managers, clinicians, patients and consumers in general) can agree are relevant to deciding how to meet the diverse needs of a covered population under reasonable resource constraints.
Revisions and appeal	There is a mechanism for challenge and dispute resolution regarding the limit-setting decisions, including the opportunity for revising decisions in light of further evidence or arguments.
Enforcement	There is either voluntary or public regulation of the process to ensure that the first three conditions are met.

Dillon, Chief Executive of NICE, explicitly committed NICE to submit itself to the principles of A4R: "NICE has adopted the principles of procedural justice – 'accountability for reasonableness' – as espoused by Daniels and Sabin (2002)" (Rawlins and Dillon, 2005b).

2.3 Methods

A qualitative study was done of NICE Technology Appraisal No. 98, "Methylphenidate, atomoxetine and dexamfetamine for attention deficit hyperactivity disorder (ADHD) in children and adolescents (Review of Technology Appraisal 13)," published in March 2006. The case analysis had descriptive, explorative, and explanatory elements. The analysis was primarily concerned with the real-life application of NICE processes and focused on the Technology Assessment Report (King et al., 2004b), since this document "is used as the basis of the appraisal" (NICE, 2004b). The resulting critique shall be presented and, hopefully, will be understood in a spirit of scientific inquiry.

First, the initial phase of the study consisted of defining a theoretical framework for the study. This included description of NICE technology appraisal processes, which fell within a period of substantial upgrade and definition of the so-called "reference case" analysis by NICE (see below, Chapter 3, *NICE Appraisal Process*). During this phase, a thematic framework was defined, comprising use of the A4R concept as a process benchmark, an in-depth critique of the technology Assessment Report underlying the appraisal, as well as a review of the clinical and economic literature on attention-deficit/hyperactivity disorder in order to incorporate the complex interrelated issues involved in this technology appraisal (cf. Chapter 1, *Introduction*).

The second phase of the study comprised data collection on a number of closely related strategies. (1) From May 2004 to publication of guidance in March 2006, the NICE website (www.nice.org.uk) was visited at intervals of less than one month each and checked for newly posted information and documents (including meeting minutes and announcements) on (a) the technology appraisal process and related methods, (b) clinical guideline development, (c) deliberations of the NICE Citizens' Council, and (d) ADHD. (2) Scientific articles cited in these documents were obtained for analysis. (3) Independent literature searches (using the PubMed and EBSCO databases as well as Google Scholar) were conducted for articles on ADHD diagnosis, treatment, compliance, cost, and cost-effectiveness, and were (4) complemented by a search for relevant abstracts presented at international meetings in the fields of clinical psychiatry, child and adolescent psychiatry, pediatrics, health economics, and pharmacoeconomics. All searches for literature fully covered the technology assessment period (from June to December 2004; cf. Table 3.2, and Chapter 4, *NICE Appraisal of ADHD Treatments*). After May 2005, no more systematic searches for scientific literature were conducted, and new papers were added to the database in an opportunistic manner only. However, searches for full economic evaluations comparing at least two treatment options for ADHD were updated in December 2006. Collected documents were indexed using categories including study type, product tested, and subject matter (e.g., treatment compliance) for further analysis and interpretation.

All key steps of the ADHD appraisal process were identified and compared with NICE process descriptions (NICE, 2004b,c). The Assessment Report (King et al., 2004b) was subjected to a critical appraisal by this author, which included an examination of design choices and justifications provided by the Assessment Group for internal and external consistency. Unless otherwise specified, citations in the following sections will refer to the Assessment Report (AR).

2.4 Limitations

The critique and discussion presented here should not be interpreted as an alternative health technology assessment of ADHD treatments. Any attempt to provide an independent systematic review would clearly exceed the limits of the present study, which is primarily interested in exposing strengths and weaknesses of the NICE process, with a view towards policy implications. On occasion, an alternative interpretation of data may be offered; however, this should be understood as a means to reveal the potential relevance of any pertinent gaps of the NICE assessment, and does not imply definite conclusions.

NICE was criticized by some observers for not paying enough attention to drug safety (Fletcher, 2000). The present analysis of the case of NICE Technology Appraisal No. 98 did confirm a strong emphasis on effectiveness and cost-effectiveness, but did not identify obvious shortcomings or substantial gaps with respect to drug safety, which would have had an impact on the economic evaluation. Correspondingly, the following critique will not provide a detailed review of safety considerations. Readers interested in this aspect of ADHD pharmacotherapy may wish to consult one of the recently published reviews of this subject, such as the papers by Wolraich et al. (2007), Pliszka (2007), Gibson et al. (2006), and Himpel et al. (2005).

As emphasized earlier in the *Introduction*, qualitative research cannot substitute for quantitative work; it is simply a complement allowing to "reach the parts other methods cannot reach" (Pope and Mays, 1995). On its own, empirical work based on a case study of one technology appraisal certainly cannot justify inductive inferences on more than 100 appraisals completed by NICE. It may, however, in a truly Popperian spirit, falsify certain unjustified assumptions and exaggerated expectations concerning the robustness of the NICE model. Then, any anomalies identified might generate hypotheses, which in turn could contribute to further improvement of technology appraisal processes.

NICE Appraisal Process

Scoping
Assessment
Appraisal
Appeal
Clinical Guidelines

Chapter 3
NICE Appraisal Process

In November 2005, NICE introduced a new single technology appraisal ("STA") process, which was created to provide faster guidance on new technologies (NICE, 2006i; Buxton and Akehurst, 2006). This process differs from "conventional" multiple technology appraisals ("MTAs") in a number of important ways, including the reliance on cost-effectiveness models submitted by manufacturers, which are subsequently scrutinized by independent assessment groups. Alongside the new process, MTAs will continue to be the standard approach by NICE. The present analysis will be restricted to the standard process and its application to the ADHD technology appraisal. Earlier, this process had been hailed by the WHO (2003) to represent the "state of the art" internationally.

In general terms, NICE (multiple) technology appraisals consist of three phases, (1) scoping, (2) assessment, and (3) appraisal. As an optional fourth phase, an appeal against a Final Appraisal Determination (FAD) by NICE may be filed by consultees and will be dealt with by an Appeal Panel. NICE has delineated this process in some detail in a series of related technical documents (NICE, 2004b,c,d,h,i,j,k; cf. Figure 3.1).

3.1 Scoping

Topics for appraisal are suggested to NICE by relevant government Ministers (Department of Health [DoH] and Welsh Assembly) – usually as part of a "wave" of topics. NICE identifies experts and stakeholders as "consultees" and "commentators" and prepares a draft scope which is provided to the Assessment Group. The Assessment Group is an independent academic group commissioned by the NHS Research and Development Health Technology Assessment Program to assist in the appraisal process.

These groups also receive from NICE the draft remit (i.e., the initial brief given to NICE). Approximately eight weeks thereafter, a scoping workshop is held by NICE. Components of the scoping procedure include a clear definition of the clinical problem (or disease) and the patient population, the technology (and its comparators) and their treatment setting, measures of health outcomes and costs, time horizon,

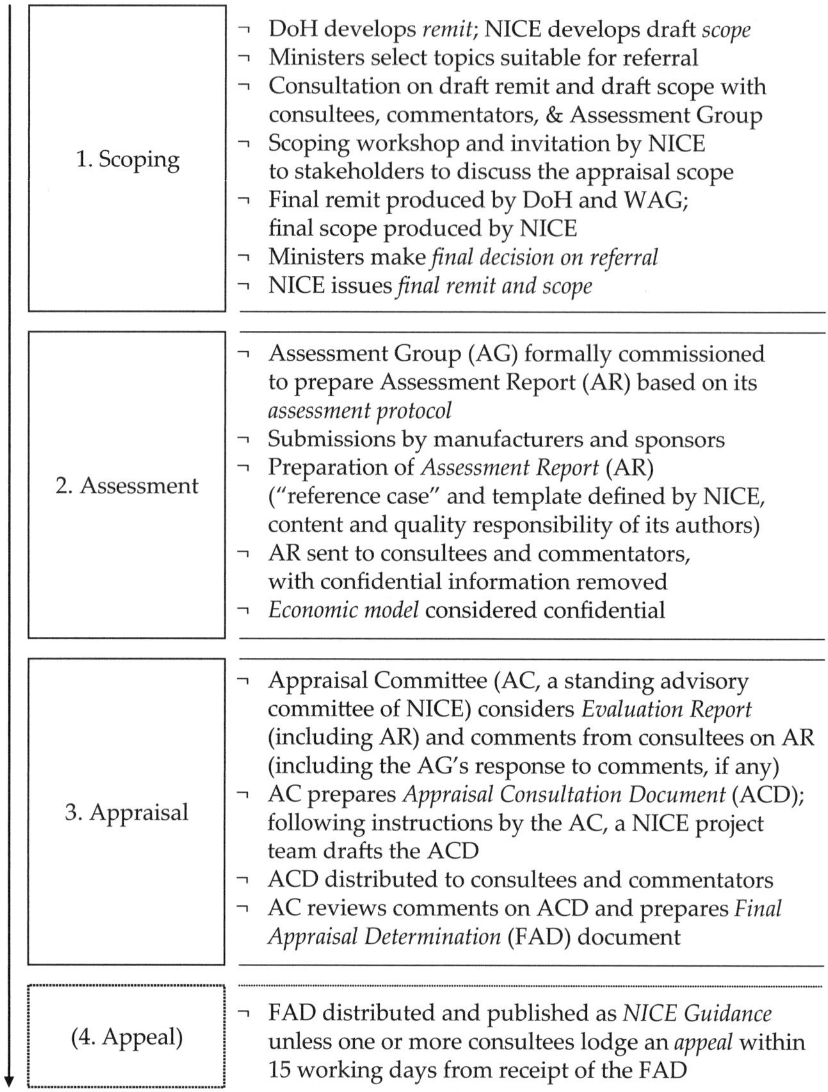

1. Scoping	¬ DoH develops *remit*; NICE develops draft *scope* ¬ Ministers select topics suitable for referral ¬ Consultation on draft remit and draft scope with consultees, commentators, & Assessment Group ¬ Scoping workshop and invitation by NICE to stakeholders to discuss the appraisal scope ¬ Final remit produced by DoH and WAG; final scope produced by NICE ¬ Ministers make *final decision on referral* ¬ NICE issues *final remit and scope*
2. Assessment	¬ Assessment Group (AG) formally commissioned to prepare Assessment Report (AR) based on its *assessment protocol* ¬ Submissions by manufacturers and sponsors ¬ Preparation of *Assessment Report* (AR) ("reference case" and template defined by NICE, content and quality responsibility of its authors) ¬ AR sent to consultees and commentators, with confidential information removed ¬ *Economic model* considered confidential
3. Appraisal	¬ Appraisal Committee (AC, a standing advisory committee of NICE) considers *Evaluation Report* (including AR) and comments from consultees on AR (including the AG's response to comments, if any) ¬ AC prepares *Appraisal Consultation Document* (ACD); following instructions by the AC, a NICE project team drafts the ACD ¬ ACD distributed to consultees and commentators ¬ AC reviews comments on ACD and prepares *Final Appraisal Determination* (FAD) document
(4. Appeal)	¬ FAD distributed and published as *NICE Guidance* unless one or more consultees lodge an *appeal* within 15 working days from receipt of the FAD

Fig. 3.1 NICE Technology Appraisal process overview
Topics for appraisal are referred to NICE in groups ("waves")

and any special considerations appropriate to the topic. Following preparation of a final remit (produced by the DoH and the Welsh Assembly Government) and a final scope (by NICE), a formal decision is made by the Ministers whether to refer the technology in question for appraisal by NICE. Once referred to NICE, the appraisal process is initiated by NICE (Figure 3.1), and the timeline (cf. Table 3.2, below) commences after NICE invites consultees and commentators to participate.

3.2 Assessment

The key activity in the assessment phase is the evaluation of the evidence relating
to the technologies in question by the Assessment Group. The most recent update
of the NICE methods guide (NICE, 2004c) is highly prescriptive of admissible
evidence, of its analysis and of the presentation of findings. Specifically, a reference
case has been defined with the objective of achieving consistency across assessments, providing a detailed description of the methods considered most appropriate
for the Appraisal Committee's subsequent deliberations (see below, *"Appraisal"*).
These include, *inter alia* and within the scope developed by NICE, the use of all
health effects on individuals as outcome measure, to determine health benefits in
terms of QALYs (using a standardized and validated generic instrument), to derive
preferences for health state valuation from a representative sample of the public
using a choice-based method (i.e., as opposed to a rating scale) for elicitation, the
use of an annual discount rate of 3.5% for both costs and health effects, and finally
"QALY egalitarianism"[1] as equity position (Table 3.1).

Table 3.1 NICE reference case definition
Major changes that NICE introduced in April 2004 included the definition of an explicit "reference
case", the abolishment of differential discounting on costs and health benefits, the mandatory use
of probabilistic sensitivity analysis to address decision uncertainty, and explicit consideration of
subgroup analyses (NICE, 2004c)

Analytic approach	Choices prescribed by NICE for reference case analysis
Problem definition	Scope from NICE
Comparator(s)	Routine therapies in NHS
Evidence on outcomes	Systematic review
Economic evaluation	Cost-effectiveness analysis (CEA)
Perspective on outcomes	All health effects on individuals
Perspective on costs	National Health Service (NHS) and personal social services (PSS)
Discount rate	3.5% p.a. on both costs and health effects
Addressing uncertainty	Probabilistic sensitivity analysis
Measure of health benefits	Quality-adjusted life years (QALYs)
Source of preference data	Representative sample of the public
Health state valuation method	Choice-based method (i.e., standard gamble [SG] or time trade-off [TTO])
Description of health states for calculating QALYs	Using a standardized and validated generic instrument
Equity position	Each additional QALY has equal value

---

[1] "QALY egalitarianism" refers to a normative assumption of the extrawelfarist school of thought,
implying that an additional QALY should receive the same weight regardless of any other characteristics of the individuals receiving the health benefit. This premise relies on the validity of the

Synthesizing evidence on outcomes should enable an unbiased estimate of clinical effectiveness. To achieve this NICE expects a systematic review and meta-analysis, requiring that an assessment of the degree of and the reasons for heterogeneity be undertaken before any statistical pooling is carried out. The need is acknowledged to construct a decision-analytical framework in order to estimate clinical and cost effectiveness relevant to the decision-making context in a clinical setting. Accordingly, modeling – "an unavoidable fact of life in economic evaluation" (Buxton et al., 1997) – is explicitly accepted and is likely to be required, among other situations, when trial populations are atypical, intermediate outcomes data from trials are used, relevant comparators have not been used in trials, or when long-term consequences extend beyond trial follow-up.

NICE further expects parameter uncertainty to be presented using probabilistic sensitivity analysis (or, where appropriate, stochastic analysis of patient-level data). Moreover, patient subgroups should be identified and clinically justified, and uncertainty in subgroup results should be fully reflected.

In addition, the Assessment Group is required to incorporate submissions from manufacturers and sponsors, alongside details of models used in these submissions. Such submissions are expected to meet the same criteria, and any electronic models need to be provided to NICE and the Assessment Group. Commercially sensitive data may be designated "commercial-in-confidence" and will remain confidential, i.e., will not be published with the Assessment Report. In order to address the debate about the use of confidential information in technology assessments (e.g., Mauskopf and Drummond, 2004), attempting to contain the practice of keeping information confidential, NICE has reached an agreement with the pharmaceutical industry defining the circumstances under which non-publication of data would be acceptable[2] (NICE, 2004g).

A time frame of 28 weeks is allowed by NICE for completion of the Assessment Report, although in practice this is reduced to 14 weeks when the deadline for receipt of external submissions is factored in (cf. Table 3.2). Thus, the timely and high-quality production of an Assessment Report represents a formidable challenge for the selected Assessment Group.

---

quality-adjusted life year as a measure capturing health-related quality of life (Rawlins and Culyer, 2004), reflects the idea that the NHS ought to maximize the health of the whole community (Culyer, 1997), and is closely related to the linear "QALY aggregation rule" (Dolan et al., 2005; Schlander, 2005a). It should be noted that, at least in theory, as Alan Williams (1996) stated, "there is nothing in the QALY approach that requires QALYs to be used only in a maximizing context," even though he was quick to add, "it is QALY maximization that is the natural interpretation of the drive for efficiency in health care" (Williams, 1996). Others have suggested that equity weights might be applied to QALYs before aggregation (e.g., Culyer, 1989). For further discussion of some of these and related issues, see also later, e.g., Chapter 5, "*Quality of Life and Utility Estimates*", Chapter 6, "*Objectives of Health Care Provision*", and also Chapter 6, "*(Almost) Exclusive Reliance on QALYs as an Outcome Measure?*"

[2] This agreement between NICE and the Association of the British Pharmaceutical Industry (ABPI) was made on October 27, 2004. This was after the September 17, 2004 deadline set for submissions by consultees for the ADHD appraisal reviewed here (cf. Table 3.2). See also Chapter 6, *Discussion and Implications*.

Table 3.2 NICE Technology Appraisal process timelines

Reconstructed using the following data sources: NICE Guidance to the Technology Appraisal Process (NICE, 2004b); Assessment Protocol (King et al., 2004a); Project History (published on NICE website, http://www.niche. org.uk/page.aspx?o=adhd, accessed repeatedly; last access at http://www.nice.org.uk/page.aspx?o=72340 and 297183, December 20, 2005); cf. also http://www.nice.org.uk/page.aspx?o=TA098, last access March 27, 2006

NICE Technology Appraisal Process in General			NICE ADHD Appraisal		
Phase	Milestone	Key Activities	Timing	Schedule	Actual
Scoping		Remit from DoH to NICE			2003 (July)
		Scope published			2003 (Aug.)
		Final Scope published			2003 (Oct.)
		[ADHD appraisal temporarily halted]	n.a.	n.a.	
		Final Scope published			2004 (May)
Assessment	Official start of appraisal	Consultees/commentators invited to participate	Week 0	2004 (June, 10)	2004 (June, 10)
		Final protocol available (from Assessment Group)	Week 3	2004 (June, 30)	2004 (June, 22)
		Consultees' meeting			2004 (June, 30)
		Deadline for submissions from consultees to NICE	Week 14	2004 (Sept., 17)	2004 (Sept., 17)
	AR Available	Assessment Report (AR) received by NICE	Week 28	2004 (Dec., 10)	2004 (Dec., 09)
		Consultees invited to comment on AR	Week 30	2004 (Dec., 24)	

(continued)

Table 3.2 (continued)

NICE Technology Appraisal Process in General

Phase	Milestone	Key Activities	Timing	NICE ADHD Appraisal Schedule	Actual
Appraisal		Comments on AR from consultees received	Week 34	2005 (Jan., 21)	2005 (February)
		Evaluation Report sent to Appraisal Committee	Week 36	2005 (Feb., 04)	2005 (February)
		First meeting of Appraisal Committee	Week 37	2005 (Feb., 11)	2005 (Feb., 15)
	ACD available	ACD produced and distributed	Week 40	2005 (March, 04)	
		ACD published on website	Week 41	2005 (March, 11)	2005 (March, 09)
		Second meeting of Appraisal Committee	Week 45	2005 (April, 08)	2005 (April, 21)
	FAD available	FAD produced and distributed	Week 51	2005 (May, 20)	
		FAD published on website	Week 52	2005 (May, 27)	2005 (June, 06)
Appeal		Appeal announcement published on website			2005 (July, 07)
		Appeal details published on website			2005 (July, 22)
		Appeal Panel meeting			2005 (Aug., 25)
		Final Decision of the Appeal Panel published			2005 (Dec., 08)
Guidance	Completion of appraisal	Expected date of issue, after appeal hearing		2005 (August)	2006 (March, 22)

The Assessment Group may produce a *de novo* economic model, which will be protected by intellectual property rights. Although it may be provided to stakeholders upon their written request, it will be supplied as a read-only copy and must not be re-run with alternative assumptions or data inputs (NICE, 2004b).

3.3 Appraisal

The Appraisal Committees are standing advisory committees of NICE whose members are appointed for a three-year term. Members are drawn from the NHS, patient and caregiver organizations, relevant academic disciplines, and the pharmaceutical and medical device industries.

The appraisal stage of the process comprises four elements.

One element is the consideration of the evidence in the Assessment Report (including confidential material) together with that submitted by other parties, the aim being to develop an Appraisal Consultation Document (ACD), with the participation of members of the independent academic Assessment Group.

The preparation of and consultation on the ACD should respect specified benchmarks for incremental cost-effectiveness ratios, and take into account the longer-term interests of the NHS in encouraging innovation in technologies that will benefit patients.

A further element of the appraisal process is the review by the Appraisal Committee of the ACD in the light of comments received during consultation.

The ultimate element of the appraisal process is the preparation of the Final Appraisal Determination (FAD). Subject to any appeal, the FAD will form the basis of the guidance by NICE on the use of the appraised technology. This process is transparent in so far as ongoing activities including meeting agendas are published on the NICE website.

Throughout the appraisal phase there are well-defined opportunities for consultees to contribute. Consultees are invited by NICE to make comments on the Assessment Report, and their comments may lead to a decision to undertake additional analyses before the Appraisal Committee meeting to develop the ACD. Consultees and commentators are given an additional opportunity to comment on the ACD within a time frame of four weeks. New data will be accepted at this stage "only if they are likely to materially affect the provisional recommendations in the ACD, and only by prior agreement" with NICE. Although key documents are made publicly available through its website, NICE does not accept unsolicited submissions, that is comments from stakeholders other than invited consultees (NICE, 2004b).

3.4 Appeal

Consultees are given 15 working days from receipt of the FAD to lodge an appeal which will be considered only if it falls within one or more of the following categories: (a) NICE has failed to act fairly and in accordance with its published procedures, (b) the FAD is perverse in light of the evidence submitted, with "per-verse" meaning that the FAD is "obviously and unarguably wrong, in defiance of logic, or so absurd that no reasonable Appraisal Committee could have reached such conclusions" (NICE, 2004d), or (c) NICE has exceeded its powers.

New evidence or simply disagreement with a FAD will "almost certainly" not be accepted in this last stage of the appraisal process (NICE, 2004d). Nor is it possible to reopen arguments and issues on which a determination by NICE has been reached. The phases of appraisal and, where applicable, of appeal also follow defined timelines (see Table 3.2). In light of the above, the whole process of tech-nology appraisals may be described as having attributes of transparency, reliability, predictability, and participation.

3.5 Clinical Guidelines

A separate role of NICE, not to be confused with technology appraisals, is the issue of clinical guidelines that provide recommendations for the treatment and care of patients by health care professionals. Clinical guidelines are normally broader in scope than technology assessments, and as a consequence any gaps in the available scientific evidence are addressed by expert opinion. Clinical guidelines are devel-oped by a Guideline Development Group comprising of health professionals and patient/caregiver representatives. Guideline Development Groups are set up by one of currently seven National Collaborating Centers, which have been established by NICE to harness the expertise of the Royal medical colleges, professional bodies and patient/caregiver organizations. Accordingly, in contrast to technology appraisals, the clinical guideline development process is predominantly administered by clini-cal experts, rather than economists (cf. Wailoo et al., 2004; Williams, 2004; Little-johns et al., 2004).

NICE Appraisal of ADHD Treatments

Scope
Assessment
Appraisal
Appeal
Clinical Guidelines

Chapter 4
NICE Appraisal of ADHD Treatments

The first appraisal of methylphenidate for "hyperactivity" (hyperkinetic disorder, HKD according to ICD-10; World Health Organization, 1992) was conducted by NICE in 2000. In October 2000, NICE issued guidance recommending the use of methylphenidate as part of a comprehensive treatment program for "severe ADHD" (NICE, 2000), which had been considered roughly equivalent to HKD[1]. The evidence basis for this appraisal was a technology review commissioned by NICE (Lord and Paisley, 2000) that drew heavily on two previously published systematic reviews, one by the US Agency for Healthcare Research and Quality (AHRQ; Jadad et al., 1999) and a second by the Canadian Coordinating Office for Health Technology Assessment (CCOHTA; Miller et al., 1998).

In addition, submissions were made by the manufacturers of the two immediate-release methylphenidate (MPH-IR) products available at that time (see Table 1.2). One UK cost-utility analysis was also available (Gilmore and Milne, 2001) based on a Wessex Development and Evaluation Committee (DEC) report (Gilmore et al., 1998) at the time of appraisal, which indicated that for methylphenidate (MPH-IR) in the treatment of hyperactivity (HKD, ICD-10) the cost per QALY estimate was £7,400 to £9,200 at 1997 prices for a 12-month time horizon (Gilmore and Milne, 2001). The NICE technology review carried an expiry date of July 2003, and the review date for the guidance was scheduled for August 2003.

4.1 Scope

In mid-2003, NICE published the scope for the imminent review, which was expanded to cover the full range of drug treatments for ADHD in children and adolescents (NICE, 2003); specifically methylphenidate(including new formulations),

---

[1] HKD according to ICD-10 criteria corresponds best to the "impaired combined subtype" of ADHD according to DSM-IV criteria – see Chapter 1, *Introduction* (cf. Tripp et al., 1999; Wolraich et al., 1998).

atomoxetine (a non-stimulant drug for ADHD that had been licensed in the US since 2002, but which was still in development in the UK at the time of the 2003 scoping), and dexamphetamine (an older stimulant drug, licensed as an "adjunct in the management of refractory hyperkinetic states in children;" BNF, 2006). The scope specified the Department of Health remit to NICE as follows:

Comparators should include placebo and usual care. Outcomes should include the incidence and severity of core symptoms, problem behaviors, educational performance, measures of depression and/or anxiety, measures of conduct/oppositional-disorder-related outcomes, adverse events, and quality of life. A recommendation was also included that consideration should be given to the impact of comorbid disorders, quality of life of other family members, and the optimal duration of treatment, where the evidence permits.

In October 2003, the appraisal process was temporarily paused "to synchronize the appraisal timelines with the anticipated licensing of one of the technologies in this appraisal" (NICE, 2005i), and it was resumed in May 2004 (cf. Tables 1.2 and 3.2).

4.2 Assessment

In June 2004, the final protocol for the technology assessment (King et al., 2004a) was provided by the Assessment Group, reflecting the scope delineated above. This was published on the NICE website in October 2004. Treatment outcomes to be included were specified confirming the scope, including incidence and severity of core symptoms, of co-existing problems (. . .), measures of depression and/or anxiety, adverse effects, and quality of life. "If evidence allows," consideration should be given to the impact of comorbid disorders. The assessment protocol stated explicitly that "studies that have used parent and teacher ratings of hyperactivity" would be assessed in the first instance; "in addition, physician ratings of clinical global impression" would be examined. Deadline for industry submissions was September 17, 2004, and the final Assessment Report was scheduled for December 9, 2004 (cf. Table 3.2). It also stated in detail the search strategy for evidence, which would include the following sources and study designs: conference proceedings, gray literature, randomized controlled clinical trials (of at least three weeks duration), full economic evaluations that compare at least two options and consider both costs and consequences, including cost-effectiveness, cost-minimization, cost-utility and cost-benefit analysis. It further explicated that "full paper manuscripts of any titles/abstracts that may be relevant" would be obtained where possible.

On December 9, 2004, the Assessment Report (King et al., 2004b) was completed by a group of ten authors, one of whom was a clinical expert. It was subsequently published by NICE on March 9, 2005, together with the Appraisal Consultation Document (ACD). The Assessment Report (AR) – comprised of 605 pages with 13 appendices – included a systematic review of the evidence and a statistical data synthesis using advanced mixed treatment comparison (MTC) techniques, a review of the submissions by manufacturers, and an economic evaluation model developed *de novo* by the Assessment Group[2]. The main conclusions of the Assessment Report were that "(i) drug therapy seems to be superior to no drug therapy; (ii) no significant differences between the various drugs in terms of efficacy or side effects were found – mainly due to *lack of evidence*; (iii) the additional benefits from behavioural therapy (in combination with drug therapy) are uncertain" and "Given the lack of evidence for any differences in effectiveness between the drugs, the [economic] model tends to be driven by drug cost, which differ considerably" (Assessment Report [AR], Executive Summary, p. 20).

More specifically, it was stated that "for a decision taken now, with current available data, *the results of the economic model clearly identify an optimal treatment strategy*" (AR, Ch. 6, p. 261; italics added) and that "this analysis showed that a treatment strategy of 1st line dexamphetamine, followed by 2nd line methylphenidate immediate-release for treatment failures, followed by 3rd line atomoxetine for repeat treatment failures was optimal"[3] (AR, Ch. 6, p. 260).

The primary economic model was based on six randomized clinical trials reporting Clinical Global Impression/Improvement (CGI-I) sub-scores after a treatment duration of three to eight weeks, one of which was "commercial-in-confidence." An unspecified number of studies excluded from the effectiveness review were said to have, nevertheless, been included in the cost-effectiveness analysis (cf. AR, Ch. 6, p. 226). Data from these studies were mathematically synthesized despite design heterogeneity. For secondary extensions of the model, further studies were included using different clinical effectiveness measures. A detailed critique of key aspects of the Assessment Report will be provided later, alongside a discussion of their relevance and of potential implications for the appraisal process as currently adopted by NICE.

4.3 Appraisal

NICE convened the first Appraisal Committee meeting on February 15, 2005, and published an Appraisal Consultation Document (ACD) on its website on March 9, 2005 (NICE, 2005a). The preliminary recommendation was in favor of all three compounds – methylphenidate, atomoxetine, and dexamphetamine – as therapeutic options within their licensed indications. It stated that the decision about which product to use should be based on the presence of comorbid conditions (for example,

---

[2] For a discussion of some critical features of the decision analytical model, see below, Chapter 5, *Critique*.

[3] Dexamphetamine in the United Kingdom is licensed as an "adjunct in the management of refractory hyperkinetic states" only (cf. above, *Scope*; BNF, 2006). Likewise, the absence of any reference to methylphenidate modified-release formulations (MPH-MR08 and MPH-MR12) is noteworthy. These formulations are mentioned in the discussion chapter of the Assessment Report only "for patients in whom a midday dose is unworkable" (AR, Ch. 7, p. 266). This is relevant for the broader issue of treatment compliance, which will be discussed in Chapter 5.3, *Efficacy, Effectiveness, and Treatment Compliance*.

tic disorders, Tourette syndrome, epilepsy), the different adverse effect profiles of each drug, specifically-identified issues regarding compliance, for example possible problems created by the need to administer a midday treatment dose at school, the risk potential for drug-diversion (where the medication is forwarded on to others for non-prescription uses) and/or misuse, and the individual preferences of the child/adolescent and/or their parent/guardian.

Compared to no treatment, estimated costs per quality-adjusted life year (QALY) gained were below £7,000 for all options evaluated. The meeting minutes provide little information about details other than mentioning that topics of the discussion included, among others, "the availability of long-term studies," and "the issue of single daily dose regimens versus multiple-dose regimens" (NICE, 2005b).

Following a second Appraisal Committee meeting on April 21, 2005 (NICE, 2005d), the Final Appraisal Determination (FAD) was issued by NICE on its website on June 06, 2005 (NICE, 2005c) and these recommendations were upheld except for two changes, viz. "*specifically identified* issues regarding compliance, for example..." was replaced by "*specific* issues regarding compliance *identified for the individual child or adolescent*, for example..." and the deletion of the word "individual" before "preferences."

The definitions of terms provided by NICE as criteria for audit confirm that the FAD recommendation of June 2005 is somewhat more restrictive than the ACD (NICE, 2005a) wording. Specifically, "issues regarding compliance" according to the ACD "could include *administration* of a mid-day dose at school," whereas the FAD (NICE, 2005c) defines that they "could include *problems created by the need to administer* a mid-day dose at school" (all italics added). This revised wording suggests that the actual manifestation of problems with a midday dose might be required prior to prescription of modified-release formulations of methylphenidate.

The Appraisal Committee considered evidence from the Assessment Report as well as submissions and comments from manufacturers/sponsors, professional/specialist and patient/caregiver groups, and commentator organizations on the draft scope, Assessment Report and ACD. Emphasis was placed by the Appraisal Committee on a total of 64 randomized controlled clinical trials that the Assessment Group had found to meet its inclusion criteria (cf. Chapter 5, *Critique*, below). One further trial, the NIMH MTA Study (MTA Cooperative Group, 1999a,b – for a review of this landmark study in clinical ADHD research, see Chapter 6, *Discussion*), was included in the evidence base that was taken into account. A substantial number of generally minor adjustments of the ACD were incorporated into the FAD, underscoring the transparent and participatory nature of the process. Few of these changes are noteworthy and need to be emphasized or discussed in the present context (see also Chapter 5, *Critique*):

First, a sentence was added to the FAD stating "the evidence from short-term randomized placebo-controlled trials suggests that methylphenidate is an effective treatment to reduce core symptoms of ADHD in children who continue to take the medication." This narrow focus upon short-term, placebo-controlled designs is potentially misleading since, at the time of assessment and appraisal, there was also compelling evidence available from two high-quality long-term studies, both demonstrating significant benefits from methylphenidate over two years

(MTA Cooperative Group, 1999a,b, 2004; Klein et al., 2004; Abikoff et al., 2004a). In fact, one of these studies (Klein et al., 2004) confirmed effectiveness of methylphenidate (average daily doses from 35.6 mg to 41.0 mg, given t.i.d., i.e., divided in three administrations which corresponds to the dosing schedule used in the MTA study), in the longer term by virtue of a 100% relapse rate during a single-blind switch to placebo after one year (Abikoff et al., 2004a); the same study showed stable treatment benefits from methylphenidate over two years (Abikoff et al., 2004a).

Second, a further sentence in the FAD stating that "most studies did not indicate statistically significant differences in terms of *effectiveness* when comparing the immediate-release and modified-release formulations with each other" raises concern about the distinction between *efficacy* and effectiveness. This issue has perpetuated from the Assessment Report and will be addressed in more detail later (Chapter 5, *Critique*).

Third, another sentence stating that "atomoxetine was normally given in a single daily dose and could also be suitable in circumstances where multiple daily dosing was impractical" (ACD, p. 17) was deleted in the FAD.

In summary, the Appraisal Committee found that, on the basis of the evidence reviewed, it was "*not possible to distinguish between the different [treatment] strategies on the grounds of cost-effectiveness*" (FAD, p. 13), and "accepted the importance of having a range of drug treatment options" (FAD, p. 17). They "concluded that all three drugs are cost-effective relative to no drug treatment" (FAD, p. 18). The Committee also noted "that there were a number of important factors to be taken into account when selecting a treatment for an individual ... with ADHD [including] ... consideration of concordance and compliance issues, particularly with respect to the timing of doses, ... previous adverse effects, comorbidities, and the preferences of patients and carers" (FAD, p. 18).

In effect, this NICE guidance ultimately provides patients, their parents/guardians, and their physicians with a very high degree of discretion regarding the choice of treatment.

4.4 Appeal

One consultee (the manufacturer of a modified-release methylphenidate product – MPH-MR12, Table 1.2) lodged an appeal against the FAD and NICE Guidance and a public hearing was convened at NICE on August 25, 2005[4]. The outcome of the appeal process was published by NICE on December 08, 2005 (NICE, 2005e, 2005h), dismissing the appeal while at the same time recognizing a failure of the Assessment Group to conform to the agreed assessment protocol.

---

[4] The document "Decision of the Panel" (NICE, 2005h) states that an Appeal Panel was convened on September 25, 2005, to consider the appeal.

The appeal was made on the grounds that NICE had failed to act fairly and in accordance with its Appraisal Procedure (see Chapter 3, *Appeal*) since a key study (referred to as LYBI[5]) had been omitted from the technology assessment report, and subsequently had not been considered when the Appraisal Committee prepared the ACD. The Appeal Panel "expressed its disappointment at the failure of the assessment group to include study LYBI in its assessment report," a clear "protocol deviation" (Decision of the Panel, p. 3f.; NICE, 2005h), but maintained that the Appraisal Committee had given the study due consideration before completing the FAD.

The appellant also alleged that NICE had prepared guidance "which is perverse in light of the evidence" (see Chapter 3, *Appeal*), as two studies (including LYBI) had shown MPH-MR12 to be more effective than the comparator, atomoxetine. Although the Appeal Panel acknowledged statistically significant differences between the effects of MPH-MR12 and atomoxetine discussed in the FAD[6], it upheld the view of the Appraisal Committee that it "had to make an overall judgement about the clinical superiority of MPH (either as IR or MR formulations) compared to atomoxetine on the totality of the available evidence" (Decision of the Panel, p. 5; NICE, 2005h). On this basis, including the observation of only extremely small QALY differences (extending only to the third decimal place) calculated by the Assessment Group, the Appeal Panel dismissed the appellant's claim that MPH-MR12 was more effective and less expensive than atomoxetine.

After the final decision of the Appeal Panel, NICE postponed the issue of guidance in order to be able to incorporate anticipated advice on the use of atomoxetine resulting from an ongoing review of its health risks and benefits by the Medicines and Healthcare products Regulatory Agency (MHRA). Final guidance (NICE, 2006b) was published by NICE March 22, 2006, and reflected the Final Appraisal Determination (FAD), obviously without deviation.

4.5 Clinical Guidelines

In parallel to the appraisal process, on June 16, 2004, the Department of Health (DoH) and the Welsh Assembly Government requested NICE to develop a clinical guideline on the "management of attention-deficit/hyperactivity disorder" (NICE, 2004f). As part of its "Tenth Wave" working program, NICE cited the remit on its

---

[5] Study "LYBI" was published by Newcorn et al. (2004, 2005).

[6] Three studies comparing MPH and ATX were discussed in the FAD: One study compared ATX and MPH-IR (Kratochvil et al., 2002), finding "no difference on subjective outcomes" (FAD, p. 11), although it had not been designed and thus not powered to detect such differences. The other two "unpublished studies" (identifiable as Kemner et al., 2004, 2005; Newcorn et al., 2004, 2005) compared ATX and MPH-MR12, both reporting significantly greater response rates with MPH-MR12 compared to ATX [FAD, pp.10–12]. For more detailed information on these studies, see Chapter 6, *Discussion*, and Table 5.15. For a comparison of effect sizes achieved with a modified-release formulation of methylphenidate (MPH-MR12) and with atomoxetine (e.g., Steinhoff et al., 2003), see also Chapter 6, *Insights from Disease-Specific Effectiveness Measures*.

website on August 11, 2004, as "to prepare a guideline for the NHS in England and Wales on the effectiveness of methylphenidate and other pharmacological and psychological interventions in combination or separately for the treatment of ADHD" and that "the guideline should apply to the treatment of children, young people and adults where evidence of treatment effectiveness is available" (NICE, 2004e).

This process will be led by the National Collaborating Centre for Mental Health and is broader in scope than the technology appraisal, intended to cover "the full range of care routinely made available by the NHS," notably including psychological interventions as well as treatment of adults (see Draft Scope, published January 31, 2006, and subsequently confirmed by the Final Scope of August 8, 2006; NICE, 2006a,j).

NICE Appraisal of ADHD Treatment Options: A Critique

Chapter 5
NICE Appraisal of ADHD Treatment Options: A Critique

As the recommendations generated by NICE are driven primarily by the Assessment Report (King et al., 2004b) – this document "is used as the basis of the appraisal" (NICE, 2004b) – the following critique will focus primarily (though not exclusively) on key issues addressed by the Assessment Group.

The review of the assessment identifies gaps related to critical issues in a number of areas, including the selection criteria (and their application) used for clinical evidence (including endpoints) considered in the economic model, the distinction between efficacy and effectiveness in light of the crucial role of treatment compliance in ADHD, the methodology behind the synthesis of data from multiple sources, the structure of the economic model developed by the Assessment Group, and the relationship between cost-utility findings of the Assessment Group and evaluations of cost-effectiveness in the public domain (cf. Chapter 6, *Discussion*).

In this critique, issues without potential influence on either the conclusions of the assessment or the NICE appraisal (i.e., the overall picture) will not be considered, despite some minor technical issues with the assessment[1].

As indicated earlier, the assessment protocol (King et al., 2004a) had been completed June 22, 2004, and the Assessment Report (AR; King et al., 2004b) was prepared during the second half of the same year (Table 3.2). This document was completed by the Assessment Group in December 2004 and comprised of 605 pages including 13 appendices. It recapitulated the scope of the assessment (NICE,

---

[1] One such example relates to the discount rates used. The annual discount rates described both in the assessment protocol (King et al., 2004a, p. 16; this document was completed in June 2004) as well as in the Assessment Report (King et al., 2004b, p. 223)–6% for costs and 1.5% for benefits – and used by the Assessment Group for an extended analysis – do *not* reflect current guidelines by the Department of Health from 2003 (Netten, 2003) and, subsequently, by NICE of April 2004 (NICE, 2004c) to use an annual discount rate of 3.5% for both costs and benefits. This is in contrast to an explicit statement in the Assessment Report (p. 223) that discount rates were applied "in accordance with NICE guidance." This anomaly is surprising given not only that the senior author of the Assessment Report mentioned this change in the latest edition of his authoritative textbook (Drummond et al., 2005, p. 111), but also the intense discussion and a wide-spread consensus among economists that equal discount rates should be used for both health outcomes and costs (Claxton et al., 2006; Keeler and Cretin, 1983).

2003) and briefly delineated the background of the health problem underlying the assessment, identifying issues related to prevalence, etiology, diagnostic criteria, and symptoms, as well as psychiatric comorbidity and social impairment, but not long-term sequelae of the disorder (AR, pp. 34ff.). A brief description of the medications studied was followed by a methods section, which covered search, data extraction, and analysis strategies for the effectiveness and the cost-effectiveness reviews. Search criteria were designed broadly to identify "ongoing and recently completed research" (AR, p. 42) by including, among others, "conference proceedings, reports, dissertations and other grey literature" (assessment protocol, pp. 2ff.; AR, pp. 41ff.; see King et al., 2004a); "economic evaluations could include cost-consequence, cost-utility, cost-effectiveness analysis, cost-minimisation and cost-benefit analyses" (AR, p. 50). Deviating from the assessment protocol, a restriction was introduced insofar as clinical studies were excluded if they had been only published as abstracts or as conference presentations (AR, p. 46). Similarly "economic evaluations reported as conference proceedings or abstracts were excluded since the data they contain *may* not be complete" (AR, p. 50, italics added; for related consistency issues, see *Appendix*).

In a recent overview, which focused on the use of clinical data in health technology assessments of rapidly evolving technologies, it was reported that all but two technology assessment groups producing evaluations on behalf of NICE used data from conference abstracts and presentations. It was further suggested that these "technology assessment teams should increase their efforts to obtain further study details by contacting trialists" (Dundar et al., 2006).

Following an effectiveness review, the Assessment Report offered "a systematic review of the health-related quality of life and cost-effectiveness literature" (AR, p. 50, pp. 177ff.) and a critical review of three submissions of product evaluations, which had been prepared by their respective manufacturers (AR, pp. 192ff.). For economic modeling, efficacy data were synthesized using advanced mixed treatment comparison methods. Utility, resource utilization, and cost data as well as assumptions were described extensively. The primary model was enhanced by a number of probabilistic sensitivity analyses designed to integrate various effectiveness measures, alternative sources of utility data and different time horizons (from one year up to age 18 years).

Although the Assessment Group discussed limitations of its model, notably including data deficiencies, the interpretation of the license of dexamphetamine, and situations where a midday dose of medication might be unworkable, it still concluded that its "evaluation clearly identified an optimal treatment strategy" (cf. AR, pp. 260ff.). The Assessment Report was subsequently published as a peer-reviewed contribution to the specialist periodical *Health Technology Assessment*, apparently unchanged (King et al., 2006), despite that the NICE appeal panel had expressed disappointment about the omission of an important clinical study (referred to as "LYBI" – Newcorn et al., 2004) in the Assessment Report (see Chapter 3, above). The appeal panel had noted that its "disappointment was increased by the fact that the original [assessment] protocol had stipulated that both published and unpublished data be included" (NICE, 2005h).

5.1 Scoping

The scope defined by NICE, and described earlier, provided the framework for the analyses commissioned to the Assessment Group and was narrower than that used for the development of clinical guidelines. It is especially notable that the role of psychological interventions remained beyond the scope of the technology appraisal, despite the importance of psychosocial interventions in clinical practice.

For instance, the traditional view in Europe has been that behavioral treatment should be preferably initiated prior to pharmacotherapy (cf. Taylor et al., 1998)[2]. In 2004 an upgrade of the European clinical guidelines for hyperkinetic disorder (HKD) was published on behalf of the European Society for Child and Adolescent Psychiatry (ESCAP), recommending that medication should be considered when psychosocial treatments alone are insufficient (Taylor et al., 2004). To date, these clinical guidelines for ADHD have not reflected the economic implications of interventions considered.

Still, a key attribute of the treatment paradigm for ADHD in clinical practice is the need to decide on the appropriate sequence of specific therapies following diagnosis, education, advice, and support. Therefore, to be optimally relevant, a health technology assessment of therapeutic interventions for ADHD might be reasonably expected to address the choice between behavioral treatment, medication management (including the specific type of drug to select), or the combination of both, by providing current data on their relative cost-effectiveness.

This narrow scope of the technology appraisal compared to guideline development could have been avoided. Earlier economic analyses had been constrained by a paucity of reliable data on the clinical effectiveness of behavioral treatment. A report commissioned in December 1998 by the Canadian Coordinating Office for Health Technology Assessment (CCOHTA), involving data from a limited number (n = 24) of evaluable subjects under psychological/behavioral therapy (Miller et al., 1998; Klassen et al., 1999) showed that from an economic perspective "pharmaceutical therapies were more attractive than psychological/behavioral therapies under all conditions" (Zupancic et al., 1998, p. 12). However, the wide confidence intervals associated with efficacy estimates derived from the meta-analysis of published trials (cf. Klassen et al., 1999) limited the conclusions that could be drawn. CCOHTA's interpretation was that sensitivity analyses did not alter the conclusion that methylphenidate dominated the alternative options assessed, including psychological/behavioral therapy and combined treatment (Shukla and Otten, 1999). The first NICE appraisal of ADHD treatments in October 2000 also focused on medication for "severe ADHD" (thought to be broadly similar to HKD as previously described), and recommended the use of methylphenidate as part of a comprehensive treatment program, although not necessarily in conjunction with specific psychological treatment such as behavioral therapy. This recommendation was made

---

[2] In contrast in the United States many clinicians have long seen drug treatment as a first-line option, with initiation of behavioral therapy considered concurrently "as appropriate" (AAP, 2001).

on the basis that the estimated cost per QALY gained was approximately £10,000 to £15,000 (Lord and Paisley, 2000; NICE, 2000).

The situation has evolved as published evidence on the clinical efficacy of psychosocial interventions has become available. The NIMH MTA Study[3] (MTA Cooperative Group, 1999a,b, 2004) provided important data over two years on the effectiveness of an intense psychosocial treatment strategy. Moreover, the New York-Montreal long-term study also provided data on another 103 subjects with ADHD treated over 24 months with methylphenidate alone or in combination with comprehensive multimodal psychosocial interventions (Abikoff et al., 2004a; Klein et al., 2004). However, consistent with the pre-defined scope of the NICE appraisal, neither the Assessment Group nor the Appraisal Committee reviewed this study.

As a consequence of the narrow scope, the appraisal does not address the massive superiority of drug therapy compared to ambitious psychosocial interventions, in terms of their effectiveness and cost-effectiveness for symptomatic treatment of (pure) ADHD. This superiority has since been further confirmed by an economic evaluation of the MTA study results, which also used symptomatic normalization of patients as the primary end point of analysis. Although the full publication was not available until September 2005 (Jensen et al., 2005) – which was after the completion of the NICE appraisal (Table 3.2) – two congress abstracts had been available in the public domain since mid-2004[4] (Jensen et al., 2004; Schlander et al., 2004a).

Further economic analyses have since been presented at international meetings. These analyses provide cost-utility estimates based upon the MTA study from a United States payers' perspective (Schlander et al., 2005a; cf. below, Chapter 6, *Discussion and Implications*) and, more recently, European analyses have been become available (Schlander et al., 2006a,b,c; cf. also below). These data indicate that the cost-effectiveness of behavioral interventions, applied alone or in combination with drug treatment, will vary as a function of co-existing disorders and therapeutic objectives. According to these analyses, for "pure" ADHD without psychiatric comorbidity, an MTA-style medication management strategy clearly represents the most attractive option on grounds of cost-effectiveness. However, in the presence of specific comorbidities and at higher levels of willingness-to-pay, intensive behavioral therapy for patients with coexisting internalizing symptoms such as anxiety and combined treatments notably for patients with co-existing conduct disorder and oppositional defiant disorder may also become cost-effective choices (Schlander et al., 2005a, 2006b,c; Foster et al., 2005, 2007). This is particularly true when broader measures of functional impairment, such as those captured by the Columbia Impairment Scale (Bird et al., 1993, 1996) are considered as relevant clinical outcomes (Foster et al., 2005, 2007; Schlander et al., 2006b,c).

---

[3] For a discussion of this study enrolling 579 children with ADHD, cf. below, Chapter 6, *Discussion and Implications*.

[4] Note that the search strategy (as described in the assessment protocol - see King et al., 2004a – cf. above, Chapter 4, *NICE Appraisal of ADHD Treatments*) included conference proceedings and specified that "full paper manuscripts of any titles/abstracts that may be relevant" would be obtained where possible.

Thus, the NICE appraisal of ADHD treatments was constrained by sub-optimal use of existing evidence. Enhanced insights might have been gained by use of a broader scope and by consideration of all the published effectiveness and cost-effectiveness data that were available at the time.

5.2 Data Selection for Assessment

The number and heterogeneity of outcome measures used in ADHD trials (Collett et al., 2003; APA, 2000) presents a real challenge to a comprehensive research synthesis of treatment effectiveness. Accordingly, the Canadian authors of a recent systematic review of "extended treatment" studies in which treatment was administered for 12 weeks or more[5] refrained from conducting a formal meta-analysis (Schachar et al., 2002). They reasoned that the substantial heterogeneity in 14 published studies arising from variations in age, comorbidity, and treatment duration in the patient populations studied together with differences in study methodology, the variety of outcome measures, and data reporting would result in a high risk of an imprecise and potentially misleading result from a quantitative meta-analysis[6](Schachar et al., 2002; Ioannidis et al., 1998). Similarly, the authors of the AHRQ systematic review of November 1999 also deemed quantitative meta-analysis, on the basis of 77 randomized clinical trials selected, "inappropriate, since associated with a greater chance of obtaining imprecise and potentially misleading results" (Jadad et al., 1999).

The general approach, as well as the specific parameters chosen for analysis of ADHD outcomes, require careful consideration in terms of the reliability and validity of measurement instruments, since the consistency of outcome measures is particularly challenging in this condition. It is widely accepted among child and adolescent psychiatrists that parents and teachers (as used as sources for the Conners' CPRS and CTRS rating scales) are the optimal informants about the symptoms and behavioral problems associated with ADHD[7] (Smith et al., 2000; Danckaerts et al., 1999), and that the Conners' Ratings Scales (CRS) as a group represent the most widely used and empirically supported instrument to assess symptoms related to ADHD (Collett et al., 2003; Conners, 2000). Following "consultation with a clinical

---

[5] In clinical ADHD treatment research, the majority of published trials to date have been "short-term" crossover studies with observation periods of less than 12 weeks (Jadad et al., 1999; Miller et al., 1998).

[6] In fact, Schachar et al. (2002) considered that the data allowed calculation of medication treatment effect sizes on core ADHD symptoms (Conners' Rating Scale) and on reading (Wide Range Achievement Test) for descriptive purposes only. For the relevance of this observation, see below, section on outcomes measures considered by the Assessment Group for cost-effectiveness evaluation.

[7] While children and adolescents with ADHD certainly are the best reporters of their subjective experience, they tend to underestimate their disease-specific problems. For example, self-reported hyperactivity has been shown to lack sensitivity and specificity (Collett et al., 2003; Danckaerts et al., 1999).

expert" and specifications documented in the assessment protocol[8], the review of clinical data (AR, Ch. 4, p. 224) used scores of the hyperactivity sub-scales of the CRS to present an effectiveness overview. Accordingly, in the quantitative systematic review commissioned by CCOHTA in 1998 (Miller et al., 1998; Klassen et al., 1999), the great majority of eligible studies (24 out of 26) used a Conners' Scale (CRS, 22; or IOWA Conners, 2). Furthermore, in the AHRQ Evidence Report of November 1999, the Conners' Scales were the most frequently used instruments in 78 studies selected for review (Jadad et al., 1999).

Thus, albeit excluding measures of inattention and impulsivity, the choice of parent and teacher rating scales of hyperactivity is eminently justifiable, though it represents a trade-off between simplicity of analysis and comprehensiveness, in contrast to other ADHD-related technology assessments, which also incorporated measures of inattention and impulsivity (e.g., Miller et al., 1998; Klassen et al., 1999).

Inspection of the clinical studies selected for technology assessment reveals two important anomalies. One is an apparent inconsistency resulting from the interpretation by the Assessment Group of the inclusion requirement that "studies must be of at least three weeks duration." To make sense out of this criterion, one would expect a minimum *treatment* duration of three weeks. Such an expectation would be consistent with the rationale for this three-week cut-off given by the Assessment Group, namely that "the effect of medication on behavior is often (not always) apparent immediately, but the impact on the social adjustment of the child may well not be apparent in the first days of therapy" (final assessment protocol; King et al., 2004a, p. 3f.; reproduced in AR, p. 45). This was justified by the Assessment Group by way of reference to the DSM-IV diagnostic manual (AR, p. 44f.).

However, despite this rationale, a minimum of three weeks *study* (not: *treatment*) duration was used by the Assessment Group as the inclusion criterion. As a consequence, more than one third[9] of the 64 (65, including the important NIMH MTA study) randomized trials selected for the clinical effectiveness review were crossover studies with observation periods shorter than three weeks per treatment arm (usually five to seven days; indeed some studies specified daily crossovers between treatment modalities[10]). Moreover, some of these crossover studies (for example, Swanson et al., 2004) had been conducted without washout phases between treatment periods, which obscured transparent statistical controls for potential carryover effects[11].

---

[8] "Studies that have used parent and teacher rating scales *of hyperactivity* will be assessed *in the first instance*" (cf. above; see King et al., 2004a, p. 4; italics added).

[9] These studies include the following: Brown and Sexten, 1988; Rapport et al., 1989; Fischer and Newby, 1991; Fitzpatrick et al., 1992; DuPaul and Rapport, 1993; Pelham et al., 1987, 1990, 1993, 1999a,b, 2001; Hoeppner et al., 1997; Manos et al., 1999; Efron et al., 1997a,b; Stein et al., 1996, 2003; Kolko et al., 1999; Swanson et al., 2004; Barkley et al., 1990, 2000; Ahmann et al., 1993; Handen et al., 1999; James et al., 2001; Tervo et al., 2002.

[10] For instance, Pelham et al., 1999a,b.

[11] If social adjustment of a child is a clinical outcome of interest, then crossover designs will be problematic due to frequent violation of the well-established requirement that "a similar baseline condition must be present at the start of each of the treatment periods." ... Not only must the

One might argue that this interpretation was formally correct, but it was clearly inconsistent with the Assessment Group's own reasoning that studies "based either on single dose administration or on treatment over a few days" had been "carried out to clarify the mode of action [...] rather than as therapeutic trials, so they should not be included in assessments of clinical value" (AR, Ch. 3, p. 45). No doubt the methodology actually applied was inappropriate for examining the clinical question raised, namely that of social adjustment.

While many very-short-term studies were included[9], at the same time high-quality double-blind trials with parallel group design and two week treatment duration were excluded from the effectiveness review (for example, Biederman et al., 2003), although these exclusions were consistent with the pre-defined protocol. Other randomized clinical trials (RCTs) were overlooked as well. This is a crucial oversight because these trials fulfilled the inclusion criteria for effectiveness (and cost-effectiveness) review. One of these (a head-to-head comparison of two of the therapeutic options considered) followed a double-blind, double-dummy parallel group design with six-week treatment duration[12] (Newcorn et al., 2004, 2005). Another study was a placebo-controlled, dose-response study by Michelson and colleagues (2001), involving 297 randomized patients. Exclusion of this study was justified on grounds that it was available as an abstract only (cf. AR, Appendix 3, p. 337) although its full publication had appeared in *Pediatrics* in November 2001.

At this point, therefore, it can be concluded that the clinical effectiveness review, a major component of an assessment setting the stage for economic evaluation, was impaired by technical anomalies. These anomalies include an incomplete search, an illicitly introduced change of pre-specified search criteria by excluding abstracts and conference proceedings from the actual assessment, and an inappropriate interpretation of the inclusion criterion for studies to document a minimum treatment period of three weeks. In total, these problems led to an idiosyncratic selection of clinical evidence. Furthermore, by design, the focus of the clinical effectiveness review was limited to measures of hyperactivity without consideration of ADHD-defining core symptoms of inattention and impulsivity.

While the issue of missed evidence[13] (such as Newcorn et al., 2004, 2005, and Michelson et al., 2001) pervades the whole technology assessment, the problem of inappropriately (as determined against provisions of the assessment protocol) included data from short-term crossover trials does not persist in the economic

---

baselines be similar, "there must not be any carry-over (i.e. residual) effects (even psychological ones) after either treatment. This means that the disease manifestations should revert to the same baseline and that the effect of treatment should disappear when either treatment is stopped" (Spilker, 1991, p. 29f.). Such problems may arise especially if and when attempts are made to interpret secondary endpoints, while trials were designed to primarily assess different effects.

[12] Study "LYBI" (Newcorn et al., 2004, 2005), referred to in the Appeal process, is particularly important because it is one out of only three studies that directly compared methylphenidate and atomoxetine.

[13] The problem of overlooked data is not limited to the clinical effectiveness review, but extends to the review of economic evaluations; see later.

model. This is the unintended consequence of a departure from the effectiveness criteria previously employed. In marked contrast to other assessments such
as the CCOHTA Technology Report (Miller et al., 1998), the cost-effectiveness
evaluation provided by the Assessment Group deviates from the approach taken
for the effectiveness review (AR, Ch. 6, cf. p. 225) in a number of important
ways.

First, it relies for its "base case" on an analysis on the clinician-rated Clinical
Global Impression improvement sub-scale (CGI-I), scores of which were transformed into "response rates"[14]. Secondary economic analyses were performed from
response rates using efficacy data from the clinician-rated Clinical Global Impression severity sub-scale (CGI-S), the parent-rated ADHD-RS, and finally the SNAP-
IV scale, but again not the Conners' Scales[15].

Second, the studies chosen as inputs for cost-effectiveness analysis do differ from
those selected for the effectiveness review. Although, at least in principle (when
abstracting from technical peculiarities, for instance regarding treatment duration
in crossover studies, as delineated earlier), the selection of studies for the effectiveness review was made in a transparent manner using a set of specified quality
criteria (AR, Ch. 3, pp. 44ff.), this does not hold for the selection of studies used for
economic modeling (Figure 5.1; cf. also below, *Selection of Clinical Effectiveness
Studies for Economic Evaluation*).

5.2.1 *Outcome Measures*

The rationale underlying the decision of the Assessment Group *not* to utilize clinical
efficacy and effectiveness data based on one of the Conners' Rating Scales for the
economic evaluations deserves scrutiny[16]. It will be shown later that the choices
made by the Assessment Group significantly reduced the clinical evidence available
for decision analytic modeling.

The Assessment Report (AR) provides a rationale for this choice based on "two
key assumptions [that] are implicit in using the CTRS as a continuous rating scale
[for cost-effectiveness analyses], that is:

---

[14] In addition to the dubious psychometric properties of this sub-scale, any artificial dichotomization of continuous variables results in an upward distortion in the apparent real variation of correlations across studies (Hunter and Schmidt, 1990; Cohen, 1988). Unless corrected for, this effect
will necessarily impede the detection of differences between interventions studied. There is no
indication in the Assessment Report that the Assessment Group was aware of this statistical effect.

[15] Note that some of the Conners' "hyperactivity" scales include inattention as well.

[16] This descriptive section does not address underlying causes, such as standards stipulated by
NICE guidelines ("reference case analysis"), which may have contributed to the observed prob-
lems. Rather, the focus here is on Assessment Group choices irrespective of constraints (see also
Chapter 6, *Discussion / Case Analysis*).

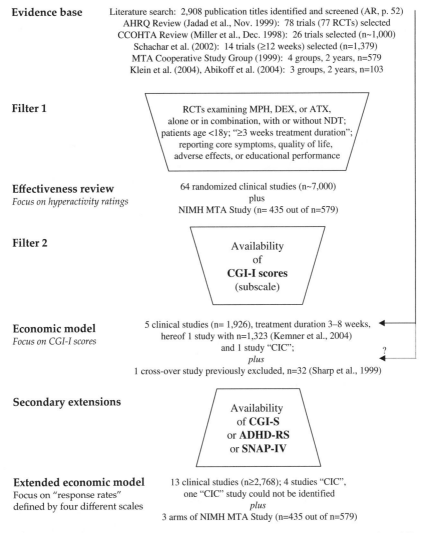

Evidence base   Literature search: 2,908 publication titles identified and screened (AR, p. 52)
AHRQ Review (Jadad et al., Nov. 1999): 78 trials (77 RCTs) selected
CCOHTA Review (Miller et al., Dec. 1998): 26 trials selected (n~1,000)
Schachar et al. (2002): 14 trials (≥12 weeks) selected (n=1,379)
MTA Cooperative Study Group (1999): 4 groups, 2 years, n=579
Klein et al. (2004), Abikoff et al. (2004): 3 groups, 2 years, n=103

Filter 1   RCTs examining MPH, DEX, or ATX,
alone or in combination, with or without NDT;
patients age <18y; "≥3 weeks treatment duration";
reporting core symptoms, quality of life,
adverse effects, or educational performance

Effectiveness review   64 randomized clinical studies (n~7,000)
Focus on hyperactivity ratings   plus
NIMH MTA Study (n= 435 out of n=579)

Filter 2   Availability
of
CGI-I scores
(subscale)

Economic model   5 clinical studies (n= 1,926), treatment duration 3–8 weeks,
Focus on CGI-I scores   hereof 1 study with n=1,323 (Kemner et al., 2004)
and 1 study "CIC";
plus
1 cross-over study previously excluded, n=32 (Sharp et al., 1999)

Secondary extensions   Availability
of **CGI-S**
or **ADHD-RS**
or **SNAP-IV**

Extended economic model   13 clinical studies (n≥2,768); 4 studies "CIC",
Focus on "response rates"   one "CIC" study could not be identified
defined by four different scales   *plus*
3 arms of NIMH MTA Study (n=435 out of n=579)

Fig. 5.1 Reduction of clinical evidence available for economic modeling after application of filters
for effectiveness review and cost-utility model
"CIC", commercial-in-confidence

- that the cost and desirability of achieving a small gain in CTRS score for many
children is assumed to be the same as the cost and desirability of achieving a
large gain in CTRS score for few children, and
- that efficacy is constant across baseline levels of ADHD severity. However, the
efficacy of stimulants [by way of generalizing, 'stimulants' may be read here as a
substitute for 'medication' or 'treatment' in the broader context of the AR] may
depend on the quality and severity of symptoms" (AR, Ch. 5, p. 186).
Further it is argued in the Assessment Report that

- "if this measure [the CTRS-H or CPRS-H] is used, a gain of 1 point on the scale is valued the same, regardless of where you begin on that scale, so the relative value of different effect sizes is not readily interpretable" (AR, Ch. 6, p. 224). Moreover,

- "no published studies were available to provide a link between mean CTRS-H or CPRS-H score and utility data. In order to identify the most optimal treatment strategy in a decision-analytic model one must be able to value the differences in outcome, and this is not currently possible with mean CTRS-H or CPRS-H score" (AR, Ch. 6, p. 224).

In order to calculate costs per QALY gained for the present economic model, response rates were preferred since they facilitate dichotomizing the effectiveness data on the grounds that they indicate an "explicitly identified clinically meaningful change" (AR, Ch. 6, p. 224). In using this approach, which implies the use of an absolute threshold (cf. Hays and Woolley, 2000), the Assessment Group discarded alternative, more sensitive ways to assess treatment effectiveness, such as cost per effect sizes on the Conners' scales as was employed by CCOHTA[17] (Miller et al., 1998). This may be seen as a "pragmatic" choice, given that currently available utility data for patients with ADHD pertain to the states of "responder" and "non-responder" (AR, Ch. 6, p. 224).

While the Assessment Group recognized that "the choice of outcome measure is a critical design issue" of an economic analysis (AR, Ch. 5, p. 178), no reference at all was made to the extensive body of scientific literature (cf. Collett et al., 2003; APA, 2000) concerning the psychometric properties, i.e., the performance characteristics of the measures used.

A recent comprehensive review of ADHD rating scales (Collett et al., 2003) provides some insights in this regard. The validity and reliability, including internal consistency, of the various versions of the Conners' scales has been extensively documented. Normative data from large, ethnically heterogeneous samples of parent and teacher ratings are available separately by gender and age groups. The recent CRS-R (Conners' Rating Scales Revised; Conners, 1997) "have become one of the standard measures of ADHD. The strengths of the CRS-R include a very large normative base, supported factor structure, and strong psychometric properties" (Collett et al., 2003, p. 1021). The widely used older version IOWA Conners (Loney and Milich, 1982) is also "surprisingly robust given its limited number of items. Its brevity and sensitivity to treatment effects support its excellent utility for treatment monitoring and other applications that require repeated administrations. Its frequent citation in the literature allows the potential user to have confidence in its validity and to appreciate its functioning in various applications. The availability and adequate functioning of the multiple informant versions allow the comparison of youths' functioning across perspectives and settings" (Collett et al., 2003, p. 1023). Importantly, the IOWA Conners' Inattentive/Overactive (I/O) sub-scale includes items comparable to the DSM-IV descriptors. Also the newer versions

---

[17] As has been noted earlier, the Conners scores were, in the opinion of Schachar and colleagues (2002), the only scores allowing (descriptive) quantitative synthesis of long-term data.

of the Conners' Scales include items specific to DSM-IV defined ADHD and its associated features.

Despite this background, it remains unclear why the Assessment Group preferred, for its secondary model extensions, to use the ADHD-RS (DuPaul, 1991; DuPaul et al., 1998) and the SNAP-IV (Swanson, 1992) *instead* of the most widely used ADHD-specific instrument, the Conners' Scales (cf. also *Appendix*). While the ADHD-RS and SNAP-IV have a number of strengths and uses, both have been less widely used than the Conners' Scales and are associated with some important limitations. Specifically, the ADHD-RS appears to demonstrate suboptimal sensitivity and specificity and, hence, carries the risk of mis-classifying symptomatology (Collett et al., 2003), and the SNAP-IV symptom scale is not fully supported by published psychometric evaluations or normative data (Collett et al., 2003). Thus, the concerns expressed by the Assessment Group in relation to the Conners' Scales seem to apply no less, or even more so, to their chosen instruments.

5.2.2 Quality of Life and Utility Estimates

The Assessment Group chose to base its primary analyses on Clinical Global Impairment (CGI) scores, or, for that purpose, on CGI-derived "response rates", following the NICE definition of the reference case for economic assessment. This was predicated on the use of a standardized and validated generic (non-disease-specific) instrument to quantify the effects of technologies in terms of health-related quality of life (HRQoL) for patients (NICE, 2004c). Other indicators of HRQoL were used (even) less frequently in ADHD treatment studies (cf. AR, Ch. 4, pp. 60–168; AR, Appendix 12, pp. 368–604). In particular, the CTRS/CPRS and the SNAP-IV scales (like the ADHD-RS, too) do not qualify as (disease-specific) HRQoL instruments as noted in the Assessment Report (p. 178); rather they should be classified as narrowband symptom orientated scales (Collett et al., 2003).

However, it is somewhat unclear how the use of CGI scores might serve to overcome the concerns voiced in relation to the use of Conners' ratings. Instead, within the framework of cost-effectiveness analysis under expected utility theory, there are a number of noteworthy issues surrounding the use of CGI scores to derive HRQoL weights for QALY calculation. Neither the Conners' scales nor the CGI have been established to represent continuous rating scales, and there is absolutely no evidence that CGI-I (global improvement) sub-scores of the CGI ("very much improved" or "much improved" defining a "responder" in the primary analysis) are independent of baseline level. Indeed the relevant CGI-I question is framed so that it explicitly refers to improvement "compared to the condition at admission to the project" (Guy, 1976), thus compounding the uncertainty about the degree of normalization achieved in "responders"[18].

---

[18] The simplistic approach taken to handle the complexities of a valid evaluation, ADHD treatment effectiveness is perhaps most evident when looking at the single CGI-I item descriptor: "Rate total improvement whether or not in your judgment it is due entirely to drug treatment. Compared to his [the patient's] condition at admission to the project, how much has he changed? 1, very much

There have been very few studies of the psychometric properties of the CGI, and their findings have been contradictory (Guy, 2000). It has been asserted that the CGI scale is unreliable (test/re-test correlations for the CGI were rather low, a finding confirmed for the CGI-I sub-scale in a second study [Guy, 2000; Dahlke et al., 1992]). Moreover, some of the items of the CGI have notably abnormal distribution properties in clinical studies, and some items are inappropriately constructed and are of doubtful clinical significance (Beneke and Rasmus, 1992).

Any proposed link between, or combination of, "response rates" based on crude (and subsequently dichotomized) CGI sub-scores and utility estimates, therefore, can be expected to result in outcomes data that may appear mathematically "precise," but will obscure the substantial uncertainty surrounding the relevance of CGI input data (Guy, 2000). Clearly, then, the CGI-I, chosen for the primary economic analysis, cannot provide normative information on a level of response that is independent from baseline. Comparing the single item descriptor of the CGI-S (severity of illness)[19], chosen for secondary economic analyses, with the health state descriptions used to generate utility estimates also reveals marked discrepancies (see below; cf. footnote 20).

There are limited data available for quantifying the differences in utility weights associated with improved HRQoL resulting from a treatment response. Earlier technology assessments had used expert estimates, suggesting a gain of $0.970–0.884 = 0.086$ (with reference to the IHRQL instrument; Gilmore and Milne, 2001) to $1.000–0.883 = 0.117$ (with reference to the EQ-5D; Lord and Paisley, 2000) per responder – or had been restricted to estimating incremental cost per effect size in the Conners' Teacher Rating Scale (CTRS) symptom scores (Miller et al., 1998). In a recent study involving 142 evaluable ADHD patients, in which parents were utilized as proxy raters, utility values based on EQ-5D ratings for patients with severe symptoms were 0.772; patients with moderate symptoms, 0.805; patients with mild symptoms, 0.838; health state "no symptom improvement," 0.773; health state "symptom improvement," 0.837 (Coghill et al., 2004). The resulting difference of $0.837–0.773 = 0.064$ was used by the Assessment Group for their primary ("base case") analysis (cf. AR, Ch. 6, p. 235).

Two further studies, both manufacturer-sponsored and based on standard gamble experiments[20], reported utility gains specific to treatment modality. Interestingly, the findings of each study contradict one another in terms of estimates in favor of the

---

improved, 2, much improved, 3, minimally improved, 4, no change, 5, minimally worse, 6, much worse, 7, very much worse" (Guy, 1976).

[19] The single CGI-S item descriptor reads: "Question: Considering your total clinical experience with this particular population, how mentally ill is the patient at this time? Answers: 1, normal, not at all; 2, borderline mentally ill; 3, mildly ill; 4, moderately ill; 5, markedly ill; 6, severely ill; 7, among the most extremely ill patients" (Guy, 1976). Note that reference to "this particular population" makes ratings context-sensitive, for instance related to comorbidity and admission selection effects in any given study center.

[20] The wording of the AR (Ch. 6, p. 235) is imprecise and potentially misleading as it implies that the estimates presented by Coghill et al. (2004) – which were used for the primary economic analysis – were based on standard gamble experiments; they were, in fact, derived from EQ-5D-based ratings (see Coghill et al., 2004).

products marketed by the respective sponsors (Price et al., 2004; Secnik et al., 2004). Despite noting some inconsistent findings in one of the company submissions, its estimates were used, after certain manipulation, for sensitivity analysis (cf. AR, Ch. 6, pp. 240ff.; Secnik et al., 2004)[21]. More importantly in the present context, none of the hypothetical health states presented to the parents as proxy raters were congruent with the simplistic CGI scales. Furthermore, the three studies mentioned above (Coghill et al., 2004; Price et al., 2004; Secnik et al., 2004) share the use of one-time interviews with parents as the basis of the evaluation, so that it remains unclear if and to what extent adaptation of patients might occur, and how precisely this phenomenon might impact the utility estimates (cf. Menzel et al., 2002; Koch, 2000; Kahneman et al., 1997; Boyd et al., 1990).

From an international perspective, a more fundamental – though separate, being related to the extrawelfarist framework adopted by NICE – *caveat* deserves consideration. The *caveat* concerns the use of the QALY maximization assumption of the NICE reference case itself[22], which has been shown to be empirically flawed with regard to social preferences (Dolan et al., 2005). Within the United Kingdom, debate on underlying value judgments has also been opened by NICE, with its Citizens Council playing an important role (Davies et al., 2005; NICE, 2005f; Rawlins and Culyer, 2004). Although transcending the scope of a single technology appraisal, this *caveat* is worthy of mention at this point. A criticism similar to that applied by the Assessment Group to the Conners' ratings (cf. above) has been made against QALYs, namely that (empirically) identical QALY differences will not be *valued* equally across the scale. There is strong evidence for a general public preference

---

[21] According to the AR (p. 240), "the review ... highlighted some concerns about the validity of these estimates, particularly the fact that the utility of a non-responder without side effects differs between treatments. For example, the utility associated with non-response to atomoxetine, without side effects, is estimated to be 0.902, which compares to an estimated utility of 0.880 associated with non-response and no medication. A difference in utility of 0.022 is relatively large in this population, particularly between health states with identical characteristics. ... so the sensitivity values analysis uses the utility of non-response associated with no medication." The other utility values, however, were used without adaptation. Interestingly, the cited study (which had been presented orally, not as a poster as erroneously stated by the Assessment Group; see AR, Ch. 5, p. 217) reported a higher utility (of 0.886) for atomoxetine "nonresponders" *with* side effects than for "responders" without medication (0.880; Secnik et al., 2004; cf. also AR, Ch. 5, p. 217). Accordingly, these sensitivity analyses using treatment-specific utility values favored those therapies presumably associated with a higher utility gain (AR, Ch. 6, p. 242). In the meantime, a series of closely related papers (Matza et al., 2004, 2005b,c; Secnik et al., 2005) has appeared in various journals, reporting details on the elicitation of those standard gamble scores. As it turns out, the description of health states (Secnik et al., 2004, 2005; cf. also AR, Appendix 10, pp. 359–366) for patients treated with stimulants with "no side effects" includes symptoms associated with insomnia – which has been listed as a "side effect" separately in the description of corresponding health states "with side effects" – which may amount to double-counting and is the only conceivable explanation for the twice as high differences in utility gains reported with non-stimulants (i.e., atomoxetine; difference, 0.06) compared to stimulants (i.e., MPH-IR; difference, 0.02; or MPH-ER, difference, 0.03). This series of experiments was conducted under contract with the manufacturer of atomoxetine and should be interpreted with caution.

[22] As explicitly stated by NICE: "The reference case specifies ... methods ... consistent with an NHS objective of maximizing health gain from limited resources" (NICE, 2004c, p. 21).

for movements starting at lower levels over equidistant improvements starting at higher levels (Dolan et al., 2005; Ubel, 1999a; Nord, 1999). In other words, in that respect the superiority of the QALY approach to measuring health gains rests on the (implicit and explicit) assumptions of expected utility theory (cf. Drummond et al., 2005), requiring cardinal properties of the quality weights used as an input. Yet, quality weights, interpreted as utility estimates reflecting HRQoL, have been shown to depend on elicitation method (notably, time trade-off and standard gamble) in a systematic way (Salomon and Murray, 2004), are prone to a variety of potential measurement errors (Dolan, 2000; Tversky and Kahneman, 1974), and have been subject to further normative questions (Schlander, 2005a; Dolan, 2000; Kahneman et al., 1997; Richardson, 1994), all contributing to uncertainty around quantitative estimates not accounted for within the decision analytic modeling approach itself.

While the approach taken for economic assessment of ADHD treatments has been conceptually in line with NICE guidance, the Assessment Group's stance "that small differences in health states can be estimated in terms of utility values" (AR, Ch. 5, p. 181) needs to be viewed in the context that "the practical problems are particularly great when the benefit from a health intervention is small" (Garber, 2000). Further, the assertion by the Assessment Group that "the preferences of children and adolescents may be most relevant" and "should be measured in patients" (AR, Ch. 5, p. 179) contradicts NICE guidelines as the NICE reference case specifies that "a representative sample of the public" should be used as the "source of preference data" (NICE, 2004c). Moreover, the Assessment Group's assertion neither reflects the tendency of patients to underestimate their disease-specific problems[23] nor normative concerns (e.g., Dolan et al., 2003; Richardson, 1994). In addition, as previously mentioned, utility weights derived from one-time elicitation may be misleading when applied to temporally-extended outcomes. A series of real-time measures of instant utility may then be preferable (cf. Menzel et al., 2002; Kahneman et al., 1997), which is a relevant consideration irrespective of the data source used.

In spite of existing problems associated with the measurement of health-related quality of life (HRQoL) in pediatric populations (De Civita et al., 2005; Griebsch et al., 2005), children and adolescents with ADHD have been reported to have substantially lower HRQoL compared to normative data (Klassen et al., 2004; Sawyer et al., 2002). HRQoL (as measured by parent-proxy EQ-5D ratings, not CGI scores) was found to be correlated with parent-reported ADHD symptom severity

---

[23] See Danckaerts et al., 2000. In general, it is known that the reliability and validity of self-report instruments of psychopathology in children is poor (Achenbach and Edelbrock, 1987). Barkley and colleagues found adolescents to rate themselves no different from normal controls on measures of conflict, though their mothers (and observers) reported more conflicts (Barkley et al., 1991). Self-report measurement with regard to hyperactivity and attention deficits is particularly controversial. For instance, Fischer and colleagues (1993) found that the accuracy of self-reports was specifically low for inattention-overactivity. Likewise, patients have been found to underestimate externalizing behaviors (Loeber et al., 1991). Also children and adolescents typically report fewer problems of inattentiveness-restlessness than are reported by their parents (Kashani et al., 1985; Stewart et al., 1973; Mannuza and Gittelman, 1986).

(Matza et al., 2005c; Klassen et al., 2004) and the presence of comorbid psychiatric diagnoses. These diagnoses include oppositional defiant disorder, conduct disorder, and other psychiatric conditions such as anxiety disorders and depression, but not learning disabilities (Klassen et al., 2004), all of which are known to co-exist frequently with ADHD as described previously (Steinhausen et al., 2006; Schlander et al., 2005b; Gillberg et al., 2004; Green et al., 1999). Despite correlations shown with symptom scores, of course, suitable HRQoL instruments would have the potential advantage of capturing a broader range of children's day-to-day functioning in multiple settings (Matza et al., 2004).

To summarize, there is no compelling evidence to support the choice of the CGI-I as a primary outcome measure for cost-effectiveness evaluation in children and adolescents with ADHD. In fact, the assessment protocol had mentioned that "*in addition* physician ratings of clinical global impression will be examined," suggesting CGI scores – not CGI-I sub-scale ratings – might be used to support findings. None of the hypothetical health states used for proxy-rating to derive utility weights were congruent with *any* one of the instruments used to determine responders.

5.2.3 Selection of Clinical Effectiveness Studies for Economic Evaluation

Another important consequence of the selection criteria is the substantial reduction of the evidence base available for economic analyses. After application of the selection criteria, notably including reports of CGI-I sub-scores, only five studies out of 65 used in the clinical effectiveness review remained for inclusion in the economic analysis (Figure 5.1; cf. AR, Ch. 4). An unintended side effect was the elimination of the crossover studies, where treatment duration per arm had been less than three weeks, which were included in the effectiveness review. The preceding problem of not identifying all relevant clinical studies further compounded this situation.

Table 5.1 provides a quantitative overview of studies selected for assessment and their patient numbers, broken down into categories as defined by the Assessment Group. Based on information provided in the Assessment Report, this illustrates the use of key measurement instruments in these studies. Further this tabulation indicates, extending Figure 5.1, the large volume of data that was not used for economic modeling, as well as the discordance between data used in the effectiveness review and that used in the cost-effectiveness analysis, both of which were performed by the (same) Assessment Group.

Earlier guidance by NICE had recommended use of methylphenidate as part of a comprehensive treatment program for severe ADHD (NICE, 2000). The underlying technology assessment had relied heavily on conclusions of systematic reviews conducted previously by the Agency for Healthcare Research and Quality (AHQR) in the United States (comprising 78 studies, 56 of which included methylphenidate)

Table 5.1 Clinical studies selected by Assessment Group for (a) effectiveness review and (b) economic modeling (overview)

Category	(Comparators)		Clinical studies (Overall)		Clinical studies with endpoints available for efficacy / effectiveness assessment										Used for CUA			
					Conners' scale		Hyperactivity		SNAP-IV		ADHD-RS		CGI (-I or -S)		BC		Ext.	
A	B		#	n	#	n	#	n	#	n	#	n	#	n	#	n	#	n
MPH-IR	**Plac.**		**43**	**2,819+?**	**24+?**	**1,243+?**	**16+?**	**832+?**	**1+?**	**312+?**	**2+?**	**126+?**	**3+?**	**400+?**	**1**	**58**	**2**	**58+?**
LD	Plac.		12	624	8	491	6	263	0	0	1	42	1	30	0	0	0	0
MD	Plac.		21	1,269	12	669	9	558	0	0	1	84	1	58	1	58	1	58
HD	Plac.		9	926	4	83	1	11	1	321	0	0	1	321	0	0	0	0
HD (CIC)	Plac.		1	CIC	?	?	?	?	?	?	?	?	?	?	0	0	1	?
IR-Comb.	**Plac.**		**5**	**148**	**5**	**148**	**1**	**40**	**0**	**0**	**0**	**0**	**0**	**0**	**0**	**0**	**0**	**0**
LD+NDT	Plac.		0	0	0	0	0	0	0	0	0	0	0	0	0	0	0	0
MD+NDT	Plac.		3	93	3	93	1	40	0	0	0	0	0	0	0	0	0	0
HD+NDT	Plac.		2	55	2	55	0	0	0	0	0	0	0	0	0	0	0	0
MPH-ER	**Plac.**		**9**	**1,246+?**	**1+?**	**19+?**	**2+?**	**331+?**	**1+?**	**312+?**	**2+?**	**94+?**	**5+?**	**774+?**	**1**	**321**	**2**	**321+?**
LD	Plac.		2	66	1	19	1	19	0	0	1	47	1	47	0	0	0	0
MD	Plac.		5	1,133	0	0	1	312	1	312	0	0	3	680	1	321	1	321
MD (CIC)	Plac.		1	?	?	?	?	?	?	?	?	?	?	?	0	0	1	?
HD	Plac.		1	47	0	0	0	0	0	0	1	47	1	47	0	0	0	0
MPH-IR	**NDT**		**8**	**396**	**8**	**396**	**3**	**260**	**0**	**0**	**0**	**0**	**1**	**86**	**1**	**86**	**1**	**86**
LD	NDT		1	30	1	30	0	0	0	0	0	0	0	0	0	0	0	0
MD	NDT		4	227	4	227	2	174	0	0	0	0	0	0	0	0	0	0
HD	NDT		3	139	3	139	1	86	0	0	0	0	1	86	1	86**	1	86**
IR-Comb.	**NDT**		**21**	**1,076**	**20**	**1,028**	**6**	**525**	**0**	**0**	**0**	**0**	**2**	**134**	**1**	**86**	**2**	**134**
LD+NDT	NDT		3	167	3	167	1	116	0	0	0	0	0	0	0	0	0	0
MD+NDT	NDT		11	507	11	507	3	232	0	0	0	0	0	0	0	0	0	0
HD+NDT	NDT		7	402	6	354	2	177	0	0	0	0	2	134	1	86**	2	134**

ER-Comb.	**NDT**	**3**	**105**	**3**	**105**	**0**	**0**	**0**	**0**	**0**	**0**	**0**	**0**	**0**	**0**	**0**	**0**
LD	NDT	2	35	2	35	0	0	0	0	0	0	0	0	0	0	0	0
MD	NDT	1	70	1	70	0	0	0	0	0	0	0	0	0	0	0	0
HD	NDT	0	0	0	0	0	0	0	0	0	0	0	0	0	0	0	0
DEX	**Plac.**	**6**	**143**	**3**	**81**	**3**	**77**	**0**	**0**	**0**	**0**	**1**	**28**	**0**	**0**	**0**	**0**
MD	Plac.	2	60	1	32	1	28	0	0	0	0	1	28	0	0	0	0
HD	Plac.	3	65	1	31	1	31	0	0	0	0	0	0	0	0	0	0
TR	Plac.	1	18	1	18	1	18	0	0	0	0	0	0	0	0	0	0
DEX-Comb.	**Plac.**	**2**	**34**	**0**	**0**	**0**	**0**	**0**	**0**	**0**	**0**	**0**	**0**	**0**	**0**	**0**	**0**
MD+NDT	Plac.	1	17	0	0	0	0	0	0	0	0	0	0	0	0	0	0
HD+NDT	Plac.	1	17	0	0	0	0	0	0	0	0	0	0	0	0	0	0
DEX-Comb.	**NDT**	**5**	**157**	**4**	**140**	**3**	**118**	**0**	**0**	**0**	**0**	**1**	**48**	**0**	**0**	**0**	**0**
MD	NDT	2	52	1	35	1	35	0	0	0	0	0	0	0	0	0	0
HD	NDT	1	48	1	48	1	48	0	0	0	0	1	48	0	0	0	0
SR	NDT	2	57	2	57	1	35	0	0	0	0	0	0	0	0	0	0
ATX	**Plac.**	**9**	**2,313**	**4**	**1,460**	**8**	**2,119**	**0**	**0**	**9**	**2,313**	**8**	**2,119**	**0**	**0**	**5**	**812**
LMD	Plac.	3	962	1	594	3	962	0	0	3	962	3	962	0	0	2	368
HD	Plac.	6	1,351	3	866	5	1,157	0	0	6	1,351	5	1,157	0	0	3	444
MPH-IR	**MPH-ER**	**4**	**331+?**	**1+?**	**19+?**	**2+?**	**331+?**	**1+?**	**312+?**	**0+?**	**0+?**	**1+?**	**312+?**	**1**	**(?)**	**1**	**(?)**
LD	LD	1	19	1	19	1	19	1	0	0	0	0	0	0	0	0	0
MD	MD	1	312	0	0	1	312	?	312	0	0	1	312	0	0	0	0
MD (CIC)	MD (CIC)	2	?	?	?	?	?	?	?	?	?	?	?	1	?***	1	?
IR-Comb.	**ER-Comb.**	**3**	**105**	**3**	**105**	**0**	**0**	**0**	**0**	**0**	**0**	**0**	**0**	**0**	**0**	**0**	**0**
MD	LD	2	35	2	35	0	0	0	0	0	0	0	0	0	0	0	0
HD	MD	1	70	1	70	0	0	0	0	0	0	0	0	0	0	0	0

(continued)

Table 5.1 (continued)

Category (Comparators)		Clinical studies (Overall)		Clinical studies with endpoints available for efficacy / effectiveness assessment										Used for CUA			
				Conners' scale		Hyperactivity		SNAP-IV		ADHD-RS		CGI (-I or -S)		Bc		Ext.	
A	B	#	n	#	n	#	n	#	n	#	n	#	n	#	n	#	n
MPH-IR	**DEX**	**3**	**202**	**3**	**202**	**2**	**154**	**0**	**0**	**0**	**0**	**0**	**0**	**0**	**0**	**0**	**0**
LD	LD	1	125	1	125	1	125	0	0	0	0	0	0	0	0	0	0
MD	MD	1	29	1	29	1	29	0	0	0	0	0	0	0	0	0	0
HD+NDT	HD+NDT	1	48	1	48	0 (1)*	0 (48)*	0	0	0	0	0 (1)*	0 (48)*	0	0	0	0
MPH-ER	**DEX**	**1**	**22**	**1**	**22**	**0**	**0**	**0**	**0**	**0**	**0**	**0**	**0**	**0**	**0**	**0**	**0**
LD+NDT	SR+NDT	1	22	1	22	0	0	0	0	0	0	0	0	0	0	0	0
MPH-IR	**ATX**	**1**	**228**	**1**	**228**	**1**	**228**	**0**	**0**	**1**	**228**	**1**	**228**	**0**	**0**	**0**	**0**
HD	HD	1	228	1	228	1	228	0	0	1	228	1	228	0			0
MPH-ER	**ATX**	**1**	**1,323**	**0**	**0**	**1**	**1,323**	**0**	**0**	**1**	**1,323**	**1**	**1,323**	**1**	**1,323**	**1**	**1,323**
MD	LMD	1	1,323	0	0	1	1,323	0	0	1	1,323	1	1,323	1	1,323	1	1,323
MTA Study	3 groups	cf. Table 5.4												–		–	435

Tabulated on the basis of information provided in the Assessment Report (AR, Ch. 4, pp. 60–163, and Ch. 6, pp. 226 and 252–254). CEA, cost-effectiveness analysis; CUA, cost-utility analysis (by Assessment Group); BC, base case analysis; Ext, extended analyses; #, number of studies; n, number of patients; MPH, methylphenidate; IR, immediate-release formulation; ER, extended-release formulation (combining both MPH-MR08 and MPH-MR12); Plac., placebo; NDT, non-drug treatment; Comb, combined treatment; DEX, dexamphetamine, ATX, atomoxetine; CIC, commercial-in-confidence data; LD, low dose (for MPH-IR, ≤15mg/d; for MPH-ER, ≤20mg/d); MD: medium dose (for MPH-IR, 15–30mg/d; for MPH-ER, 20–40mg/d; for DEX, 10–20mg/d); LMD, low-to-medium dose (for ATX, <1.5mg/kg/d); HD, high dose (for MPH-IR, >30mg/d; for MPH-ER, >40mg/d; for DEX, >20mg/d; for ATX, ≥1.5mg/kg/d); SR, sustained-release formulation (DEX);TR, time-release formulation (DEX); ?, data not available, normally related to "commercial-in-confidence" (CIC) information. Note that both trials comparing ATX with MPH randomized patients in an unbalanced way: Kemner et al. (2004) compared a group of 850 patients treated with MPH-MR12 with 473 patients treated with ATX, whereas Kratochvil et al. (2002) compared a group of 184 patients treated with ATX with 44 patients treated with MPH-IR. A further study comparing MPH-MR12 and ATX is not listed here since it was not included by the Assessment Group (Newcorn et al., 2004, 2005). Note also that some studies may appear more than one time, e.g., Klein and Abikoff (1997) compared high-dose MPH-IR, MPH-IR+NDT, and NDT + placebo in a three-arm parallel-group design and their study is listed twice. Another study designated "commercial-in-confidence" and used for the primary ("base case") economic analysis could be identified in the public domain (Steele et al., 2004, 2006); for details, cf. Table 5.7. The numbers presented in the Table have been calculated using data from various tables of the Assessment Report (AR, Ch. 4). For determining studies used for economic analysis, information has been taken from Tables 6.2, 6.14, 6.16, and 6.17, and the studies by Quinn et al. (2003) – data designated "commercial-in-confidence" (AR, Appendix 12, p. 597; Celltech submission to NICE) and by Elia et al. (1991; also published by Castellanos et al., 1997) have been added (cf. AR, Ch. 6, p. 254).

and by CCOHTA in Canada (comprising 26 Studies, 8 of which were relevant to the comparison of methylphenidate with placebo – cf. Lord and Paisley, 2000).

However, as illustrated in Table 5.1, in the *present* NICE assessment out of 43 clinical studies comparing methylphenidate immediate-release products (MPH-IR) with placebo, involving a total of over 2,800 patients, only one study comprising 58 patients – 20 of whom had received MPH-IR – was left for the primary (base case) economic evaluation[24] (Pliszka et al., 2000). Based on these 20 patients, the MPH-IR response rate of 65% derived from CGI-I scores is associated with a binomial 95% confidence interval from 41% to 85%. The treatment duration of three weeks in this study barely met the specified minimum requirement for inclusion in the effectiveness review. (One further placebo-controlled study including 32 girls in a three-week crossover design was added later as to have *any* data on dexamphetamine: Sharp et al., 1999; see below.) Two additional studies comparing MPH-IR with placebo were integrated in secondary, "extended" economic analyses. One of these studies was designated "commercial-in-confidence"[25], and for this reason it remains unclear which endpoints had been documented in this trial and how these were "synthesized" in the "final analysis" (cf. AR, Ch. 6, p. 254, and Chapter 5 below, *Economic Model*). The other study (Elia et al., 1991; Castellanos et al., 1997), comprised of 48 boys with ADHD diagnosed according to DSM-III criteria, reported CGI results in graph form only. This data presentation confounded tabulation of these results in the context of the present paper. Of note, the Assessment Group faced the same difficulty and admitted that it could not reproduce the results in a table (cf. AR, Ch. 4, p. 156).

The overview provided in Tables 5.1, 5.2, 5.7 and 5.8 reveals in detail that all treatments under investigation, beyond immediate-release methylphenidate, were affected by a massive shrinkage of their effectiveness database available for economic modeling.

The greatest data attrition was in studies involving dexamphetamine (DEX). Although 13 studies with a total of 334 patients had been integrated in the effectiveness review (of which, 7 studies with 221 patients reported Conners' ratings), no effectiveness data remained after application of both filters (Figure 5.1). The Assessment Group addressed this problem of complete data absence for dexamphetamine by recurring to a study published by Sharp and colleagues (1999)[26] that had been eliminated from the effectiveness review earlier in the selection, on grounds of "inadequate data presentation" (AR, Appendix 3, p. 338). The Assessment Report accounts for this anomaly by stating that "a number of studies excluded from the

---

[24] For further information on those clinical trials that were included in the economic model, see Tables 5.7 and 5.8, below.

[25] In the AR, this study is referenced as Quinn et al. (2003), the source identified is a "Celltech integrated study report" (AR, reference no. 86, p. 276). No information is available on number of patients enrolled.

[26] The data used for evaluation were drawn from a publication reporting on ADHD in girls; they relate to a threefold crossover trial (MPH-IR, DEX, placebo) enrolling 32 girls (no boys); cf. also Table 5.7. See also discussion in main text, below. It remains unclear from the Assessment Report whether the data on MPH-IR were integrated from this study into the analysis, too.

Table 5.2 Clinical studies selected by Assessment Group for (a) effectiveness review and (b) economic modeling (complete list of selected long-term studies with observation periods ≥12 weeks)

| Category | (Comparators) | Clinical studies (Overall) | | Clinical studies with endpoints available for efficacy / effectiveness assessment | | | | | | | | | | Used for CUA | | | |
| | | | | Conners' scale | | Hyperactivity | | SNAP-IV | | ADHD-RS | | CGI (-I or -S) | | BC | | Ext. | |
A	B	#	n	#	n	#	n	#	n	#	n	#	n	#	n	#	n
MPH-IR																	
HD	Plac.	1+?	166+?	?	?	?	?	?	?	?	?	?	?	0	0	0+?	?
	Plac.	1	166	?	?	?	?	?	?	?	?	?	?	0	0	1?	?
HD (CIC)	Plac.	1?	CIC	?	?	?	?	?	?	?	?	?	?	0	0	1?	?
IR-Comb.	Plac.	1	40	1	40	1	40	0	0	0	0	0	0	0	0	0	0
MD+NDT	Plac.	1	40	1	40	1	40	0	0	0	0	0	0	0	0	0	0
MPH-ER	Plac.	1?	?	?	?	?	?	?	?	?	?	?	?	0	0	1?	?
MD (CIC)	Plac.	1?	?	?	?	?	?	?	?	?	?	?	?	0	0	1?	?
MPH-IR	NDT	4	290	4	290	3	260	0	0	0	0	0	0	1	86	1	86
LD	NDT	1	30	1	30	0	0	0	0	0	0	0	0	0	0	0	0
MD	NDT	2	174	2	174	2	174	0	0	0	0	0	0	0	0	0	0
HD	NDT	1	86	1	86	1	86	0	0	0	0	1	86	1	86*	1	86*
IR-Comb.	NDT	7	555	7	555	6	525	0	0	0	0	1	86	1	86	1	86
LD+NDT	NDT	2	146	2	146	1	116	0	0	0	0	0	0	0	0	0	0
MD+NDT	NDT	3	232	3	232	3	232	0	0	0	0	0	0	0	0	0	0
HD+NDT	NDT	2	177	2	177	2	177	0	0	0	0	1	86	1	86*	1	86*
DEX	Plac.	4	98	3	81	2	49	0	0	0	0	0	0	0	0	0	0
MD	Plac.	1	32	1	32	0	0	0	0	0	0	0	0	0	0	0	0
HD	Plac.	2	48	1	31	1	31	0	0	0	0	0	0	0	0	0	0
TR	Plac.	1	18	1	18	1	18	0	0	0	0	0	0	0	0	0	0
DEX-Comb.	Plac.	2	34	0	0	0	0	0	0	0	0	0	0	0	0	0	0
MD+NDT	Plac.	1	17	0	0	0	0	0	0	0	0	0	0	0	0	0	0
HD+NDT	Plac.	1	17	0	0	0	0	0	0	0	0	0	0	0	0	0	0

DEX-Comb. NDT	1	17	0	0	0	0	0	0	0
MD	1	17	0	0	0	0	0	0	0
ATX Plac.	1	416	416	416	416	416	416	416	416
Plac.	1	416	416	416	416	416	416	416	416
MPH-ER MPH-IR / MD (CIC)	1?	?	?	?	?	?	?	?	?
HD	1?**	?	?	?	?	?	?	?	?
MTA Study	3 groups	cf. Table 5.8						1	435

Tabulated on the basis of information provided in the Assessment Report (AR, Ch. 4, pp. 60–163, and Ch. 6, pp. 226 and 252–254). CUA, cost-utility analysis (by Assessment Group); BC, base case analysis; Ext., extended analyses; #, number of studies; n, number of patients; MPH, methylphenidate; IR, immediate-release formulation; ER, extended-release formulation (combining both MPH-MR08 and MPH-MR12); Plac., placebo; NDT, non-drug treatment; Comb., combined treatment; DEX, dexamphetamine; ATX, atomoxetine; CIC, commercial-in-confidence data; LD, low dose (for MPH-IR, $\leq$20mg/d); MD: medium dose (for MPH-IR, 15–30mg/d; for MPH-ER, 20–40mg/d; for DEX, 10–20mg/d); LMD, low-to-medium dose (for ATX, <1.5mg/kg/d); HD, high dose (for MPH-IR, >30mg/d; for MPH-ER, >40mg/d; for DEX, >20mg/d; for ATX, $\geq$1.5mg/kg/d); SR, sustained-release formulation (DEX); TR, time-release formulation (DEX). Note that some studies may appear more than one time, e.g., Klein and Abikoff (1997) compared high-dose MPH-IR, MPH-IR+NDT, and NDT + placebo in a three-arm parallel-group design and their study is listed twice (marked by an asterisk*; note that in the AR the study is often referred to as "Klein et al., 1997"). Further to this, with active treatment periods of 8 weeks (and an observation period of 12 weeks), one could argue that this study does not fulfill criteria for "long-term" studies. Indeed, Schachar et al. (2002) in their review did not include this study. **Another study designated "commercial-in-confidence" and used for the primary ("base case") economic analysis could be identified in the public domain (Steele et al., 2004, 2006); this study does not fulfill criteria for "long-term" trials. The numbers presented in the table have been calculated using data from various tables of the Assessment Report (AR, Chapter 4). For determining studies used for economic analysis, information has been taken from Tables 6.2, 6.14, 6.16, and 6.17, and the study by Quinn et al. (2003) – data designated "commercial-in-confidence" (AR, Appendix 12, p. 597; Celltech submission to NICE) has been added (cf. AR, Ch. 6, p. 254).

effectiveness review, for reasons of data presentation, were nevertheless found to provide information on response rate. These studies were, therefore, included in the calculation of response rates for the cost-effectiveness analysis" (AR, Ch. 6, pp. 225f.). Again it remains entirely unclear which studies in addition to this dex-amphetamine trial (Sharp et al., 1999) might have been added to the database, and what criteria exactly were used in their selection. Of note, the Assessment Report does not provide relevant information – neither about other trials included in the economic analysis that had not been part of the cost-effectiveness review, nor about the particular study mentioned (Sharp et al., 1999) – except (for the latter study) for treatments tested (MPH-IR, DEX, and placebo) and number of patients per treat-ment group (32 per group).

The ultimate inclusion of this study (Sharp et al., 1999) is noteworthy because, in the absence of any other data on dexamphetamine, it drove both the efficacy synthesis as well as the withdrawal rate assumptions underlying the conclusion of the economic modeling exercises undertaken (cf. below, *Economic Model*, and Figure 5.2, p. 101), namely, that an ADHD treatment strategy starting with first line DEX was optimal[27].

Upon review of the original publication it turns out that treatment duration was three weeks in a crossover design[28]. Moreover, all study subjects were girls (see also Table 5.7), which is an important consideration as gender differences in ADHD are well documented (though perhaps less well understood; cf. Arcia and Conners, 1998, and Arnold, 1996) and influenced by referral bias in some studies (Bieder-man et al., 2005). The authors of the study themselves quote "substantial evidence of normative sex differences that influence the manifestation of ADHD" (Sharp et al., 1999, p. 40), described by the participants of a National Institute of Men-tal Health (NIMH) conference on the subject (Arnold, 1996). Gender differences have been found to include overall prevalence (boys being affected three to ten times more often; Faraone et al., 2003a; Scahill and Schwab-Stone, 2000), comor-bidity patterns (boys being more likely to manifest disruptive behavior disorders and learning disabilities; Faraone et al., 2003a; Abikoff et al., 2002; Scahill and Schwab-Stone, 2000), and neurobiological findings such as dopamine receptor den-sity, which may be relevant in light of the dopaminergic mechanism of action of stimulants (Andersen and Teicher, 2000).

In this study the response rates of 84% (27/32 for dexamphetamine) and 81% (26/32 for MPH-IR) based on CGI-I scores in this small all-female sample are associated with binomial 95% confidence intervals from 67% to 95% (for DEX) and 64% to 93% (for MPH-IR), respectively; results that were indistinguish-able, with exception of a significant mean loss in body weight associated with

---

[27] "For a decision taken now, with current available data, the results of the economic evaluation clearly identify an optimal strategy" (AR, Ch. 6, p. 260f. and reiterated again on p. 266).

[28] Apparently there were no washout phases between treatment periods. "None of the ... pairwise comparisons ... yielded significantly different results on carryover analysis" (Sharp et al., 1999, p. 44), but carryover effects were tested by comparing the teachers' ratings of hyperactivity during the first week of each treatment phase, not by assessing CGI scores (Sharp et al., 1999, p. 42). The section of the paper describing "statistical analysis" mentions "extreme outliers."

dexamphetamine, but not methylphenidate. Interestingly, the investigators concluded that their data "provide additional support for the usual clinical practice of beginning with MPH [-IR]" (Sharp et al., 1999, p. 46).

A total of six clinical studies were selected to inform the primary ("base case") cost-effectiveness analysis, based upon CGI improvement scores (of 1 or 2) that were considered to define a treatment responder. These studies collectively comprise 1,958 patients (with one open-label study [Kemner et al., 2004, 2005] contributing 1,323 of these patients); 1,727 of whom had been observed for the minimum period of three weeks only. No clinical effectiveness data beyond eight weeks treatment duration were available in this group of studies (see Table 5.2).

However, long-term treatment effectiveness and cost-effectiveness are of particular interest because ADHD, as a chronic condition, is associated with potentially harmful long-term sequelae, including underachievement in school, poor occupational functioning, abnormalities in personality development, antisocial behaviors, risk of accidents, substance abuse, and delinquency (see Chapter 1, *Introduction*; e.g., Mannuzza and Klein, 2000).

Unfortunately, most ADHD treatment studies have been short-term, often crossover trials (Jadad et al., 1999; Miller et al., 1998). Thus it might appear logical that, for the primary economic evaluation, the Assessment Group indeed used no studies with treatment duration in excess of eight weeks. One study (Klein and Abikoff, 1997) is cited as 12 weeks duration in the Assessment Report (AR, Ch. 4, p. 102 and p. 112), but in fact this was the time span during which clinical outcomes were assessed and the active treatment period was eight weeks in each of its three parallel arms, comprising a total of 86 patients.

For the secondary ("extended") economic model, the MTA Study (MTA, 1999a,b) was also used, although it remains unclear exactly how these data were integrated (cf. Chapter 6.1.1, *Insights from Clinical Long-Term Data*).

As a point of reference in regard to long-term clinical data, Schachar and colleagues (2002) identified 14 randomized clinical trials (RCTs) with 1,379 subjects in their systematic review of extended ADHD treatment studies. In all of these studies treatment was administered for at least 12 weeks. Five studies involved 774 patients and followed patients for more than 26 weeks. It is noteworthy (cf. above, *Outcome Measures*) that, again, the most frequently used outcome measure was one of the versions of the Conners' Rating Scale. Out of the 14 studies covered in the review, only the 14-month duration MTA Study included information on all 20 clinically relevant elements selected *a priori* for extraction from the articles. Data spanning a follow-up of 24 months in the MTA Study have since become available (MTA Cooperative Group, 2004; Arnold et al., 2005). Apart from the MTA Study, none of the (other) trials included in the review by Schachar et al. (2002) were incorporated into the database used for economic modeling by the Assessment Group.

Results of a further two-year study involving 103 children, conducted at two sites (New York and Montreal) between 1990 and 1995, were also published in July 2004 (Klein et al., 2004; Abikoff et al., 2004a,b) and although this study was primarily designed to assess the impact of multimodal psychosocial treatment added to MPH-IR administered three times daily (t.i.d.), it also provided information that was relevant to the NICE appraisal. Children switched to placebo after 12 months of treatment with methylphenidate relapsed without exception. For a more detailed discussion of this study, see Chapter 6.1.1, *Insights from Clinical Long-Term Data*.

To recap these observations briefly, the endpoints selected for economic evaluation are difficult to justify from a clinical perspective, and the choices made for assessment were not supported by a review of the relevant literature. The proposed superiority of CGI-I scores over the most widely used Conners' Rating Scales is, at best, speculative. Using these scores as inputs, in conjunction with utility weights estimated for "responders" according to a different definition, in order to calculate QALYs cannot realistically be expected to meet the requirements of expected utility theory. Taking normative concerns related to the QALY concept into account, the preference for CGI-I sub-scale scores over Conners' Rating Scale scores is unsafe at best. Yet, in combination, as has been shown, the two resulting quality filters applied by the Assessment Group led to a dramatic reduction of the clinical evidence base available for economic modeling.

5.3 Efficacy, Effectiveness, and Treatment Compliance

The distinction between *efficacy* (typically measured in randomized clinical trials, RCTs) and *effectiveness* (real-world outcomes associated with an intervention) has long been recognized, accepted and understood. Whereas RCTs follow an explanatory orientation ("*can* the intervention work?"), economic evaluations – to be meaningful – require a pragmatic orientation ("*does* the intervention work?" – Schwartz and Lellouch, 1967; see also Weinstein et al., 2003, CRD, 2001; Cook and Campbell, 1979). Efficacy data collected during clinical trials deliberately and necessarily exclude naturalistic effects associated with a normal clinical practice setting. Effectiveness, on the other hand, may be influenced by a number of external factors, including poor treatment compliance by the patient, with consequential implications for the cost-effectiveness of the treatment under study. Inadequate compliance may also result in direct waste of resources when, for example, prescriptions are filled but not used.

Sometimes, practical difficulties arise from the fact that "compliance" is a term with an imprecise definition. It requires, among other issues, a clear distinction to be made between "adherence" and "persistence." In general, early discontinuation of treatment (lack of "persistence") is a common occurrence, and "an intriguing but unanswered question is whether the transition from punctual to erratic compliance (i.e., non-adherence) is a precursor to discontinuation" (Métry, 1999), although each share a number of common features. In the absence of reliable data a pragmatic approach may be to assume that many patients are likely to begin missing a portion of their medication, while some others may suddenly discontinue treatment. Reduced "adherence" can be considered a significant contributor to treatment discontinuation due to perceived lack of efficacy (Métry, 1999).

Instead of addressing these issues with respect to their relevance for ADHD treatment, the Assessment Group states: "The exploration of the effects of non-compliance would involve a number of assumptions: the assumption that RCT data capture *none* of the effects of compliance; the application of a selected estimate of compliance from a source outside of the clinical trials; and an assumption regarding the distribution of reduced compliance between morning, lunchtime and evening doses of medication. It was *felt* that these modeling assumptions would not be reasonable given the lack of available data, which would render the results of *any* sensitivity analysis around compliance uninformative to decision-makers" (AR, Ch. 6, p. 233; italics added). Apparently there was a prevailing belief that compliance would be adequately captured in controlled clinical trials and this is evident from statements in the Assessment Report that "intention-to-treat analyses are favoured in assessments as they mirror the noncompliance ... that [is] likely to occur when the intervention is used in practice" (AR, p. 28)[29], and "in our base case analysis it is assumed that the trial data adequately captures the effect of compliance on response to treatment" (AR, Ch. 6, p. 232). Consequently, the Assessment Group claims that "the effect of compliance on response rates to IR-MPH and ER-MPH is reflected in the model" (AR, Ch. 6, p. 250). In a sensitivity analysis on the subject (AR, Ch. 6, pp. 250ff.; see also below, "*Economic Model*"), non-compliant patients were simply assumed to be a subset of non-responders identified in the clinical study database used (cf. above).

The approach to the problem of treatment compliance is a major issue pervading the assessment, with potentially far-reaching implications for its conclusions, because it entails comparisons between different drug regimens with different administration schedules. The approach taken by the Assessment Group, therefore, requires some further illumination.

5.3.1 Internal Versus External Validity of Clinical Trials

It is commonly accepted that the high internal validity of RCTs is achieved at the expense of their external validity (i.e., generalizability), the reason being, besides other issues such as patient and investigator selection effects, careful monitoring of study subjects designed "to 'control' the environment ... under a strict research protocol," as the senior author[30] of the Assessment Report explained elsewhere

---

[29] Efficacy trials have usually been short-term, and non-compliant patients have been discontinued. As child and adolescent psychiatrist Margaret Weiss from Vancouver, British Columbia, noted, "Although in an intent-to-treat analysis the ratings of the last visit are carried forward as an endpoint, the ratings may have been obtained while the patients were still in the study and on medication. *This method of preserving data does not reflect how the patient is doing off medication at the point in time when the study is complete*" and, "The process of selecting consenting patients for research studies is also biased in that most studies demand families who are motivated, English speaking, able to get to the appointment, and sophisticated enough to understand potential risks. The intervention of just being in a protocol is rarely studied as a therapy in its own right..." (Biederman et al., 2006b; italics added; cf. Weiss et al., 2006). See also note in the main text about "Hawthorne effects", Chapter 5, below.

[30] The senior author explicitly assumed "overall responsibility for the cost-effectiveness section of the report" (Assessment Report, p. 3).

(Drummond et al., 1997, pp. 233ff.). The same author has reiterated that "great efforts are typically made in the conduct of a clinical trial to ensure that patients consume their prescribed medications. ... To the extent that patients do not comply with the prescribed therapy, there may be a dilution of the treatment effect originally observed in the trial" (Drummond et al., 2005, p. 251; cf. also Drummond et al., 1997, p. 239), and "the health outcomes to be included in an economic analysis [...] should not be limited to efficacy and safety as demonstrated in randomized clinical trials, but should also consider overall treatment effectiveness as observed in real-world settings" (Drummond, 2003).

As a consequence there has been a call for more pragmatic clinical trials with minimal quality assurance and study management in psychiatry, intended to provide generalizable answers to important clinical questions without bias (March et al., 2005). Only recently this has been echoed in child and adolescent psychiatry, where a need was recognized for more "naturalistic-observational studies in the framework of ADHD health care" (Rothenberger et al., 2006).

Accordingly, members of a recent ISPOR Task Force on "Good Research Practices for Cost-Effectiveness Analysis Alongside Clinical Trials" agreed that "it is generally acknowledged that pragmatic effectiveness trials are the best vehicle for economic studies," and expressed the view that "artificially enhanced compliance" in RCTs is a threat to their external validity (Ramsey et al., 2005)[31]. In a recent informative review on the subject of non-compliance, Hughes and colleagues (2001) concluded that "A prime reason for this [note added: *the difference between efficacy in RCTs and effectiveness in the real world*] is the difference in patient compliance which is generally better within the context of controlled clinical trials." Evidence for this phenomenon is apparent from studies of antihyperlipidemic and antihypertensive medications. Andrade and colleagues (1995; cf. Table 5.3) found a substantially higher risk of discontinuation of treatment (i.e., non-persistence) at two health maintenance organizations (HMOs) compared with that reported in RCTs (see Table 5.3).

Moreover, compliance rates found in open-label trials were similar to those in the HMOs. These lower compliance (persistence) rates in a real world (HMO) setting were due to a variety of reasons. It is noteworthy that the differences were also compound-specific. These findings were further consistent with discontinuation rates reported in studies of therapy for other chronic diseases. In long-term clinical trials in hypertension, discontinuation rates have been reported at approximately 30%, whereas community-based studies with one or more years of follow-up have reported drop-out rates of approximately 50% (Andrade et al., 1995). Caro et al. (1999a,b) also reported a high proportion of patients who stopped their antihypertensive medication under real-world conditions within a relatively short time and

---

[31] The view that "clinical trials are artificial treatment environments, and do not provide all the economic information needed by decision-makers," was further endorsed by the senior author of the present Assessment Report, in an editorial accompanying the ISPOR Task Force Report (Drummond, 2005). More recently he criticized "out-of-date methods" that may "lead to a sub-optimal assessment of the cost-effectiveness of a new drug in a given setting. For example, an insistence on data only from RCTs may mean that some of the advantages of a product cannot easily be demonstrated" (Drummond, 2006).

Table 5.3 Compliance (one-year persistence) rates
differ between the "exploratory" setting (cf. Schwartz and Lellouch, 1967) of randomized
controlled trials (RCTs) and the real-world situation encountered in health maintenance
organizations, HMOs (Andrade et al., 1995):

Drug (Class)	One-Year Probability of Discontinuation	
	HMOs (in brackets, 95% confidence intervals)	RCTs summary estimates (in brackets, 95% confidence intervals)
Bile acid sequestrants	41 (38–44) %	31 (30–33) %
Niacin	46 (42–51) %	04 (03–05) %
Lovastatin	15 (11–19) %	16 (15–17) %
Gemfibrozil	37 (31–43) %	15 (13–16) %

stated that "Whether a patient stopped treatment seemed to depend on the class of antihypertensive drug prescribed initially," and "persistence was inversely related to therapeutic turbulence" (Caro et al., 1999b). These authors sought to explain this observation in terms that "Perhaps patients [note added: *compared to study subjects*] are less forgiving of therapeutic trial and error." The potential implications for ADHD treatment are obvious and will be discussed later. Here it may suffice to emphasize that compliance effects cannot be studied properly in the "pure" context of RCTs because of the limitations imposed to increase the internal validity of efficacy comparisons.

By definition, RCTs require strict adherence to a specified treatment protocol, and procedures are implemented to keep patients on that specified treatment regimen and to minimize the risk of non-compliance. A further aspect is the greater medical awareness of patients participating in clinical trials (Revicki and Frank, 1999). This has the effect of creating a situation consistent with more general changes in behavior seen in humans who are aware of being observed ("*Hawthorne effect*"). In this regard it has been reported that the contact interval between physician and patient does have an influence on patient compliance. In addition, Wasson et al. (1992) reported a 29% reduction in aggregate health resource consumption when the frequency of contact between physician and patient was increased by means of between-visit phone calls by the physician. This puzzling finding, which was confirmed in a RCT, is probably due to the fact "that more frequent contact makes it possible to identify and resolve early certain problems that would be more difficult and costly to resolve if not discovered until later" (Urquhart, 1999). A special variant of this phenomenon is known in compliance research as the "*white coat effect*" (Feinstein, 1990), in which poor or partial compliers tend to improve their compliance around the time of scheduled follow-up visits, an effect that appears to be limited to two to three days on either side of the visit (Kass et al., 1986; Cramer et al., 1990). This can lead to confusion because it tends to drive such variables that are drug-influenced (in the short-term) into desirable ranges[32], hence giving a clinical impression that the patient is being treated effectively. In RCTs with

---

[32] As will be discussed later, the specific pharmacokinetic and pharmacodynamic (PK/PD) properties of methylphenidate make this compound a potential candidate for such effects.

frequent diagnostic work-ups, this effect may exert a – sometimes "welcome" from an *exploratory* perspective – positive influence on "efficacy" while simultaneously obscuring real "effectiveness," therefore necessarily reducing the "external validity" of RCT findings.

5.3.2 Quantitative Evidence on Treatment Compliance

Compliance, then, remains a challenge even within the experimental context of RCTs. For instance, non-compliance, if undetected and not corrected for, may lead to inconclusive or misleading results of dose-finding and other clinical studies. Against this background, much effort has been devoted to the measurement of compliance.

The use of medication event monitoring systems (MEMS) is considered to represent the current gold standard in compliance measurement. Compliance rates revealed with MEMS are more accurate and consistently lower than those estimates generated through self-reporting by patients (or caregivers), blood-level monitoring, prescription refills, or pill counts. This in turn implies that data derived from these other measurement methods will tend to overestimate compliance (Métry, 1999). Even the use of medication event monitoring systems (MEMS) may result in under-reporting of non-compliance, because there is no guarantee that opening the EM device to remove a tablet means that the dose was actually taken.

A recent systematic review (Claxton et al., 2001) of 76 clinical studies employing electronic monitoring devices (MEMS) – all of which had been published in peer-reviewed journals – confirmed earlier findings about the inverse relationship between number of daily doses required and rate of compliance, which was statistically significant ($p<0.001$) among dosing schedules.

These data provide quantitative information about the extent that compliance may be negatively influenced by more complex dosing regimens across a variety of medical conditions (Table 5.4). Most studies defined compliance as the proportion of days in which the appropriate number of doses were taken ("dose-taking compliance"), although this is not a universal definition. In addition, for the purpose of the review, dose-timing compliance – a measure of intake of medication within the prescribed time frame – was defined as within 25% of the dosing interval (e.g., twice-daily doses should be taken 12 + 3 hours apart). Dose-timing compliance is particularly important for drugs with a duration of action of less than 24 hours (cf. below: "*non-forgiving drugs*").

The clinical impact of non-compliance is dependent on the condition treated as well as the medication in question. For example, in immunosuppressive treatment after organ transplantation or in oral contraception, there may be important sequelae when the level of active drug has fallen below the minimum therapeutic index for efficacy. In other treatment situations, however, a single missed dose may be inconsequential (Meredith, 1999). Besides the dose-response relationship, the time-dependency of drug action is of relevance since therapeutic coverage will also depend on PK/PD behavior in relation to the recommended dosing interval,

Table 5.4 Treatment compliance (adherence)
is correlated with the complexity of dosing regimens, as exemplified by the number of daily doses
that need to be taken (Claxton et al., 2001). Overall, compliance declined as the number of doses
increased (p<0.001 among dose schedules). The following differences of dose-taking compliance
in-between dosing schedules were statistically significant: o.a.d. vs. t.i.d., p<0.008; o.a.d. vs. q.i.d.,
p<0.001; b.i.d. vs. q.i.d., p≤0.001. For dose-timing compliance, there were too few studies for
statistical comparisons. Abbreviations used: o.a.d., once daily administration; b.i.d., administration
divided in two daily doses; t.i.d., three daily doses; q.i.d., four daily doses. MEMS, medication
event monitoring system

| Compliance Dosing Regimen | Systematic Review of MEMS Studies (Claxton et al. 2001) | | | |
| | Dose-Timing Compliance | | Dose-Taking Compliance | |
	Mean (s.d.)	Range	Mean (s.d.)	Range
1 dose / 24 h (o.a.d.)	74% (31%)	27%–89%	79% (14%)	35%–97%
1 dose / 12 h (b.i.d.)	58% (23%)	22%–79%	69% (15%)	38%–90%
1 dose / 8 h (t.i.d.)	46% (08%)	40%–55%	65% (16%)	40%–91%
1 dose / 6 h (q.i.d.)	40% (n.a.)	n.a.	51% (20%)	33%–81%

i.e., the relationship between pharmacokinetics (PK) and pharmacodynamic (PD)
actions. On this basis, non-compliance forgiving drugs can be differentiated from
non-forgiving drugs, the latter being characterized by clinical sequelae arising from
the absence of therapeutic coverage as a consequence of missed or delayed doses
(Meredith, 1999; Peck, 1999).

Before turning to issues related to treatment compliance *specific* to ADHD, key
aspects need to be reiterated. RCTs cannot be expected to capture the full impact of
non-compliance in real-world situations. The magnitude of the difference between
both settings will be influenced, among other factors, by the specific treatment
modalities in question. Many factors that impact treatment persistence also affect
compliance (adherence), and a causal relationship between non-adherence and subsequent non-persistence appears likely. Dissatisfaction with treatment (e.g., arising
from inconvenience, side effects, and/or perceived lack of efficacy) may precede
discontinuation. The clinical consequences of non-adherence depend greatly on the
particular disease and on characteristics of the specific drug in question. Pharmaceuticals may be characterized as "forgiving" or "non-forgiving" with regard to
non-compliance on grounds of underlying characteristics such as dose response
relationship, time-dependency of action, and therapeutic coverage resulting from
their PK/PD behaviors.

5.3.3 Treatment Compliance of Patients with ADHD

The authors of the Assessment Report (AR) state that "In our base case analysis
it is assumed that the trial data [note added: *referring to double-blind, double-
dummy ADHD trials*] adequately captures the effect of compliance on response
to treatment" (AR, Ch. 6, p. 232). It is evident from the foregoing description

that this assumption is grossly inappropriate[33]. Disease-specific factors that may be expected to contribute to non-compliance (Swanson, 2003) have not been adequately addressed in the assessment. These factors include individual and/or parental attitudes towards (psychotropic) medication that encompass potential concerns about safety and long-term treatment, as well as social stigma, particularly in association with a midday dose in children who may become the target of school-yard bullying (aside from the potential risk of diversion to peers of short-acting stimulant medications; cf. Wilens, 2004; Graff Low and Gendaszek, 2002). Further factors also include disease-defining symptoms such as inattention (including their rapid recurrence 3–4 hours after the last dose of conventional MPH-IR, cf. below), and the presence of comorbidity – externalizing disorders such as oppositional and defiant disorder and/or internalizing ones such as anxiety and depression (Table 5.5). Indeed, depression has also been shown to be significantly correlated with non-compliance, with depressed patients being three times more likely than non-depressed patients to be non-compliant with therapy (DiMatteo et al., 2000).

The issue of non-compliance is arguably more relevant in ADHD than in some other chronic diseases. In light of the evidence, it is unclear why the authors of the Assessment Report retreated to the position that "none of the studies in the systematic review of compliance [note added: *by Claxton et al., 2001 (Table 5.4)*] looked specifically at ADHD" (AR, Ch. 6, p. 233). If anything, the apparently more pronounced impact of multiple daily dosing on "dose timing compliance" – in contrast to "dose taking compliance" – would indicate the compound magnitude of the problem relevant to ADHD, as a delay of intake would be associated with rapid recurrence of disease-defining symptoms, which include easy distractibility, poor self-regulation, and oppositional and defiant behavior (cf. Swanson, 2003, p. 122) – all of which are likely to exacerbate compliance problems.

Table 5.5 Disorder-specific factors affecting compliance
with attention-deficit/hyperactivity disorder (ADHD) treatment (modified after Swanson, 2003):

Reluctance to take medication
• Social stigma associated with taking medication for a psychiatric disorder
• Embarrassment, resulting in teasing and bullying by peers
• Parental (and/or individual) attitudes to psychostimulant medication
• Concerns over long-term safety and treatment effects
Inadequate supervision
Disorder-related factors
• Oppositional and defiant behavior
• Easy distractibility
• Poor self-control
• Coexisting depression

---

[33] The simplistic calculation put forward on p. 232 of the Assessment Report, in particular, indicates a rather mechanistic interpretation of human behavior, ignoring both monitoring efforts and the multiple psychological factors associated with a clinical trial setting. As shown above, it also contradicts statements of the senior author of the Assessment Report made elsewhere, including the authoritative textbook that he co-authored (Drummond et al., 2005; cf. Appendix, *Consistency Issues*).

The pharmacokinetic (PK) profile of conventional immediate-release methyl-phenidate formulations (MPH-IR) is characterized by rapid absorption, low plasma protein binding, and rapid extracellular metabolism (Patrick et al., 1987). Plasma half-life is about 2.0 to 3.0 hours, and has been described to be somewhat shorter for generics compared to the brand name product (Vitiello and Burke, 1998). Effects on behavior appear during absorption, typically begin 30 minutes after ingestion, last for 3 to 4 hours, and dissipate rapidly thereafter. Thus the pharmacokinetic profile of a given dose of methylphenidate determines its pharmacodynamic effects, with the time course of both essentially matching each other. Maximum effects occur 1.5 to 2.0 hours after dosing. Due to marked individual variability in the dose-response relationship of methylphenidate, dosage must be titrated for optimal effect and avoidance of toxicity in each child (Kimko et al., 1999).

A phenomenon called "clockwise hysteresis" has been identified, referring to the disappearance of the concentration-enhancing and activity-reducing effects of MPH before the medication leaves the plasma (Cox, 1990). Hence, multiple doses of MPH-IR are required to maintain effectiveness throughout the day. Accordingly, owing to its PK/PD relationship, methylphenidate constitutes a prototypical example of a non-forgiving compound (Swanson et al., 1978; Greenhill, 1992; Greenhill et al., 2001b).

This fact implies that, *ceteris paribus*, even in otherwise poorly controlled clinical trials the mere occurrence of white coat effects could, in real life, be sufficient to mislead *clinical* judgment of effectiveness.

This fact further implies that doses administered under supervision of caregivers (i.e., in particular morning doses) can be expected to be at a much lower risk of non-compliance than a midday dose to be taken by patients themselves in school, not necessarily under adequate supervision. It is noteworthy that the plasma level troughs tend to occur at the most unstructured times of the day, such as lunchtime, recess, or during the bus ride home from school (Pelham et al., 2000). This leaves little room for doctors to tailor the timing of MPH-IR administration to enhance compliance, for instance by pairing medication doses with typical family activities as advocated by Weinstein (1995).

The clinical relevance of these observations is broadly endorsed not only by expert consensus (e.g., Banaschewski et al., 2006; Wolraich et al., 2005; Wilens and Dodson, 2004; Steinhoff, 2004; Olfson, 2004; Coghill, 2003; Swanson, 2003; AACAP, 2002), including the clinical expert who contributed to the assessment (cf. Banaschewski et al., 2006; Taylor, 2006), but also by empirical evidence.

Although the review by Claxton et al. (2001) was limited to studies employing the current gold standard of compliance measurement (i.e., MEMS) and did not identify ADHD-specific studies, there is empirical evidence from studies in ADHD using other methods of compliance measurement. In light of their methodology, these studies on psychotropic medication compliance are likely to underreport the extent of the problem in ADHD. These data were reviewed by Hack and Chow (2001), and their key findings are summarized in Table 5.6. A review of related literature led these authors to suspect that, "because compliance rates are lower for children as compared to adults and psychiatric patients as compared to medical

Table 5.6 Long-term compliance (persistence) rates
in children and adolescents with ADHD treated with stimulants (from Hack and Chow, 2001);
m, months. Note that as yet there have been no studies in child and adolescent psychiatry using
electronic monitoring devices (MEMS) for compliance measurement

Authors	Medication	Compliance Measurement	Number of Subjects	Compliance (after_months)
Kauffman et al. (1981)	MPH (and amphetamine)	Urine testing; *pill count*	n = 12	67% (4¼ m) *87% (4¼ m)*
Firestone (1982)	MPH	Parent report	n = 76	56% (10m)
Sleator et al. (1982)	Stimulants	Teacher & parent report; *child report*	n = 52	35% (12m) *60% (12m)*
Brown et al. (1985)	MPH	Pill count	n = 30	77% (3m)
Brown et al. (1987)	MPH	Pill count; *parent report*	n = 58	75% (3m) *88% (3m)*
Johnston and Fine (1993)	MPH	Verbal reports	n = 24	80% (3m)

patients [. . .] children with psychiatric illness may be at great risk for poor medication compliance" (Hack and Chow, 2001).

Extrapolating these data to a full 12-month period gives an estimated non-compliance ("non-persistence") rate after one year of 61% (weighted average; range: 34%–70%). The Technology Report by CCOHTA of December 1998 (Miller et al., 1998) refers to a Methylphenidate Survey from British Columbia, which indicated that only 35% and 15% of school-aged children, respectively, continue to have prescriptions filled six and 12 months following the initial prescription (Zupancic et al., 1998, p. 6f.). This study confirmed enormous variability and often-occurring low rates of persistence with methylphenidate therapy (Miller et al., 1998, 2001, 2004).

Another Canadian study – a telephone survey commissioned by the manufacturer of an extended release formulation of MPH (Hwang et al., 2003) – revealed that 75% of parents reported that their children (ADHD patients treated with immediate-release methylphenidate divided in three daily doses, "MPH-IR t.i.d.") missed doses "from time to time" and that 55% reported missing doses in the past two weeks. According to these data the third daily dose was the dose most often missed. These non-compliance rates were considered likely underestimates, as there is reason to believe that an important degree of non-compliance exists once a patient reports missing any doses (Sackett et al., 1991).

Database analyses from the United States extend these findings, consistently demonstrating higher persistence rates among patients receiving modified-release methylphenidate with a 12-hour duration of action compared to those receiving mixed amphetamine salts (MAS) or immediate-release methylphenidate (Kemner and Lage, 2006a,b; Sanchez et al., 2005; Marcus et al., 2005; Lage and Hwang, 2003, 2004; cf. below, Chapter 6, *Insights from Disease-Specific Effectiveness Measures*, and Table 6.3).

A first analysis of administrative data from the National Managed Care Bench-mark Database, covering more than 17 million insured lives, had been presented in 2003 and published as a full paper in 2004 (Lage and Hwang, 2003, 2004). It identified n = 344 children age 6–12 years receiving MPH-IR t.i.d., and n = 1,431 receiving a modified-release preparation of methylphenidate with a dura-tion of action of 12 hours (MPH-MR12) once daily (o.a.d.). Patients receiving MPH-MR12 were significantly less likely to discontinue (47% versus 72% among patients receiving MPH-IR over one year), less likely to switch (37% versus 59%), and more likely to persist (12% versus 1%), with non-persistence in this study defined as the occurrence of treatment gaps greater than 14 days (Lage and Hwang, 2004).

Retrospective evaluations of administrative data typically do not allow differ-ential analysis of reasons for treatment discontinuation and may be distorted by effects such as patient selection bias, and therefore it would appear conceivable that MPH-MR12 prescriptions might be associated with higher grades of impairment, which might contribute to higher rates of chronic treatment among such patients. Thus it is remarkable that the use of MPH-MR12 in this analysis was associated with significantly fewer emergency room and general practitioner visits and with a significantly lower accident and injury rate (Lage and Hwang, 2003, 2004), while at the same time these patients had a higher mean number of prior diagnoses, chronic medications, and prior total medical costs (Lage and Hwang, 2004). Further anal-yses used the same database and therefore overlapping source data (Kemner and Lage, 2006a,b). These studies extended the findings of the first analysis on the basis of 5,939 individuals age 6 years or older, who were treated either with MPH-IR (t.i.d.; n = 1,154) or MPH-MR12 (o.a.d.; n = 4,785). There were again a higher number of prior diagnoses among patients receiving MPH-MR12 (3.44 versus 2.96 for patients receiving MPH-IR, $p<0.001$) but no significant differences between the two groups regarding the incidence of comorbid conditions associated with ADHD (Kemner and Lage, 2006b). Use of MPH-MR12 was associated with a mean length of treatment of 199 days (compared to 108 days for MPH-IR; Kemner and Lage, 2006b), less hospitalizations (Kemner and Lage, 2006b), and again less emergency room visits (Kemner and Lage, 2006a).

Two independent Medicaid claims database studies add further empirical sup-port to these issues, both of which indicated low levels of treatment compli-ance in ADHD. In a Texas Medicaid-sponsored retrospective analysis of 9,549 patients, Sanchez and colleagues found significantly higher persistence rates among patients receiving modified-release methylphenidate with a 12-hour duration of action (MPH-MR12) compared to those receiving mixed amphetamine salts or MPH-IR (Sanchez et al., 2005). In a California Medicaid claims database study supported by the manufacturer of MPH-MR12, a significantly longer mean duration of treatment was reported for patients initiating MPH-MR12 compared to MPH-MR08 (8-hour duration of action), with the lowest persistence rates found in patients treated with MPH-IR (Marcus et al., 2005).

Collectively, these data illustrate the importance of the compliance problem asso-ciated with ADHD treatment, notably with short-acting psychostimulants. As men-tioned earlier, the Assessment Report did not address this issue and its undeniable implications and sequelae in relation to a meaningful economic evaluation of alternative treatment options. This enigmatic shortcoming is difficult to comprehend as two broadly accepted approaches are available to address the problem[34]. These are (1) the use of models to assimilate existing information from various sources combined with appropriate sensitivity analyses, and (2) the use of information from randomized pragmatic trials capturing the "real-world" situation (Freemantle et al., 2005; Hughes et al., 2001; Baltussen et al., 1999; Revicki and Frank, 1999). The latter approach was endorsed for the economic evaluation of a novel antipsychotic drug by the senior author of the present Assessment Report. This author even suggested that his approach might serve as a model for future economic assessments in a wider context (Drummond et al., 1998). He explicitly acknowledged that the design of such studies "is inevitably a compromise between control and pragmatism" (Drummond et al., 1998) – a fact that should be reflected in quality rating criteria for trials included in formal reviews. In the context of the present assessment, this approach is relevant because pragmatic randomized real-world effectiveness studies were available, one of which (Steele et al., 2004, 2006) comprised a direct comparison of MPH-IR and MPH-MR12 (see Tables 5.7 and 5.9)[35]. This raises the question of how the data from this trial were integrated for analysis.

In summary at this point, the Assessment Group did not adequately address the entire range of problems surrounding the distinction between efficacy and effectiveness and the role of treatment non-compliance, especially in ADHD.

5.4 Data Synthesis Across Endpoints and Studies

The focus on CGI-I scores as the clinical effectiveness criterion for primary economic evaluation resulted in an evidence base of only six studies available for analysis, with a total of 1,958 patients. One open-label study contributed a disproportionate number of patients (1,323), and another trial was reinstated after previously being discounted on the grounds of quality concerns (Table 5.7; cf. AR, Ch. 6, p. 226, Table 6.2)[36]. This evidence base is both qualitatively and quantitatively insufficient to assess the relative value of six alternative interventions, i.e.,

---

[34] Of course, the general issue of how to deal with the impact of non-compliance on the cost-effectiveness of medical treatments is not unique to ADHD.

[35] Ironically, the discussion in the Final Appraisal Determination (FAD; NICE, 2005c) – but not in the Appraisal Consultation Document (ACD; NICE, 2005a) – warned that "this study was open-label and so should be interpreted with caution" (FAD, Section 4.1.2.4; cf. below).

[36] From the Assessment Report (p. 226) it is not transparent whether one additional "commercial-in-confidence" study referred to as "Quinn et al. 2003" might have been included, too. No published information on this trial is available. From the AR (cf. p. 93 and p. 146), however, it is possible to infer that this study was designed to compare MPH-MR08, MPH-IR, and placebo. The study was commissioned by the manufacturer of MPH-MR08 (cf. Table 1.2 above and AR, p. 276, quoting a "Celltech integrated study report").

Table 5.7 Synopsis of clinical studies

selected by Assessment Group for primary ("base case") data synthesis and economic evaluation

All patients defined by DSM-IV diagnostic criteria. Subtypes: C, combined; I, inattentive; H, hyperactive. AR, Assessment Report, MPH, methylphenidate, MPH-IR, methylphenidate immediate-release; MPH-MR08, MPH-MR12, methylphenidate modified-release with a duration of action of 8 or 12 hours, respectively; ATX, atomoxetine, DEX, dexamphetamine, MAS, mixed amphetamine salts, trade name Adderall (not available in Europe); PG, parallel-group; ODD, oppositional-defiant disorder; CD, conduct disorder; CIC, commercial-in-confidence; NDT, non-drug treatment; Plac., placebo; RR, response rate; o.a.d., one does per day; b.i.d., divided in two doses per day; t.i.d., divided in three doses per day; mg/d, average dose in milligrams per day; mg/kg/d, average dose in milligrams per kilogram bodyweight and day; w, week(s); [1] mean doses at study end; [2] definition of "response": reduction in mean ADHD-RS score >30%; [3] Table 6.2 of AR gives a figure of 83%; [4] according to inclusion criteria "relatively free of anxiety, depression, and conduct disorder"; [5] psychiatrist CGI-I ratings after 8 weeks of treatment, not 12 weeks as implied in Table 4.26 of AR

Clinical Study		Patients						Treatments			Clinical Endpoints					Comments
Authors	Design	n	Gender [Male]	Age [Mean/Range]	Subtypes	Comor-bidity		Modality		NDT	Duration	CGI-I [RR]	CGI-S [RR]	ADHD-RS[RR]	SNAP-IV[RR]	
								Drug	Dose[1]							
Sharp et al., 1999	3X Cross-over	32	Girls only	?	C: 100% (?)	?					3m	Yes	?	No	No	Excluded in AR from effectiveness review (for reason of "inadequate data presentation"); no further data provided in AR; inclusion in AR
		32	0	?	C: 100% (?)	?		MPH-IR b.i.d.	1.28 mg/kg/dose	"recreation	3w	81%	?	–	–	
		32	0	?	C: 100% (?)	?		DEX b.i.d.	0.64 mg/kg/dose	therapy activities"	3w	84%	?	–	–	"initially" based on DSM-IIIR, "later" combined DSM-IV, combined type
		32	0	?	C: 100% (?)	?		Plac.	n.a.		3w	16%	?	–	–	
Greenhill et al., 2002	RCT, double-blind, PG (1:1), 32 sites	314	257 (82%)	9 (5–15)	?	None (?)				None (?)	3w	Yes	No	No	No	Primary endpoint: Conners' Teacher Global Index; study listed among
		155	128 (83%)	9 (6–15)	?	None (?)		MPH-MR08 o.a.d.	40.7 mg/d	None (?)	3w	81%	63%	–	–	MPH-ER medium dose group in AR
		159	129 (81%)	9 (5–14)	?	None (?)		Plac.	n.a.	None (?)	3w	50%	26%	–	–	

(continued)

Table 5.7 (continued)

Clinical Study		Patients					Treatments			Duration	Clinical Endpoints				Comments
Authors	Design	n	Gender [Male]	Age [Mean/Range]	Subtypes	Comorbidity	Modality Drug	Dose[1]	NDT		CGI-I [RR]	CGI-S [RR]	ADHD-RS[RR]	SNAP-IV[RR]	
Kemner et al., 2004, 2005. Note that "Kemner et al., 2004" is quoted in the AR as "CIC"	RCT, open-label, PG (2:1), "multiple sites"	1,323	982 (74%)	8.9 ± 2.1 (6–12)	C: 75% I: 14% H: 12%	ODD: ?			None (?)	3w	Yes	?	Yes	No	"CIC" (no data provided in AR); primary endpoint: ADHD-RS improvement (change in mean score): MPH-MR12 superior to ATX; adherence >92% in both groups
		850	630 (74%)	8.8 ± 2.0 (6–12)	C: 74% I: 13% H: 13%	ODD: ?	MPH-MR12 o.a.d.	32.7 mg/d	None (?)	3w	69%	?	76%[2]	–	
		473	352 (74%)	9.2 ± 2.1 (6–12)	C: 75% I: 15% H: 10%	ODD: ?	ATX o.a.d. or b.i.d.	36.7 mg/d	None (?)	3w	53%	?	63%[2]	–	
Steele et al., 2004, 2006. Note that "Steele et al., 2004" is quoted in the AR as "CIC"	RCT, open-label, "real-world" design, PG (1:1)	145	121 (83%)	9 (6–12)	C: 79% I: 19% H: 2%	ODD: 41%; CD: 1%			None (?)	8w	Yes	Yes	No	Yes	"CIC" (no data provided in AR); primary endpoint: SNAP-IV (18/26 items, parent ratings); real-world effectiveness trial; MPH-MR12 superior to MPH-IR
		73	60 (82%)	9.1 ± 1.8 (6–12)	C: 79% I: 19% H: 1%	ODD: 38%; CD: 0%	MPH-IR t.i.d. (61% of patients)	33.2 mg/d	None (?)	8w	62%	"CIC" mean change available only	–	16%	
		72	61 (85%)	9.0 ± 2.1 (6–12)	C: 79% I: 18% H: 3%	ODD: 43%; CD: 1%	MPH-MR12 o.a.d.	37.8 mg/d	None (?)	8w	85%[3]	–	–	44%	

Study	Design	N		Age		Comorbidity	Treatment	Dose		Duration					Primary endpoint
Pliszka et al., 2000; cf. also Faraone et al., 2001	RCT, double-blind, PG (1:1:1)	58	?	8.1 ± 1.4	?	ODD, CD, anxiety			None (?)	3w	Yes	No	No	No	Primary endpoint: IOWA Conners' ratings
		20			?	ODD, CD, anxiety	MPH-IR o.a.d.-t.i.d.	25.2 mg/d	None (?)	3w	65%	–	–	–	
		20			?	ODD, CD, anxiety	MAS o.a.d or b.i.d.	12.5 mg/d	None (?)	3w	90%	–	–	–	
		18			?	ODD, CD, anxiety	Plac.	–	None (?)	3w	28%	–	–	–	
Klein and Abikoff, 1997	RCT, double-blind, PG (1:1:1)	86	81 (94%)	7.8 ± 1.4 (6–12)	?	None (?)[4]			None	8–12w	Yes	No	No	No	Primary endpoints: CTRS, CPRS; multiple further assessments
		29			?	None (?)[4]	MPH-IR b.i.d. or t.i.d. (?)	1.55 mg/kg/d	Yes	8w[5]	79%[5]	–	–	–	
		29			?	None (?)[4]	MPH-IR b.i.d. or t.i.d.(?)	1.48 mg/kg/d	Yes	8w[5]	97%[5]	–	–	–	
		28			?	None (?)[4]	Plac.	–	Yes	8w[5]	50%[5]	–	–	–	

Table 5.8 Synopsis of clinical studies added by Assessment Group for secondary ("extended") data synthesis and economic evaluation

For abbreviations used, cf. legend to Table 5.7; int.: internalizing comorbidity (anxiety, depression), ext.: externalizing comorbidity (CD, ODD). [1]Spencer et al. (2002) reported on two randomized trials; some data are provided only for both trial populations combined; [2]for the NIMH MTA Study, cf. *Discussion*; note that ADHD-RS response definitions varied across trials: response definition in the study by Weiss et al. (2004, 2005) was "20% reduction in the ADHD-RS-IV Teacher: Inv total score" (l.c., p. 650), whereas Elia et al. (1991) used different diagnostic criteria; this study was listed as a 9-weeks-study in the AR though treatment modalities were tested for 3 weeks each. Response definitions also varied between studies for SNAP-IV scores

Clinical Study		Patients					Treatments				Clinical Endpoints				Comments
Authors	Design	n	Gender [Male]	Age [Mean/Range]	Subtypes	Comorbidity	Drug	Dose[1]	NDT	Duration	CGI-I [RR]	CGI-S [RR]	ADHD-RS [RR]	SNAP-IV [RR]	
Kelsey et al., 2004	RCT, double-blind, PG (2:1), 12 sites	197	139 (71%)	9.5 (6–12)	C: 69% I: 27% H: 4%	ODD: 35.0%; CD: 4.1%			No	8w	Yes	No		No	Primary endpoint: ADHD-RS total score
		133	94 (71%)	9.5 ± 1,8 (6–12)	C: 70% I: 26% H: 4%	ODD: 37.6%; CD: 5.3%	ATX o.a.d.	44.5 mg/d	None (?)	8w	–	27%	63%	–	
		64	45 (70%)	9.4 ± 1,8 (6–12)	C: 67% I: 30% H: 3%	ODD: 29.7%; CD: 1.6%	Plac.	–	None (?)	8w	–	5%	33%	–	
Michelson et al., 2002	RCT, double-blind, PG (1:1), 9 sites	171		? (6–16)	C: 58% I: 41% H: 2%	ODD 20%; few others			None (?)	6w	No	Yes	Yes	No	Primary endpoint: ADHD-RS total score; other scores including CTRS and parent ratings of behavior, besides CGI-S

Study	Design													Comments
		85	60 (71%)	? (6–16)	C: 55% I: 41% H: 4%	ODD: 18.8%; few others	ATX o.a.d.	Not reported (1.0–1.5 mg/kg/d)	None (?)	6w	–	29%	60%	–
		86	60 (71%)	? (6–16)	C: 60% I: 40% H: 0%	ODD: 21.1%; few others	Plac.	n.a.	None (?)	6w	–	10%	31%	–
Weiss et al., 2004, 2005 Note that "Weiss et al., 2004" is quoted in the AR as "CIC"	RCT, double-blind, PG (2:1), 11 sites (USA, Canada, Puerto Rico)	153	123 (80%)	9.9 + 1.3 (8–12)	C: 73% I: 27% H: 1%	ODD 33%; learning disorders (LD): 30%; others: <5%				7w	Yes	Yes	Yes	No → "CIC" (no data provided in AR); primary endpoint: ADHD-RS total score (by teachers); further endpoints including CPRS and Conners' Global Index
		101	83 (82%)	9.9 + 1.4	C: 74% I: 26% H: 0%	ODD: 33%; LDs: 29%	ATX o.a.d.	1.33 mg/kg/d		7w	?	21%	69%	–
		52	40 (77%)	9.9 + 1.3	C: 69% I: 29% H: 2%	ODD: 35%; LDs: 31%	Plac.	n.a.		7w	?	10%	43%	–

(continued)

Table 5.8 (continued)

Clinical Study			Patients					Treatments					Clinical Endpoints				Comments
								Modality									
Authors	Design	n	Gender [Male]	Age [Mean/Range]	Subtypes	Comorbidity		Drug	Dose[1]	NDT	Duration	CGI-I [RR]	CGI-S [RR]	ADHD-RS [RR]	SNAP-IV [RR]	
Spencer et al., 2002 (I)[1]	RCT, double-blind, PG (1:1), multi-center	147 (20 MPH-treated - no data)	201/253 (79%)[1]	(7–13)[1]	C: 80%[1] I: 19%[1] H: 1%[1]	ODD: 38.7%; phobias: 11.5%; some others[1]				None (?)	9w	No	No	Yes	No	Primary endpoint: ADHD-RS total score; further endpoints including subscales, CPRS, CGI-ADHD-Severity; an MPH arm comprising 20 patients was included "to validate study design in the event that ATX failed to separate from placebo"; no MPH results are reported.
		65	98/129 (76%)[1]	9.7 + 1.6 (7–13)[1]	C: 80.6%[1] I: 19%[1] H: 1%[1]	ODD: 41.1%; pho-bias: 12.4%; some others[1]		ATX b.i.d., t.i.d.	Not reported (< 2.0 mg/kg/d or <90 mg/d)	None (?)	9w	–	–	65%	–	
		62	103/124 (83%)[1]	10.0 + 1.5 (7–13)[1]	C: 79%[1] I: 19%[1] H: 2%[1]	ODD: 36.3%; phobias: 10.5%; some others[1]		Plac.	–	None (?)	9w	–	–	24%	–	
		20	?	?	?	?		MPH	?	?	9w (?)	?	?	?	?	

Spencer et al., 2002 (II)[1]	RCT, double-blind, PG (1:1), multi-center	126(144 ? - not clear: MPH)	201/253 (79%)[1]	(7–13)[1]		C: 80%[1] I: 19%[1] H: 1%[1]	ODD: 38.7%; phobias: 11.5%; some others[1]			None (?)	12w	No	No	Yes	No		Primary endpoint: ADHD-RS total score; further endpoints including subscales, CPRS, CGI-ADHD-Severity
		64	98/129 (76%)[1]	9.7 + 1.6 (7–13)[1]		C: 80.6%[1] I: 19%[1] H: 1%[1]	ODD: 41.1%; phobias: 12.4%; some others[1]	ATX b.i.d., t.i.d.	Not reported (< 2.0 mg/kg/d or <90 mg/d)		12w			–	59%		–
		62	103/124 (83%)[1]	10.0 + 1.5 (7–13)[1]		C: 79%[1] I: 19%[1] H: 2%[1]	ODD: 36.3%;phobias: 10.5%; some others[1]	Plac.	–		12w			–	44%		–

(continued)

Table 5.8 (continued)

Clinical Study		Patients			Subtypes	Comorbidity	Treatments			Duration	Clinical Endpoints				Comments
Authors	Design	n	Gender [Male]	Age [Mean/Range]			Modality / Drug	Dose[1]	NDT		CGI-I [RR]	CGI-S [RR]	ADHD-RS [RR]	SNAP-IV [RR]	
Swanson et al., 2001; cf. also MTA Cooperative Group, 1999a,b	RCT, open-label, PG (1:1:1:1), 6 sites	579	465 (80%)	8.5 + 0.8 (7–<9.9)		Internalizing 14.0%; externalizing 29.5%; both: 24.7%			See below	14m (24m)	No	No	No	Yes	MTA Study[2] A variety of endpoints was studied, including SNAP-IV, CTRS, CPRS, CIS SNAP-IV-based response rates were calculated using parent and teacher ratings, including all 26 items of the scale (Swanson et al., 2001)
		144	118 (82%)	8.6 + 0.8 (7–<9.9)		Int: 13.9%; Ext: 27.8%; Both: 26.4%	Medication Management: MPH-IR t.i.d.	75%: MPH-IR 37.7 mg/d	None	14m (24m)	–	–	–	56% (14m)	Results for NDT alone (behavioral treatment arm) "omitted from evaluation" by the assessment group "as not relevant to this review" (AR, p. 254)
		145	114 (79%)	8.4 + 0.8 (7–<9.9)		Int: 13.1%; Ext: 24.8%; Both: 25.5%	Combination Treatment: MPH-IR t.i.d.	75%: MPH-IR 31.2 mg/d	Yes	14m (24m)	–	–	–	68% (14m)	

Quinn et al., 2003[cf. AR, p. 93, p. 146, p. 276]	146	119 (82%)	8.5 + 0.8 (7–<9.9)	Int.: 13.0%; Ext: 37.0%; Both: 21.1%	Community Comparison	58%: MPH-IR 22.6 mg/d, mean 2.3 doses/d	Partly	14m (24m)	–	–	–	25% (14m)
	144	114 (79%)	8.3 + 0.8 (7–<9.9)	Int.: 16.0%; Ext: 29.2%; Both: 25.0%	None (Behavioral Management)	–	Yes	14m (24m)	–	–	–	34% (14m)
("CIC")	?	?	?	?	?	?	?	?	?	?	?	?
	?	?	?	?	MPH-IR	"High dose": >30 mg/d	?	?	?	?	?	?
	?	?	?	?	"MPH-ER"; presumably MPH-MR08	"Med. dose": 20–40 mg/d	?	?	?	?	?	?
	?	?	?	?	Plac.	–	?	?	?	?	?	?

"CIC" (no data provided in AR); source quoted: "Celltech Integrated Clinical Study Report"

(continued)

Table 5.8 (continued)

Clinical Study		Patients						Treatments				Clinical Endpoints				Comments
Authors	Design	n	Gender [Male]	Age [Mean/Range]	Subtypes	Comorbidity	Modality Drug	Dose[1]	NDT	Duration	CGI-I[RR]	CGI-S[RR]	ADHD-RS[RR]	SNAP-IV[RR]	
Elia et al., 1991; see also Castellanos et al., 1997	3x crossover design	48	48 (100%)	8.6 + 1.7 (6–12)	DSM III No data on subtypes reported	ODD: 25.0%; CD: 20.8%; specific development disorders 22.9%	DEXb.i.d.	<1.3 mg/kg/d	Yes	9w		"CGI results were presented in graph form only and could not be reproduced in a table." (AR, p. 156)	No	No	This study used DSM-III diagnostic criteria and defined response as a score of 1, 2, or 3 on CGI-I; primary endpoint not specified
									Yes	3w			–	–	
							MPH-IRb.i.d.	<2.5 mg/kg/d	Yes	3w			–	–	
							Plac.	–	Yes	3w			–	–	

atomoxetine, dexamphetamine, methylphenidate in three formulations (MPH-IR, MPH-MR08, MPH-MR12), and a hypothetical "Do Nothing" alternative represented by placebo controls – especially when considering the heterogeneous impact of treatment intensity (including but not limited to dosing), concomitant, non-drug interventions and the incidence and severity of co-existent problems, including comorbidity, peer relationships, and educational performance (cf. above, Chapter 4, *NICE Appraisal of ADHD Treatments*). In an attempt to address these limitations, the Assessment Group pursued two approaches; (a) the synthesis of response rates across different effectiveness measures, and (b) the use of statistical mixed treatment comparison (MTC) techniques that enable integration of direct and indirect evidence.

5.4.1 Data Synthesis Across Endpoints

In order to broaden the data basis available for analysis, the Assessment Group extended its primary analyses of response rates by importing data from additional trials that reported different outcome measures, specifically CGI-S, ADHD-RS, and SNAP-IV scores. This resulted in the addition of seven trials involving 822 patients (plus an unknown number of subjects included in the commercial-in-confidence study "Quinn et al. 2003"[37]) over observation periods of 3 to 12 weeks (see Table 5.8). The NIMH MTA Study (MTA Cooperative Group, 1999a,b; Swanson et al., 2001) provided a further 579 patients, although not all data from the MTA Study were used and the Assessment Report is enigmatic in this regard[38]. While the Assessment Group asserted that "the nature of the treatment received in the community comparison arm of the MTA is still unclear, and as a result this data is omitted from the analysis" (AR, Ch. 6, p. 254), the Assessment Report (AR, Table 6.17, also p. 254) in fact omits information on the behavioral treatment arm rather than that on the community comparison group. It is also unclear how the analysis dealt with the different nature of the MTA trial, which compared treatment *strategies*, not specific medications (cf. below, *Economic Model*).

The inclusion of data from an increasing number of separate and disparate sources in response to data paucity in the selected studies raises important questions about the validity of the overall findings, which have not been addressed in the Assessment Report. One of these questions relates to the synthesis of efficacy

---

[37] Assuming that this study had not already been included in the base case analysis, this remains unclear from the Assessment Report (King et al., 2004b).

[38] The Assessment Report provides incomplete and contradictory information on their use. It is particularly noteworthy that the Assessment Group stated that it could incorporate the MTA data only "by assuming that the medical management group [...] represents treatment with MPH-IR" (AR, Ch. 6, p. 253). Given the administration regimens as well as the substantive efforts to manage protocol adherence in this trial, one could argue that the medication management arm might more appropriately have been used as a proxy for the effectiveness of modified-release methylphenidate under routine care conditions. See also Chapter 6, *Insights from Clinical Long-Term Data*.

data derived from different outcome measures based on the implicit assumption of similar effects of the various treatments tested across the various measures used. Most likely, this assumption is flawed (cf. Gilbody et al., 2003; APA, 2000).

For the CGI scale, it has been shown that changes in its improvement ("CGI-I") and severity ("CGI-S") sub-scale scores show only a moderate correlation ($r \sim -0.47$ to 0.66), "where one would expect a high correlation" (Guy, 2000).

Furthermore, CGI-I ratings appeared to be independent of side effect ratings, while CGI-S ratings were only moderately correlated with side effect ratings. These observations cast meaningful doubt on the appropriateness of any single sub-scale (CGI-I or CGI-S) as a composite measure of treatment success, and they fail to support the synthesis of sub-scale ratings as described by the Assessment Group. Likewise, the Assessment Report does not provide scientific justification for the chosen approach to synthesize all clinician-rated response data.

The issue of heterogeneous outcome measures is further compounded when clinical global impressions (CGI scores) are combined with scores obtained from narrow band symptom scales such as the ADHD-RS and the SNAP-IV[39]. Robust correlations between symptom scales have not been established, which is not surprising given the paucity of direct comparisons between the various symptom scales (Collett et al., 2003). Moreover, definitions of response involving the same scales varied across the studies used in the analysis. For example, response rates on the basis of the parent-rated ADHD-RS were defined in the Assessment Report as a score reduction of 25% or greater (AR, Ch. 6, p. 225), whereas Kemner et al. (2004), for their study involving 1,323 patients, used a 30% reduction (Kemner et al., 2005) and Weiss et al. (2005) used a 20% reduction to define treatment response (cf. Tables 5.7 and 5.8). The study by Elia et al. (1991), which was one of the trials added for secondary analyses, used yet another definition of "response," namely a score of 1, 2 or 3 on the CGI-I, as opposed to scores of 1 or 2 used elsewhere for assessment. In addition patient inclusion criteria in this study differed as a diagnosis of ADHD was based on DSM-III criteria.

Similarly, it remains unclear from the Assessment Report whether SNAP-IV derived "remission" rates defined by Steele and colleagues (2004) corresponded to the SNAP-IV "near normalization" criterion used in the MTA analyses (MTA Cooperative Group, 1999a,b, 2004; Swanson et al., 2001)[40].

A further aspect concerns potential confounding effects between outcome measures and treatments. For instance, response rate estimates based upon the

---

[39] Matza et al. (2004) reported correlations between ADHD symptoms and psychosocial domains of HRQoL "in the moderate range," confirming "that HRQoL and symptom measures capture related but distinct constructs" (l.c., p. 172).

[40] Review of the original publications reveals the following definitions of "response:" (a) Steele et al., 2006, pp. e59: a score of 0 or 1 ("no" or "very mild" severity) on *every* item of the *18 item* ADHD sub-scale of the SNAP-IV 26 scale based on the *parent's* perception of their child (with *no* inclusion of teacher rated scales). (b) In contrast, SNAP-IV "normalization" in the MTA Study (Swanson et al., 2001, pp. 170f.) was defined by an *overall* score ≤ 1 based on *parent and teacher* ratings, comprising *also items 19–26*, which represent DSM-IV criteria for oppositional-defiant disorder.

ADHD-RS scale were derived from six randomized studies involving 2,097 patients. Five of those studies were double-blind comparisons of atomoxetine with placebo (774 patients), while the sixth study was an open-label comparison of atomoxetine and modified-release methylphenidate (MPH-MR12) involving 1,323 patients. The SNAP-IV scale was used (with substantially different response definitions[40]) solely in the "*real-world*" trial by Steele et al. (2004, 2006) and in the MTA Study (Swanson et al., 2001), which compared predominantly MPH-IR based treatment *strategies* following a design different from all other trials (see below, Chapter 6, *Discussion*). The possibility of confounding has not been addressed or mentioned in the Assessment Report.

5.4.2 Data Synthesis Across Clinical Studies

For both the primary and the extended analyses, the Assessment Group faced a problem commonly encountered in health technology assessments, which is a paucity of study data to enable quantitative comparisons across the complete range of treatment options. For primary analysis, six studies were left after application of the selection criteria chosen by the Assessment Group. The Group resorted to indirect comparisons of treatment, a tactic that is increasingly being used in situations when there is insufficient direct evidence from head-to-head randomized trials. Although direct comparisons of treatments should be sought in the first instance (Bucher et al., 1997), indirect comparisons represent an appropriate and now well-accepted approach based upon advanced statistical methods that were developed to overcome some of the limitations of conventional meta-analyses. This approach facilitates the synthesis of direct and indirect evidence in mixed treatment comparisons (MTCs). MTCs are designed to use information derived from direct comparisons of different interventions (e.g., A vs. B and B vs. C) to synthesize an indirect comparison between interventions used in different studies (A vs. C). This indirect approach allows analyses to "borrow strength" (Higgins and Whitehead, 1996) and make inferences about the differences between A and C to support information contained in direct comparisons of A and C, where available.

As such, MTCs can be useful and sometimes represent the only alternative for multi-treatment decision-making. However, the validity of MTCs critically depends on the internal validity and similarity of the contributory trials (Song et al., 2003). As with any conventional meta-analysis, a fundamental assumption is that the relative treatment effects are consistent across trials ("fixed effects"), and that the trial-specific treatment differences follow a common distribution ("random effects"). MTCs also require that, if C had been observed in the A vs. B trials and if A had been observed in the B vs. C trials, then the true differences between A and C in these studies would be the same, or at least reflect the same common distribution as the true A/C differences found in direct A vs. C trials (Lu and Ades, 2004).

These requirements are violated whenever there are differences between the design of the studies from which data are taken for an MTC, such as (for example) $A_{TrialBased}$ in some comparative studies and $A_{RealWorld}$ in some others. Any adjustments that do not take this distinction into account will obscure the differences between $A_{TrialBased}$ and $A_{RealWorld}$. In other words, without differentiating between the two As (and, if and when applicable, Bs, Cs, and so on), the MTC approach will implicitly "assume away" – or "bias to the null" (Petitti, 2000) – any difference between them, with the effect of introducing error instead of "borrowing strength."

Relating this to the present assessment, the MTC approach chosen by the Assessment Group will inevitably conceal any potential effects of improved compliance, such as a greater difference between immediate-release methylphenidate (MPH-IR) and atomoxetine (which is usually administered once daily) or modified-release methylphenidate (MPH-MR08 or MPH-MR12), in real-world situations compared to experimental settings, from which the majority of data were taken. Obviously, providing its existence, such a greater difference would be found in (appropriately designed) pragmatic studies only. Therefore, this approach creates a heterogeneity problem, in the present case related to a critical design feature of studies that violates a fundamental assumption of any meta-analysis. For comparison, the assessment protocol had explicated that data would "only be pooled when this is statistically and clinically meaningful" (King et al., 2004a).

This theoretical expectation is consistent with a comparison of results from the pragmatic real-life study by Steele and colleagues (2004, 2006) with those of the meta-analysis ("mixed treatment comparisons," MTCs) by the Assessment Group (Table 5.9). Differences in effects were invariably greater in the real-world study by Steele et al. (2004, 2006), which can be assumed to better reflect *effectiveness*[41], than in the combined MTC analysis, which comprised predominantly data from efficacy trials.

As Petitti (2000) observed, "including disparate treatments [e.g., with regard to dosing] or outcomes [i.e., different clinical endpoints, cf. section above] in the same meta-analysis [or, for that purpose, MTC] may result in over-generalization of the results of the meta-analysis" (l.c., p. 84). The consequence is a *systematic error* due to neglect of the effects of treatment compliance, which introduces a distortion manifesting as "*bias*" (cf. Petitti, 2000, p. 73).

Specifically addressing issues in the quantitative synthesis of ADHD treatment effectiveness, Stephen Faraone (2003) noted that "it would be a mistake to compare effect sizes between studies without acknowledging the main limitation of this method, [which] ... only makes sense if we are certain that the studies being compared are reasonably similar on any design features that might increase or decrease the effect size." He explicated that "comparing effect sizes between studies is questionable if the studies differ substantially on design features that might plausibly influence drug-placebo differences" (Faraone, 2003). In particular, differences in

---

[41] Unfortunately, the study by Steele and colleagues (2004, 2006) is impaired by the absence of teacher-reported outcome ratings. A further concern relates to the fact that 39% of the patients in the MPH-IR group were dosed twice daily (b.i.d.), which may be considered an unfair comparison. This concern was addressed by *post hoc* subgroup analyses, which confirmed a statistically significant difference in favor of MPH-MR12 (with remission rates at study endpoint of 44% for MPH-MR12 versus 24% for MPH-IR given thrice daily [t.i.d.], based on SNAP-IV symptom scores). The study was supported by the Canadian subsidiary of the manufacturer of MPH-MR12.

Table 5.9 Pooling of efficacy and effectiveness trials

resulted in a compression of the "real-world" effectiveness differences between MPH-MR12 o.a.d. ("MPH-OROS") and MPH-IR t.i.d: Data synthesized by Assessment Group were predominantly efficacy data from controlled clinical studies; data in right columns integrate various endpoints. MPH, methylphenidate; IR, immediate-release formulation; MR12, modified-release formulation with a duration of action of 12 hours; NNT, number needed to treat; MTC, mixed treatment comparison (technique used by Assessment Group for data synthesis ("meta-analysis"), ext. MTC, secondary extensions of data synthesis using mixed treatment comparison technique. All differences between treatment arms observed by Steele et al. (2006) were statistically highly significant (p<0.001). The Assessment Group stated only that "the estimated response rates were subject to large uncertainty" (AR, p. 236)

Data Source	CGI-I "Real World"	CGI-I "MTC"	CGI-S "Real World"	SNAP-IV "Real World"	CGI-S and -I "synthesized" ("CGI-I baseline") "ext. MTC"	CGI-S and -I "synthesized" ("CGI-S baseline") "ext. MTC"	All "synthesized" ("ADHD-RS baseline") "ext. MTC"	All "synthesized" ("CGI-I baseline") "ext. MTC"
	Steele et al. 2006	AR, p. 236	Steele et al. 2006	Steele et al. 2006	AR, p. 253	AR, p. 253	AR, p. 255	AR, p. 255
Response Rates								
MPH-IR	62%	68%	49%	16%	76%	53%	74%	64%
MPH-MR12	83%	75%	77%	44%	85%	65%	85%	79%
Absolute Difference	21%	7%	28%	28%	9%	12%	11%	15%
Relative Difference	+ 34%	+ 10%	+ 57%	+175%	+ 12%	+ 23%	+ 15%	+ 23%
NNT (per additional responder)	4.8	14.3	3.6	3.6	11.1	8.3	9.1	6.7

effect size had been found to be considerable between double-blind studies and open-label trials (Faraone et al., 2003b).

Interestingly, the authors of the Assessment Report recognized that "the economic model rests on the assumption that the relative treatment effects will be the same across trials" (AR, Ch. 6, p. 227). Although assessment of the potential for bias should always be part of quantitative synthesis in systematic reviews (Lau et al., 1997), no such discussion is made in the Assessment Report.

In fact, there are other important sources of potential bias, including (but not limited to) the small number of studies selected (notwithstanding the contentious issues surrounding the correct application of pre-specified study selection criteria), small patient numbers and short observation periods in most of these studies (3 to 9 weeks in at least 10 out of 13 trials, including the 14-months NIMH MTA Study), heterogeneity between studies (such as gender, diagnostic criteria, comorbidity, and treatment modalities, including dosing schedules and concomitant non-drug therapies), and confounding factors between clinical endpoints and treatment strategies (cf. Tables 5.7 and 5.8). These issues were not appropriately addressed in the Assessment Report despite a wide range of sensitivity tests applied to the economic model.

In conclusion, data synthesis in the Assessment Report was based on a small number of studies and was limited by substantial heterogeneity problems, notably including study designs (pragmatic real-world versus double-blind controlled) and endpoints (clinical global impressions versus narrow-band symptom scales, data from all of which were transformed into "response rates"). In this way, any existing differences in treatment effectiveness due to compliance differences were assumed away.

5.5 Economic Model

The Assessment Group motivated the *de novo* development of its own economic model with a critical review of the quality of life and cost-effectiveness literature on ADHD (cf. AR, Ch. 5, pp. 177ff.). Again use of "a plethora of instruments" (AR, Ch. 5, p. 178) in this area was noted, followed by an incomplete and partially incorrect description of these instruments. Neither the SNAP-IV scale nor the Conners' Teacher and Parent Rating Scales (CTRS/CPRS) qualify as disease-specific instruments to measure health-related quality of life (HRQoL) in ADHD, contrary to their erroneous interpretation in the Assessment Report (AR, Ch. 5, p. 178)[42]. These scales are, in fact, narrow-band symptom scales (Collett et al., 2003). Following some speculative statements on their sensitivity (referring to an alternative outcome analysis of the NIMH MTA Study, cf. Conners et al., 2001, but not to the literature on measurement instruments), a distinction was introduced between "a

---

[42] In fact, the references given in the AR (p. 178) refer to applications of these scales in clinical studies, whereas throughout the AR no reference is made to the scientific literature on ADHD-specific outcome instruments (see *Appendix A*).

clinical perspective" (for which "reporting outcomes in a disaggregated way may be useful") and "a decision-making perspective," requiring "an overall summary score" (AR, Ch. 5, p. 179; cf. also below, Chapter 6, *Discussion*). This reasoning was used to justify an exclusive focus on quality-adjusted life years (QALYs) as an outcome measure, which goes beyond NICE guidance. While NICE reference case analysis (cf. above, Table 3.1; NICE, 2004c) requires the use of cost-utility analysis, NICE also recognizes that "other form of cost-effectiveness analysis [. . .] may have a role to play" (NICE, 2004c; cf. Chapter 6, *Discussion*). Since parent ratings (based on the generic EQ-5D scale) were actually used for the assessment (Coghill et al., 2004), the problematic assertion by the Assessment Group that the use of patient preferences were preferable (AR, Ch. 5, p. 179) did not exert a negative impact on the economic model[43]. The relevant NICE guidelines stipulate that patient preferences may be used exceptionally (in addition) "if they can be justified and they markedly alter the results compared with the reference case" (NICE, 2004c).

5.5.1 Literature Review

Like the clinical effectiveness part of the Assessment Report, the review of the ADHD cost-effectiveness literature provided by the Assessment Group reveals significant gaps. Only five presumably relevant evaluations were identified in the published literature, including the previous NICE Technology Appraisal (Lord and Paisley, 2000), the Canadian assessment of CCOHTA that used CTRS scores as effectiveness measure (Zupancic et al., 1998), and the analysis published by Gilmore and Milne (2001) on the basis of a prior Wessex DEC report from 1998 (Gilmore et al., 1998).

As previously described (see above, *Outcome Measures*), the use of the CTRS was criticized because of two "implicit assumptions," i.e., that it is "a continuous rating scale, that is that the cost and desirability of achieving a small gain in CTRS scores for many children is assumed to be the same as the cost and desirability of achieving a large gain in CTRS scores for few children, and that efficacy is constant across baseline levels of ADHD severity" (AR, Ch. 5, p. 186). It has been shown above that both concerns apply with (at least) equal validity against the use of CGI-I scores and so-derived QALYs as an outcome measure (cf. above, *Quality of Life and Utility Estimates*).

Two further studies – one from the United States (Marchetti et al., 2001) and one from the perspective of the NHS (Vanoverbeke et al., 2003) – were reviewed, although they did not meet criteria of a full economic evaluation since they did not compare (incremental) costs and effects. However, in light of the Assessment

---

[43] It was noted earlier that children with ADHD are known to underestimate their disease-specific symptoms and behavioral problems (cf. Danckaerts et al., 1999). Child preference ratings have not been published.

Group's own approach, it is noteworthy that the American study was criticized on the grounds of "the approach to estimating the response rate for each comparator was unusual in the sense that the results of different outcome measures to assess response rate were pooled" (AR, p. 353). Other cost of illness studies (or recent reviews, e.g., Leibson and Long, 2003, and Matza et al., 2005a) were not been mentioned in the Assessment Report.

More importantly in the given context, the Assessment Report does not provide any reference to cost-effectiveness publications that are directly concerned with interventions evaluated. These omitted publications include at least two US cost-effectiveness analyses based on SNAP-IV-derived normalization rates from the NIMH MTA Study (n = 579; MTA Cooperative Group, 1999a,b; Swanson et al., 2001) that had been in the public domain, which reported probabilistic findings from patient-level data over 14 months both for the overall study population and for sub-groups defined by comorbidity (Jensen et al., 2004; Schlander et al., 2004a)[44] and two cost-effectiveness analyses comparing MPH-MR12 and MPH-IR from the perspectives of Canadian third party payers (Annemans and Ingham, 2002) or the NHS in the United Kingdom (Schlander, 2004b), respectively.

Further studies explored willingness-to-pay for new drugs (De Ridder and De Graeve, 2002) or had been concerned with the cost-effectiveness of atomoxetine in Canada (Iskedjian et al., 2003). Had the search strategy delineated in the original protocol (King et al., 2004a) been applied appropriately and covered relevant international economic and psychiatric conferences[45], the Assessment Group might have identified these analyses.

5.5.2 Structure of the Model

The new economic model developed by the Assessment Group was designed to consider alternative sequences of treatments (see Table 5.12, below; cf. AR, Ch. 6,

---

[44] Additional analyses have since become available addressing the impact on cost-effectiveness ratios of diagnostic criteria (Schlander et al., 2005a) and alternative clinical endpoints (Foster et al., 2005, 2007). Also European cost-effectiveness evaluations on the basis of the NIMH MTA Study are now available (Schlander et al., 2006a,b,c). Like the full publication of the primary cost-effectiveness analysis on the basis of the MTA (Jensen et al., 2005), these data appeared *after* the Assessment and thus have to be considered separately from the critique of the Assessment Report.

[45] In contrast to the original search strategy, which had indicated that both published and unpublished data be included, the final Assessment Report contains a statement that "economic evaluations reported as *conference proceedings or abstracts* were excluded since the data they contain *may* not be complete" (AR, Ch 3, p. 50; italics added). The Assessment Group had, however, full access to the comprehensive data of at least one analysis (Schlander, 2004b, which had been presented first in May 2004) by November 2004, and it quotes *personal communication* with another health economist to support its dismissal of the Conners' Scales as an effectiveness criterion (cf. AR, Ch. 5, p. 188, and reference no. 127 of Assessment Report, p. 279).

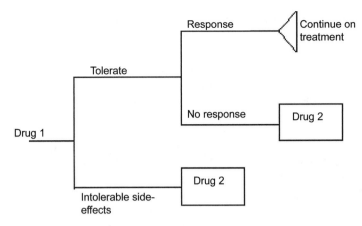

Fig. 5.2 Modular structure of economic model
Reproduced from King et al. 2006, with kind permission

pp. 220ff.) over a time period of one year[46]. Figure 5.2 illustrates the modular structure of the economic model. Pharmacotreatment of patients is assumed to begin with a titration period lasting for one month, during which response to treatment and adverse events will guide individual dose-finding for the first-line option (either DEX, MPH-IR, MPH-MR08, MPH-MR12, or ATX). Patients experiencing a response and tolerating treatment will continue with the first-line treatment. Patients who have not responded to treatment by the end of the titration period, and patients who have withdrawn from treatment for intolerable side effects, are assumed to move to the next treatment in sequence. Responders are assumed to remain on therapy and continue to be responsive for the one-year period modeled (AR, Ch. 6, p. 222).

To simulate so-defined treatment pathways, the economic model had to be populated with data on withdrawal rates and on response rates. For the primary evaluation ("base case analysis"), response rates were estimated on the basis of six randomized clinical trials (Table 5.7, above; cf. AR, Table 6.2, p. 226). The criteria for study and clinical endpoint selection were discussed earlier.

Given the structure of the economic model, withdrawal rates should capture the frequency of tolerability problems leading to treatment discontinuation, independent from non-response to treatment. This requirement created a number of serious problems.

Ten clinical trials were selected by the Assessment Group to provide information on treatment-specific withdrawal rates (Table 5.10; cf. AR, Table 6.3, p. 231). This information was also used unchanged in all subsequent extensions of the primary model (described as "sensitivity analyses" by the Assessment Group). As for the response rate synthesis, the crossover trial in 32 girls reported by Sharp and colleagues (1999), which had been excluded from the clinical effectiveness review

---

[46] A secondary analysis extended the time horizon to 12 years (from age 6 to age 18), see below.

for "inadequate data presentation" (AR, p. 338), was the only source of data on dexamphetamine and resulted in a raw data input of a zero withdrawal rate for this compound (Table 5.10).

A major concern relates to the fact that "patients withdrew from treatment for many reasons, including lack of efficacy," as recognized by the Assessment Group (AR, Ch. 6, p. 230). As a consequence, "the withdrawal rates for the model were calculated to include all reported withdrawals, regardless of the reason given" (AR, Ch. 6, p. 230). Justified in order "to maintain consistency," this approach necessarily resulted in double counting of non-responders which could not be quantified. Since the effect of double counting of non-responders can be expected to be most pronounced for those treatments with high withdrawal rates reported in clinical studies (see Tables 5.10 and 5.11), this structural phenomenon does constitute an important source of undetected bias throughout the economic model and its extensions. The Assessment Group noted four (out of ten) studies thought to be problematic in this respect (Kelsey et al., 2004; Steele et al., 2004; Weiss et al., 2004; Pliszka et al., 2000), because "a proportion of withdrawals were attributed to non-response" (AR, Ch. 6, p. 230). It is evident from higher withdrawal rates on placebo compared to active treatment that further studies were affected by this problem as well (e.g., Greenhill et al., 2002; Klein and Abikoff, 1997; see Table 5.10 and AR, Table 6.3, p. 231).

From the Assessment Report (section 6.1.6, Adverse events, pp. 229ff.) it can be inferred that no attempt was made to allow for this bias. This was justified by stating that "none of the four trials [mentioned above] calculated response in an intent-to-treat analysis" (AR, Ch. 6, p. 230), although in fact Kelsey et al. (2004) as well as Greenhill et al. (2002) used a last observation carried forward approach for intent-to-treat analysis, Steele et al. (2004, 2006) performed effectiveness analyses on an intent-to-treat sample, and Weiss et al. (2004, 2005) provided efficacy data also for patients who withdrew (according to their report, six out of 17 patients who withdrew from atomoxetine treatment did so because of adverse events). The parallel group study published by Pliszka et al. (2000) is more difficult to interpret in this regard since it enrolled only 18 to 20 patients per treatment arm, and the authors mentioned one patient who dropped out during the first study week, without providing further detail. Also Klein and Abikoff (1997) do not provide details about three drop-outs in their parallel group study, which also comprised less than 30 patients per treatment arm. The Assessment Report does not offer any hint whether per-protocol effectiveness analyses might have been considered for their potential to elucidate, at least in part, the magnitude of this apparent bias.

Finally, it remains enigmatic from the Assessment Report whether the synthesis of withdrawal rates was performed adequately. As mentioned earlier, although intended to reflect the impact of adverse events on treatment discontinuation, the withdrawal rates derived from some of the studies were higher for placebo than for active treatment (Kelsey et al., 2004; Greenhill et al., 2002; Pliszka et al., 2000; Klein and Abikoff, 1997). Nevertheless, "the probability of withdrawal was calculated in the same way as the response rates" (AR, Ch. 6, p. 230, and AR, Appendix, p. 358). As described earlier (cf. above, *Data Synthesis Across Clinical Studies*), response rates were synthesized applying a model (cf. AR, Ch. 6, p. 227). MTC

Table 5.10 Clinical data used to estimate withdrawal rates

Note that the Assessment Report does neither provide information on confidence intervals nor discuss treatment duration or other sources of heterogeneity. Spencer et al. (2002) reported data from two studies. For further details on these studies, see Tables 5.7 and 5.8 above. Abbreviations used: w, weeks; +NDT, in combination with non-drug treatment (behavioral therapy), CI, confidence interval. Source: AR, Table 6.3, p. 231, and publications cited

Treatment		Study	Treatment duration	Patient number (in treatment group)	Withdrawals in trial	
					Absolute number	Percent (exact 95% CI)
DEX		Sharp et al., 1999	3w	32	0	0.0% (0.0%–8.9%)
MPH-IR		Sharp et al., 1999	3w	32	1	3.1% (0.1%–16.2%)
		Steele et al., 2004	8w	74	12	16.2% (8.7%–26.6%)
		Pliszka et al., 2000	3w	20	1	5.0% (0.1%–24.9%)
		Klein and Abikoff, 1997	8w	31	1	3.2% (0.1%–16.7%)
	+NDT	Klein and Abikoff, 1997	8w	29	0	0.0% (0.0%–9.8%)
MPH-MR08		Greenhill et al., 2002	3w	158	20	12.7% (7.9%–18.9%)
MPH-MR12		Kemner et al., 2004	3w	850	41	4.8% (3.5%–6.5%)
		Steele et al., 2004	8w	73	12	16.4% (8.8%–27.0%)
ATX		Kemner et al., 2004	3w	473	26	5.5% (3.6%–8.0%)
		Kelsey et al., 2004	8w	133	26	19.6% (13.2%–27.3%)

(continued)

Table 5.10 (continued)

Treatment	Study	Treatment duration	Patient number (in treatment group)	Withdrawals in trial	
				Absolute number	Percent (exact 95% CI)
	Michelson et al., 2002	6w	85	12	14.1% (7.5%–23.4%)
	Weiss et al., 2004	7w	101	17	16.8% (10.1%–25.6%)
	Spencer et al., 2002	9w/12w	129	8	6.2% (2.7%–11.9%)
Placebo	Sharp et al., 1999	3w	32	0	0.0% (0.0%–8.9%)
	Greenhill et al., 2002	3w	163	32	19.6% (13.8%–26.5%)
	Pliszka et al., 2000	3w	18	2	11.1% (1.4%–34.7%)
	Kelsey et al., 2004	8w	64	17	26.6% (16.3%–39.1%)
	Michelson et al., 2002	6w	86	11	12.8% (6.6%–21.7%)
	Weiss et al., 2004	7w	52	4	7.7% (2.1%–18.5%)
	Spencer et al., 2002	9w/12w	124	7	5.7% (2.3%–11.33%)
+NDT	Klein and Abikoff, 1997	8w	29	2	6.9% (0.9%–22.8%)

models rely on relative treatment effects – in the case of withdrawal rates, this approach implies a synthesis of relative effects. Then, however, the implied meaning of the observed differences between treatment and placebo in some of the studies could only be a higher adverse event rate on placebo! To say the least, this sophisticated modeling approach is difficult to interpret. Although the Assessment Group was aware of the problem, they applied the resulting data to all analyses within their model (Figure 5.2), "regardless of definition of response" (AR, Ch. 6, p. 230), i.e., also for extensions and sensitivity analyses. Since reported and calculated withdrawal rates differed between studies and treatments (Tables 5.10 and 5.11), this modeling approach was not consistent (as claimed), but a source of bias. While this bias cannot be quantified on the basis of the information provided in the Assessment Report, it almost certainly worked in favor of dexamphetamine (which had the lowest "withdrawal rates" in the model, cf. Table 5.11 and also Table 5.10).

As described earlier in some detail, a meaningful exploration of the effects of non-compliance was rejected since "it was *felt* that [the required] modelling assumptions would not be reasonable given the lack of available data, which would render any sensitivity analysis around compliance uninformative to decision-makers" (AR, Ch. 6, p. 233). This assertion reflects the absence of a review of the existing literature on treatment compliance (cf. above and *Appendix*, below) and is associated with the decision to pool data from efficacy and effectiveness trials without distinction between the trial methodologies for data accrual (cf. above). Instead it was simply assumed that the phenomenon of non-compliance could be captured as a *subset of non-responders* reported in short-term, predominantly well-controlled efficacy studies, and on this basis it was claimed that "the effect of compliance on response rates

Table 5.11 Synthesized response and withdrawal rates for primary economic analysis
For sources of input data used for synthesis (MTC model for meta-analysis by Assessment Group), cf. Tables 5.7 and 5.10, above. The Assessment Report does not offer a discussion of the identical standard deviations for DEX and MPH-MR12 despite the difference in patient numbers. Note that the patient numbers given in the Assessment Report (Ch. 6, p. 236) slightly deviate from those calculated on the basis of original study publications (see also AR, Table 6.2, p. 226). There is however no indication that (or if so, which) additional studies might have been used for the synthesis of response rates (contrary to an enigmatic statement in the Assessment Report – cf. AR, Ch. 6, pp. 225ff., and AR, Appendix 3, pp. 333ff.). Standard deviations as reported by Assessment Group. Source of response and withdrawal rates: AR, Table 6.6, p. 236

Treatment	Response rate (standard deviation) reported by Assessment Group	Number of patients (input for treatment; from n clinical studies)	Withdrawal rate (standard deviation) reported by Assessment Group	Number of patients (input for treatment, from n clinical studies)
DEX	75% (32%)	32 (from 1 study)	2% (5%)	32 (from 1 study)
MPH-IR	68% (30%)	154 (from 4 studies)	9% (5%)	157 (from 4 studies)
MPH-MR08	57% (33%)	155 (from 1 study)	8% (6%)	158 (from 1 study)
MPH-MR12	75% (32%)	923 (from 2 studies)	12% (4%)	923 (from 2 studies)
ATX	67% (37%)	473 (from 1 study)	11% (6%)	921 (from 6 studies)
Placebo	28% (4%)	209 (from 3 studies)	11% (2%)	539 (from 8 studies)

to MPH-IR and MPH-ER is reflected in the model" (AR, Ch. 6, p. 250), although no allowance was made in the model for treatment non-persistence due to compliance problems (AR, Ch. 6, p. 246). Thus, all responders were assumed to remain on treatment for the one-year time period of the model. Accordingly, despite the compliance data and the data from the real-world study by Steele and colleagues (Steele et al., 2004, 2006), it was concluded that there was "little evidence of a statistically significant difference in the effectiveness [not: "*efficacy*"] of MPH-IR and MPH-ER" (AR, Ch. 7, p. 263). Without doubt, this approach involved a potential bias against all long-acting medications evaluated by NICE, i.e., MPH-MR08, MPH-MR12, and ATX (Schlander, 2007d).

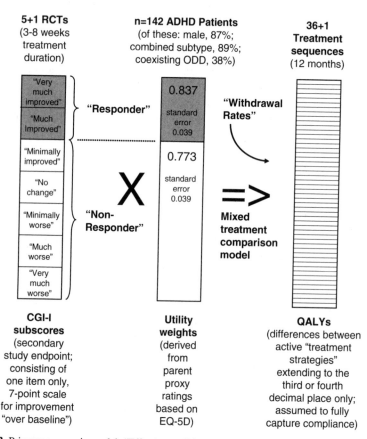

Fig. 5.3 Primary economic model: "Effectiveness" inputs and outputs
For patient numbers and some information on heterogeneity of randomized clinical trials (RCTs) used to estimate CGI-I- based response rates, see Table 5.7. For source of information on withdrawal rates, see Tables 5.10 and 5.11

5.5.3 Economic Model Results

On this basis, 37 possible treatment strategies (sequences) were defined for evaluation (Figure 5.3 and Table 5.12; cf. AR, Appendix 8, p. 355), none of which accommodated a switching scenario between MPH formulations (cf. AR, Ch. 6, p. 221). These were subsequently reduced to 19 strategies for analysis, without considering combination therapy. The Assessment Group correctly noted that this maneuver led to underestimation of decision uncertainty associated with its model (AR, Ch. 6, p. 221).

Informed by utility values ascribed to responders and non-responders, health outcomes were expressed in terms of quality-adjusted life-years (QALYs). Calculated QALY differences between active treatment strategies (excluding the "no treatment" option) were generally limited to the third or fourth decimal place (cf. AR, Table 6.7, p. 237, and AR, Table A.1, p. 355).

Table 5.12 Treatment sequences modeled by Assessment Group
The Assessment Group's new economic model featured 37 different treatment strategies (each of those listed below with and without non-drug treatment, NDT), which were subsequently reduced for "simplicity" to 19 treatment sequences. From the model description, it remains either unclear whether, or can be excluded that (AR, p. 266), heterogeneity in terms of NDT (i.e., combination therapy versus medication alone), treatment intensity (medication doses and, for MPH-IR [b.i.d. versus t.i.d.] and ATX [o.a.d. versus b.i.d.; or t.i.d. in Spencer et al. (2002)], administration schedules), as well as different patient populations (age, gender, subtypes studied, co-existent conditions – cf. Tables 5.7 and 5.8, above), and – for the secondary extensions ("sensitivity analyses") clinical effectiveness criteria, as well as confounding effects between those, were addressed adequately. None of the scenarios allowed for switching between different formulations of MPH (for instance, from MPH-IR to MPH-MR), and it was assumed that treatment response would be independent from prior treatment received. (See AR, Table 6.1, p. 222, Table 6.7, p. 237, and pp. 355ff.)

Treatment sequence	1st line	2nd line	3rd line	4th line
1	MPH-IR	ATX	DEX	No treatment
2	MPH-MR08	ATX	DEX	No treatment
3	MPH-MR12	ATX	DEX	No treatment
4	ATX	MPH-IR	DEX	No treatment
5	ATX	MPH.MR08	DEX	No treatment
6	ATX	MPH-MR12	DEX	No treatment
7	MPH-IR	DEX	ATX	No treatment
8	MPH-MR08	DEX	ATX	No treatment
9	MPH-MR12	DEX	ATX	No treatment
10	ATX	DEX	MPH-IR	No treatment
11	ATX	DEX	MPH-MR08	No treatment
12	ATX	DEX	MPH-MR12	No treatment
13	DEX	MPH-IR	ATX	No treatment
14	DEX	MPH-MR08	ATX	No treatment
15	DEX	MPH-MR12	ATX	No treatment
16	DEX	ATX	MPH-IR	No treatment
17	DEX	ATX	MPH-MR08	No treatment
18	DEX	ATX	MPH-MR12	No treatment
19	No treatment	No treatment	No treatment	No treatment

Resource utilization data came from expert estimates, with the average medi-cation doses taken from the trials used for modeling. Unit costs were calculated from the perspective of the NHS using the PSSRU compendium of the University of Kent, Canterbury (Netten and Curtis, 2004). Primary ("base case") analyses used data from six studies reporting CGI-I scores, and secondary extensions included synthesized response rates generated from CGI-S, ADHD-RS and SNAP-IV scores (cf. above). Within this framework, probabilistic analyses were employed to pro-duce cost-effectiveness acceptability curves for a variety of assumptions. This model indicated, both in its base case analysis as well as in its various extensions (AR, Ch. 6, pp. 236ff.), that a strategy consisting of first-line dexamphetamine, second-line methylphenidate (immediate-release formulations, MPH-IR), and third-line atom-oxetine was optimal.

The approach pursued (Figure 5.2 and Figure 5.3) led to the inability of the Assessment Group to differentiate treatment sequences on grounds of efficacy. This is nicely illustrated by a number of inconsistent QALY rankings of treat-ment sequences produced by the primary analysis (Table 5.13) which were not discussed in the Assessment Report. Likewise, the size of the differences between active treatment, e.g., "treatment sequence 13" (DEX initially, followed by MPH-IR, ATX, and no treatment), and "no treatment" ("strategy 19") appears very large. Given the utility weights applied, it would require an overall response difference between both "strategies" of 88 percentage points maintained over the 12-months time frame. This seems especially remarkable given the double counting of non-responders described earlier (which, however, affected the effectiveness estimates for DEX less than those for the other treatments, cf. Table 5.11), and it can only be explained by the opposite impact of two other assumptions, namely, that response to treatment would be independent from response to prior medication (AR, Ch. 6, p. 226), and that all patients would continue treatment over a full year (AR, Ch. 6, p. 222). (As discussed earlier, both assumptions are not justified by empirical data.)

Although the inconsistent QALY rankings disappeared after pooling of different effectiveness criteria in secondary model extensions (AR, Table 6.20, p. 258), the differences between treatment strategies remained very small, extending to the third or fourth decimal place only. Another "sensitivity analysis" used different utility weights, despite concerns about their validity (see above, *Quality of Life and Utility Estimates*).

A further "sensitivity analysis" extended the time period to 12 years (from age 6 to age 18). This extension is potentially misleading because a time period of 12 years – to be meaningful – would have to incorporate an economic evaluation of long-term sequelae associated with ADHD such as academic impairment, increased risk of injuries and accidents as well as encounters with the criminal justice system, etc. Current evidence of beneficial treatment effects on these sequelae is limited, and the relationship between short-term symptomatic and functional improvement and long-term outcomes has yet to be established (cf. Wilens and Dodson, 2004, and many others).

Aside from a casual note (AR, Ch. 6, p. 247: "the model also does not include long-term benefits of treatment, which could perhaps be avoidance of jail, lower

Table 5.13 Some consistency issues associated with the primary economic analysis

The primary or base case economic analysis resulted in inconsistent QALY rankings (cf. AR, Table 6.7, p. 237). Furthermore, the difference between strategy 13 (identified as "dominant" by the Assessment Group) and "no treatment" of (0.8289–0.7727)= 0.0562 QALYs compares to utility weights of 0.837 for responders and 0.773 for nonresponders (giving a difference of 0.064), which were used as inputs for the quantitative analysis (see Figure 5.3; AR, Ch. 6, p. 235). To hold given the structure and assumptions of the economic model, this difference in QALYs would require a difference in response rates between the dominant strategy and no treatment of 88% points, to be maintained over the 12 months time horizon

Treatment sequence	1st line	2nd line	3rd line	4th line	QALYs	Notes
2	MPH-MR08	ATX	DEX	No treatment	0.8273	Compare 2 vs. 3
3	MPH-MR12	ATX	DEX	No treatment	0.8278	with 11 vs. 12
7	MPH-IR	DEX	ATX	No treatment	0.8283	Compare 7 vs. 9
8	MPH-MR08	DEX	ATX	No treatment	0.8277	with 10 vs. 12
9	MPH-MR12	DEX	ATX	No treatment	0.8284	
10	ATX	DEX	MPH-IR	No treatment	0.8281	
11	ATX	DEX	MPH-MR08	No treatment	0.8281	
12	ATX	DEX	MPH-MR12	No treatment	0.8278	
13	DEX	MPH-IR	ATX	No treatment	0.8289	"dominant strategy"
16	DEX	ATX	MPH-IR	No treatment	0.8288	Compare 16 vs. 17
17	DEX	ATX	MPH-MR08	No treatment	0.8288	with 7 vs. 8
19	No treatment	No treatment	No treatment	No treatment	0.7727	

numbers of exclusions from school and improved peer relations") and the criticism of previous reviews (e.g., AR, Ch. 5, p. 192) and company submissions to NICE that they did not address long-term effects of medication (e.g., AR, Ch. 5, p. 201, p. 219), the Assessment Report does not provide any hint that the importance of this issue was recognized. There is no discussion (beyond the note on p. 247) in the Assessment Report of this limitation of currently available clinical and economic evaluations of ADHD, despite a statement that "long-term outcomes associated with ADHD" would be "discussed in [...] the report" (AR, Ch. 6, pp. 220 and 221). In particular, the issue of long-term sequelae is mentioned neither in the Executive Summary (AR, pp. 14ff.) nor in the concluding Discussion section (AR, Ch. 7, pp. 263ff.) of the Assessment Report. Consequently, the Assessment Group did not address this important need for further research (cf. AR, Ch. 7, p. 267f.), except for the generic *caveat* that "new data on long-term outcomes could change the analysis significantly" (AR, Ch. 6, p. 261; cf. also AR, Executive Summary, p. 20).

This gap appears relevant against the background that Porzsolt and colleagues (2005) identified "a serious problem" in "HTA reports which [...] express limitations in the discussions (read by many scientists), but not in the conclusions (read mainly by policy-makers)." Indeed a working group including the senior author of the NICE Assessment Report considered it "best practice" to report in scientific summaries the aspects of an assessment for which information is lacking or uncertain (Busse et al., 2002), and the NHS Centre for Reviews and Dissemination (CRD) recommended a framework for the discussion section of reviews, which should explicitly include an appraisal of the quality of the review, and address potential biases in both the primary studies and the review, as well as unanswered questions and implications for future research (CRD, 2001).

In addition to these limitations, the long-term extension of the economic model must have been particularly prone to bias from the factual exclusion of compliance issues, since these were assumed to be fully captured by the short-term studies selected for analysis. Another peculiar observation is the use of discount rates deviating from NICE guidance", despite an explicit statement to the contrary ("in accordance with NICE guidance", AR, Ch. 6, p. 223). The long-term model extension again produced inconsistent QALY rankings (Table 5.14).

As an interim summary of the above, the economic model was impaired by technical anomalies and prone to bias in various ways. For example, treatment strategies were unequally affected by the phenomenon of double counting non-responders. Further to this, the model effectively excluded *any* consideration of compliance problems. Given the limitations in enabling differentiation between treatment strategies on grounds of their "effectiveness" (actually, their "efficacy") as determined primarily on the basis of CGI (sub)scores and so derived QALY calculations, the results generated by the Assessment Group were ultimately driven by drug cost differences. Opportunities were missed to gain insights from disease-specific measures (such as Conners' ratings; cf. below, Chapter 6, *Discussion*). Owing to the incomplete search for published data, the results of two published cost-effectiveness studies using other outcome measures (Conners' ratings of inattention and overactivity) as clinical endpoints were not considered. Although the Assessment Group did mention a number

Table 5.14 Some consistency issues associated with the long-term extrapolation model
Like the 12-months model, also the sensitivity analysis extrapolating the economic model to when the hypothetical cohort of ADHD patients reaches 18 years of age is characterized by internal inconsistencies of the synthesized effectiveness results. Data source: AR, Table 6.11, p. 247

Treatment sequence	1st line	2nd line	3rd line	4th line	QALYs	Notes
1	MPH-IR	ATX	DEX	No treatment	9.2403	Compare 1 vs. 7 with 10 vs. 16
7	MPH-IR	DEX	ATX	No treatment	9.2597	
8	MPH-MR08	DEX	ATX	No treatment	9.2590	Compare 8 vs. 9 with 17 vs. 18
9	MPH-MR12	DEX	ATX	No treatment	9.2597	
10	ATX	DEX	MPH-IR	No treatment	9.2594	
16	DEX	ATX	MPH-IR	No treatment	9.2412	
17	DEX	ATX	MPH-MR08	No treatment	9.2409	
18	DEX	ATX	MPH-MR12	No treatment	9.2393	
19	No treatment	No treatment	No treatment	No treatment	8.8896	

of *caveats*, these limitations did not prevent them from claiming that their model "clearly identified an optimal treatment strategy" (e.g., AR, Ch. 7, p. 266).

5.6 Appraisal and Appeal Process

In a meeting on February 15, 2005, the NICE Appraisal Committee met with representatives of the Assessment Group to discuss "the clinical effectiveness and cost effectiveness of methylphenidate, atomoxetine and dexamfetamine – ADHD (in children and adolescents) on the basis of the evidence before them" (NICE, 2005b). A core piece of the evidence was the Assessment Report. The meeting minutes provide little information about details other than that none of the present members of the Assessment Group declared any relevant conflicts of interest[47], and that topics of the discussion included, among others, "issues such as variations in measures of efficacy across trials," "the availability of long-term studies," "the issue of single daily dose regimens versus multiple-dose regimens."

The resulting Appraisal Consultation Document (ACD; NICE, 2005a; for a summary of recommendations, cf. above, Chapter 3) indicated the Committee recognized that "ADHD is defined by the core signs of inattention, hyperactivity and impulsiveness," while the effectiveness review provided by the Assessment Group had focused exclusively on improvements in hyperactivity. The Committee also noted differences between ICD-10-defined "hyperkinetic disorder" (HKD) and DSM-IV-defined ADHD, with the severe combined subtype of ADHD being most similar to HKD, and the frequent co-existence of other conditions such as oppositional defiant disorder, conduct disorder, anxiety, depression and some others – although the Assessment Report had not addressed clinical and therapeutic implications of subtypes and comorbidity. From the sections of the ACD on clinical effectiveness and cost-effectiveness it becomes evident to what extent the Appraisal Committee relied on the Assessment Report. In particular, notable gaps left by the Assessment Report were not filled but carried forward. Regarding the effectiveness review, one important gap concerned the study by Newcorn and colleagues (2004, 2005) later referred to as "LYBI." Gaps in the cost-effectiveness review concerned recent cost-effectiveness studies (Jensen et al., 2004; Schlander et al., 2004a; Schlander, 2004b; Iskedjian et al., 2003; Annemans and Ingham, 2002; De Ridder and De Graeve, 2002). In addition, the anomalies of the Assessment Report were not revealed but carried forward, such as the inappropriate interpretation of the "three weeks duration" cut-off for study inclusion, the pooling of efficacy and effectiveness studies in the data synthesis process, or the idiosyncratic way response and withdrawal rates were estimated to populate the model. These observations under-

---

[47] This declaration confirms an earlier, similar statement in the Assessment Report (AR, p. 3): "None of the research team has any conflicts of interest to declare."

score the crucial importance of the Assessment Report as the core of the appraisal process[48].

However, the Appraisal Committee departed from the Assessment Group's conclusions on one key point. Largely on the basis of one crossover study in 32 females and a duration of each treatment period of three weeks, that had failed to qualify for the effectiveness review, the Assessment Group had claimed that, "for a decision taken now, ... the results of *the economic evaluation clearly identified an optimal treatment strategy* ... that is, dexamphetamine first-line. .." (e.g., AR, pp. 19; italics added). In contrast, the Appraisal Committee concluded that "Given the limited data used to inform response and withdrawal rates and the small differences in QALY gains generated, *it is not possible to distinguish between the different strategies on the grounds of cost effectiveness*" (ACD, section 4.2.5).

As all economic models converged in indicating incremental cost-effectiveness ratios (ICERs) versus no treatment well below £20,000/QALY gained (indeed, for all strategies assessed, below £7,000 per QALY gained in the Assessment Group's model), the Committee found that "all strategies were cost-effective" (ACD, section 4.2.5). Further considerations of the Committee (ACD, section 4.3) demonstrate substantial sensitivity to individual clinical situations, including compliance problems (even though these had not been included in the economic evaluation of the Assessment Group). Its final proposal for implementation and audit was "if there is a choice of more than one appropriate drug, the drug with the lowest cost is prescribed" (ACD, section 7.3.4). Therefore, this final proposal can only be interpreted as a consequence of the Comittee's inability to differentiate treatment options on grounds of effectiveness or cost-effectiveness (cf. ACD, Section 4.2.5).

The Appraisal Committee convened again on April 21, 2005 to prepare the Final Appraisal Determination (FAD) document in consideration of comments on the ACD received from consultees. From the meeting minutes (NICE, 2005d) it can be seen that the discussions included "randomized trials comparing atomoxetine with methylphenidate" and "the cost of atomoxetine when given in twice-daily regimens." Relatively minor changes in guidance compared to the ACD have been briefly described earlier (cf. Chapter 4, *NICE Appraisal of ADHD Treatments*). Aside from the deficiencies of the Assessment Report (as previously described) being carried forward, two major issues can be identified following the hints from the (otherwise not very informative) meeting minutes.

1. In the FAD, section 4.1 on clinical effectiveness was modified in relation to the corresponding section in the ACD. The contents of the discussion of comparative studies between MPH-IR and MPH-MR were amended to reflect the "real-world" comparison by Steele et al. (2004, 2006), which was briefly summarized although not quoted as a source. Rather than acknowledging its value as a pragmatic trial reflecting clinical practice (cf. above, regarding external versus internal validity of clinical studies, i.e., the distinction between efficacy and effectiveness), a remark

---

[48] It is not transparent from the documents published by NICE whether consultees had commented on (some of) these issues; however, based on the appeal decision and its explanation (cf. main text below), one might speculate this to be the case.

was added that "this study was open-label and so should be interpreted with caution," and the overall conclusion remained unchanged.

A further amendment was made in the section of the FAD devoted to comparative trials between atomoxetine and methylphenidate. It is clear from the data provided that study "LYBI" (Newcorn et al., 2004, 2005) was now added, which had been omitted in error from the Assessment Report. (This omission had also been carried forward into the ACD.) This was a six-week, double-blind comparison between atomoxetine (b.i.d.) and modified-release methylphenidate (MPH-MR12) once daily, co-authored by three employees of (and sponsored by) the manufacturer of atomoxetine, and showed statistically significant superiority of the efficacy of MPH-MR12 over atomoxetine using ADHD-RS scores as the clinical endpoint (cf. Table 5.15). As such it supported results from an earlier open-label study (sponsored by the manufacturer of MPH-MR12) comparing both treatment options (Kemner et al., 2004, 2005).

Correspondingly, the summary "consideration of the evidence" was modified. Whereas the conclusion ("the Committee was not able to differentiate between the drugs on the grounds of clinical effectiveness") remained unchanged, reference was now made in the FAD for the first time to "statistically significant differences in measures of effectiveness between drugs" (FAD, section 4.3.2; NICE, 2005c).

It was argued that methodological flaws in these studies (i.e., the trials by Steele et al., 2004, 2006; Kemner et al., 2004, 2005; and Newcorn et al., 2004, 2005) limited their persuasive value. However the "flaw" in Steele et al. (2004, 2006) of being open-label might in fact be an essential component of its key strength, namely increasing the external validity of its results.

As to the studies by Kemner et al. (2004, 2005) and Newcorn et al. (2004, 2005), it was specifically argued that the exclusion (by design or in effect) of patients who had not previously responded to stimulants may have biased the comparison between atomoxetine and methylphenidate. This is a valid concern, urging to exercise the utmost caution regarding any "superiority" claim in favor of methylphenidate on this basis.

On a separate but minor note, the introduction of this argument at this phase of the appraisal added to the inconsistencies of the prior assessment phase, since no such exclusion criterion had been applied to studies for inclusion in the effectiveness review or cost-effectiveness modeling (cf. also below, appeal by the manufacturer of MPH-MR12)[49]. It also remains unclear whether (and if so, to what extent) inclusion of the "LYBI" study (or, more relevant in this context, given the inclusion and exclusion criteria of the study, its sub-group analysis based on stimulant-naïve patients – cf. Newcorn et al., 2005; see Table 5.15) in the meta-analysis by means of

---

[49] For economic modeling, a number of assumptions had to be made. In the present context it should be noted that these included "that the treatment effects are independent of treatments previously received. In other words, the response rate to MPH-IR is the same if it is received as 1st line therapy as when it is received following failure on dexamphetamine or atomoxetine" (AR, Ch. 6, p. 226).

Table 5.15 Randomized clinical studies comparing atomoxetine and methylphenidate in children and adolescents with attention-deficit/hyperactivity disorder (ADHD)

[1] "% red.", percent reduction in ADHD-RS score; criterion used for definition of "response"

	Kratochvil et al., 2002		Kemner et al., 2004, 2005		Newcorn et al., 2004, 2005		
Randomization	4:1		1:2		3:3:1		
Patient number	228 (male, 211)		1,323 (male, 982)		516 (male, n.a.)		
Age	7–15		6–12		6–16		
Duration	10 weeks		3 weeks		6 weeks		
Study design	Open-label, parallel groups		Open-label, parallel groups		Double-blind, parallel groups		
Analysis plan			Powered to show superiority		Powered to show non-inferiority		
Sponsor	Manufacturer of ATX		Manufacturer of MPH-MR12		Manufacturer of ATX		
Active drug	ATX	MPH-IR	ATX	MPH-MR12	ATX	MPH-MR12	Placebo
Administration	b.i.d.	b.i.d/t.i.d.	o.a.d.	o.a.d.	b.i.d.	o.a.d.	n.a.
Patient number	184	44	473	850	222	220	74
Response Rate(ADHD-RS: baseline score reduction of 30, 40, or 50%, respectively)	n.a.	n.a.	63% (30% red.[1]) 41% (50% red.[1])	76% (30%red.[1]) 57% (50% red.[1])	45% (40% red.[1])	56% (40% red.[1])	24% (40% red.[1])
Statistical significance	Study not designed to reveal differences; no difference reported		Differences statistically significant (p<0.003)		Difference statistically significant (p = 0.016)		
Response Rate for stimulant naïve subgroup	No subgroup analyses reported				57% (40% red.[1])	64% (40% red.[1])	
Statistical significance					Difference not statistically significant (p = 0.423)		

mixed treatment comparison might have changed the effectiveness estimates used for economic modelling.[50]

2. The second hint "hidden" in the meeting minutes (NICE, 2005d) refers to administration schedules of atomoxetine employed in clinical studies. Indeed in some trials (e.g., that reported by Spencer et al., 2002) patients took atomoxetine twice daily (with the effect of doubling NHS acquisition costs compared to once daily administration; cf. Table 1.2). It is not transparent from the published data whether this had been adequately reflected by an adjustment that the Assessment Group had introduced in its economic model, accounting for approximately 10% of atomoxetine patients being treated b.i.d. (cf. AR, Ch. 6, p. 235; Table 6.5). However, a new paragraph was added to the FAD explicating that the Committee "noted that since the unit cost of a dose of atomoxetine is the same regardless of the strength, twice-daily dosing could double the cost of treatment with this drug" (FAD, section 4.3.7). Also section 4.3.4 of the FAD (NICE, 2005c) was altered by *deletion* of a sentence from the earlier ACD version, which had referred to once-daily dosing and had read: "The Committee noted that atomoxetine was normally given in a single daily dose and could also be suitable in circumstances where multiple daily dosing was impracticable."

Given the above, the manufacturer of MPH-MR12 lodged an appeal against the FAD, and the resulting proceedings can be traced more easily than the appraisal process itself since the "Decision of the Appeal Panel" published by NICE (NICE, 2005h) provides much more detailed information. One of the grounds for appeal related to the omission of study "LYBI" (Newcorn et al., 2004, 2005) from the assessment process and its subsequent different treatment during the Appraisal Committee's development of the FAD, due to its quality rating according to the study exclusion criterion "prior failure to respond to stimulants"[51]. Another ground for appeal was, in essence, related to the appellant's claim that MPH-MR12 had been shown to be more effective and less costly than – and hence dominating – atomoxetine. The appeal apparently did not relate to the lack of attention paid to the distinction between efficacy and effectiveness trials by the Assessment Group, and subsequently the Appraisal Committee, nor to the inappropriate integration in the MTC-based data synthesis of the pragmatic "real-world" study by Steele and colleagues (2004, 2006). As described earlier (see Chapter 4, above), the appeal was dismissed.

---

[50] In the documentation of the decision of the Appeal Panel (NICE, 2005h), it is confirmed that study "LYBI" had been omitted in the assessment; it is merely stated that the Appraisal Committee had "fully considered" the study when developing the Final Appraisal Determination. However, the Appraisal Committee usually does not perform quantitative analyses.

[51] As noted above (section on *Economic Model*), this created an inconsistency.

Discussion and Implications

The Case Study
Case Analysis: Symptoms and Underlying Problems
NICE Accountability for Reasonableness
NICE Technology Appraisal No. 98 – A Unique Outlier?
Implications for International Health Care Policy-Makers

Chapter 6
Discussion and Implications

There can be little doubt that the National Institute for Health and Clinical Excellence and, in particular, its Appraisal Committee and the Assessment Group, were presented with a challenge in synthesizing clinical data and generating economic evidence relating to the treatment of attention-deficit/hyperactivity disorder (ADHD). The reasons why this was a challenging task include the potential impact of diagnostic criteria, co-existing conditions ("comorbidity"), the variation of patient populations (e.g., age and gender) studied, the broad range of clinical outcome measures, and the number of clinical studies often of limited scale and duration. Due to this complexity, the ADHD technology appraisal may serve as an attractive case study to explore how well the specific processes adopted by NICE serve their purpose to provide health care policy-makers with objective, reliable, timely, and valid information useful for rational priority setting. This question is of international interest at a time when many jurisdictions perceive NICE as a prominent role model for transparent health technology appraisals, including the application of advanced economic methods.

6.1 The Case Study

Despite (or, perhaps because of) the strong face validity attributed by many observers to the approach adopted by NICE (e.g., Buxton, 2006; Pearson and Rawlins, 2005; Neumann et al., 2005a; WHO, 2003; Towse and Pritchard, 2002; Maynard, 2001b), notwithstanding some inevitable concerns, and in light of the substantial resources invested into the assessment and appraisal process, the results of this technology appraisal can only disappoint.

The findings of the critique above must cast doubt on the robustness of the NICE technology appraisal process. Specifically, the review of Technology Appraisal No. 98 revealed a variety of issues related to (1) its narrow scope, including substantive gaps in scope between the technology appraisal and the related development process of clinical guidelines, (2) the search for and selection of evidence for assessment, (3) the distinction between efficacy and effectiveness and the role of treatment compliance in ADHD, (4) data synthesis across heterogeneous effectiveness measures and study types, (5) an economic model prone to distortion and bias, double-counting non-responders and extrapolating long-term outcomes on the basis of a small number of short-term studies, and (6) some process-related issues, which will be discussed later in more detail, notably concerning certain aspects of its transparency and relevance (Table 6.1; see also Table 6.8, below). The ADHD health technology assessment therefore is open to critique regarding all four essential components of a review question (CRD, 2001), namely the population studied, the choice of interventions, the clinical and economic outcomes criteria used, as well as the study designs and selection criteria.

As noted earlier, the Final Appraisal Determination (NICE, 2005c) and guidance (NICE, 2006b) by NICE did not endorse the "clear conclusions" of the technology assessment but stated that "given the limited data used to inform response and

Table 6.1 Summary critique of NICE ADHD appraisal

Narrow scope
- Excluding psychosocial interventions and persistence of ADHD into adulthood
- Role of diagnostic criteria and co-existing conditions not addressed
- (although included in scope)

Data selection for assessment
- Search strategy deviating from assessment protocol
- (idiosyncratic interpretation and/or violation of specified search criteria)
- Reliance on CGI-I subscores for primary economic analysis
- (economic model departing from clinical effectiveness review)
- Reliance on short–term data (3–8 weeks in primary model)
- to extrapolate long-term outcomes (one year, extensions up to 12 years)

Efficacy versus effectiveness distinction
- Compliance issues assumed to be captured by randomized controlled trials (RCTs),
- with implications for the valuation of long-acting medications
- Real-world evidence not covered, although suggestive of substantial impact
- of non-adherence and non-persistence on ADHD treatment effectiveness

Data synthesis across studies and endpoints
- Remaining evidence base (after application of selection criteria)
- insufficient to assess relative value of treatment options assessed
- Synthesis of response rates derived from heterogeneous endpoints
- (e.g., pooling of clinical global impressions and narrow-band symptom scales)
- Synthesis of data from heterogeneous studies
- (e.g., pooling of data from pragmatic open-label studies and double-blind RCTs)

Economic model
- Not transparent, partially enigmatic description (e.g., inclusion of studies)
- Double counting of non-responders as a potential source of bias
- Interpreting narrow-band symptom scales as "quality of life instruments"
- Exclusive focus on cost per quality-adjusted life year (QALY) gained
- (and incomplete discussion of cost-effectiveness models in the public domain)
- Extended time horizon of 12 years without considering long-term sequelae
- (confounded by technical anomalies, e.g., discount rates applied)

Appraisal process
- Moderated the "clear conclusions" suggested by assessment report
- (despite some caveats mentioned in the assessment report)
- Could not compensate for the gaps of the technology assessment report

withdrawal rates, it is not possible to distinguish between the different strategies on the grounds of cost-effectiveness" (NICE, 2005c, 2006b). Thus the two-stage technology appraisal process adopted by NICE, separating assessments from appraisals, enabled NICE to moderate the putatively "clear conclusions" of the Assessment Report. It could not, however, compensate for the gaps of the technology assessment.

As no differences between the various treatments for ADHD were found in terms of effectiveness, the economic model and differences in cost-effectiveness were driven by drug cost (cf. AR, Ch. 7, pp. 263ff.). The Final Appraisal Determination (FAD, section 4.3.7) followed this line as the Appraisal Committee "considered that for the majority of potential users, where there is a choice of more than one appropriate product on clinical grounds, the product with the lowest cost (taking into account the cost per dose and the number of daily doses) should be prescribed." Thus the economic evaluation of this technology appraisal has added little to the drivers of rational prescribing choice beyond clinical parameters (indication, contraindications, adverse event profiles of the products, plus some general considerations related to the specific treatment setting and "individual preferences") and drug cost (minimization).

Most likely many clinicians, patients, and parents/guardians will, nevertheless, welcome the recommendations, as they are broad enough to provide maximum discretion in choice of treatment. The question remains, however, whether the economic evaluation in the NICE appraisal has been utilized to its full potential, i.e., to provide meaningful information about the relative cost-effectiveness of treatment alternatives and to support the most efficient use of scarce NHS resources. This is because it can be argued that presenting opportunities to differentiate between treatment options (beyond cost comparison) have indeed been missed during the NICE appraisal process.

A number of observations raise doubt whether this missed opportunity was purely attributable to the complexities of the problem at hand and/or the limitations of the available evidence.

Abstracting from technical anomalies of the Assessment[1], a candid explanation of the failure to differentiate between treatment alternatives is the restrictive use of clinical data and the dependence of the primary economic model on CGI-I sub-scale scores from only six studies with limited treatment durations ranging from three to eight weeks. Secondary model extensions were problematic because of the substantial heterogeneity of "response" criteria (alongside other variable constraints across studies, such as co-existing conditions, doses administered, treatment duration, concomitant psychosocial interventions, and others), and potential confounding effects between clinical endpoints and treatment alternatives. These predominantly short-term quantitative data were combined with an array of assumptions to construct and model different sequences of (long-term) treatment alternatives, a process notably

---

[1] The term "technical anomalies" here relates to deviations from the NICE "reference case" (NICE, 2004c) and to a range of consistency problems identified in the *Critique*, Chapter 5, above. See also *Appendix*.

distinct from the decisions related to clinical pathways that ultimately should be informed by the analysis. In their broadest sense, two critical choices by the Assessment Group can be interpreted as reflecting NICE technical guidance, stipulating an exclusive focus on QALYs "derived from a standardised generic (non-disease-specific) instrument" to value health effects (hence the selection of the CGI-I), and the aim to provide quantitative synthesis of such data. NICE guidance, however, does acknowledge that there may be situations "where the analysis may have to be restricted to a qualitative overview" because "sufficient relevant and valid data are not available" (NICE, 2004c).

The potential for misleading findings of quantitative meta-analyses is well-established (Egger and Smith, 1995), and there have been some important publicized cases where large trials did not confirm results from prior meta-analyses that were based on a limited number of relatively small studies (Petitti, 2000; Egger and Smith, 1995; Borzak and Ridker, 1995; Chalmers et al., 1987a). This has driven some concern about the replicability of meta-analyses (Petitti, 2000; Chalmers et al., 1987b) in light of the realization that the output quality of any type of data synthesis cannot exceed the quality of its input[2].

In the present case, the quality of the input was largely determined by the psychometric properties of the CGI-I sub-scale score (cf. above, Chapter 5, *Quality of Life and Utility Estimates*), which had been transformed into response rates on the basis of small patient numbers (for dexamphetamine, derived from a study previously excluded for quality concerns) resulting in large binomial confidence intervals (for dexamphetamine, 67% to 95%)[3]. In none of the studies, CGI scores had been the primary endpoint, and their dichotomization led to additional statistical distortions (Hunter and Schmidt, 1990). Considering the properties of this outcome measure, it is not surprising that sensitivity analysis in the form of model extensions using other definitions of response (thereby adding heterogeneity) did not alter the inability of the synthesis to differentiate between alternatives. In this situation the general conclusion applies that meta-analysis is "essentially explorative analysis, not a substitute for conduct of large trials" (cf. Petitti, 2000, p. 271; Borzak and Ridker, 1995; Peto et al., 1995).

The exclusive pursuit of a QALY-focused approach by the Assessment Group, which essentially followed NICE guidance (NICE, 2004c), led to the exclusion of important sources of some information on ADHD treatment effectiveness. The exploitation of these additional sources would have not necessarily constituted *an alternative* to the use of cost-utility evaluation but could well have been used as *complementary* information (thereby avoiding a departure from the theoretical

---

[2] Eysenck (1978) provocatively called meta-analysis "an exercise in mega-silliness," stating: "'Garbage in – garbage out' is a well-known axiom of computer specialists; it applies here with equal force."

[3] Standard deviations after data synthesis by the Assessment Group are provided in Table 5.11 (cf. also AR, Ch. 6, Table 6.6, p. 236; Table 6.15, p. 253; Table 6.18, p. 255). Interestingly, despite substantial differences in patient numbers and a dichotomous endpoint, standard deviations reported by the Assessment Group did not differ between dexamphetamine and methylphenidate, especially MPH-MR12 (see Table 5.11; AR, Table 6.6, p. 236).

framework adopted by NICE – see also Chapter 7, *Which Way Forward?*). Assuming that the acceptability of the treatment options evaluated had been established in principle (either by cost-utility analysis or by another explicit criterion, *for instance* "fair innings"-type reasoning[4] as proposed by Alan Williams in 1997, alone or in some combination), then cost-effectiveness analysis using endpoints other than QALYs might have provided an appropriate tool "to identify the most cost-effective treatment strategy for children and adolescents with ADHD, once [...] a need for medical management" has been established (the Assessment Group used this wording to describe the scope of its review, see AR, Ch. 6, p. 220)[5].

6.1.1 Insights from Clinical Long-Term Studies

As indicated earlier (cf. Chapter 5, *Scoping*), a number of long-term clinical trials were available at the time of the assessment. Among these studies, the NIMH-initiated 14-months Multimodal Treatment Study (MTA) is of particular relevance (MTA Cooperative Group, 1999a,b). Meanwhile, 36-months follow-up data have become available from this study (MTA Cooperative Group, 2004; Arnold et al., 2005). The MTA contributed 42% of the 1,379 patients included in the review by Schachar et al. (2002), and in that review it was the only trial that provided information on all 20 clinically relevant elements selected *a priori* for extraction. Also in the AHRQ systematic review by Jadad and colleagues (1999), the MTA Study was the one trial that received the maximum quality score.

Since these reviews another important long-term study (conducted in New York and Montreal) of 103 children treated over 24 months has been published[6], comparing methylphenidate treatment alone or in combination with two different psychosocial interventions (Klein et al., 2004). These investigators found "no support for adding ambitious long-term psychosocial interventions to improve ADHD and oppositional defiant disorder symptoms" for stimulant-responsive children with ADHD (Abikoff et al., 2004a). Benefits from methylphenidate (administered at average daily doses of 36 mg divided in three administrations ["36 mg/d t.i.d."] at the end of year 1 and 38 to 41 mg per day at the end of year 2, accompanied

---

[4] The idea of "fair innings" is mentioned here merely as an example of an alternative and should not be misunderstood as an endorsement of this approach. It has been suggested by health economists that NICE might be doing better if it accepted and explicitly incorporated a rule of rescue or a fair innings approach (Freemantle et al., 2002) – cf. Chapter 7, *Which Way Forward?*

[5] Drummond and colleagues, in their highly respected textbook (2005), note "cost-effectiveness analysis is of most use when a decision maker ... is considering a limited range of options within a given field" (Drummond et al., 2005, p. 103).

[6] The Assessment Report does not mention this trial even though the observed stability of benefits over time (confirmed by a placebo substitution phase after one year of treatment; Klein et al., 2004; Abikoff et al., 2004a) provides additional insights extending the evidence base related to methylphenidate treatment of ADHD. It seems conceivable that the exclusion of this study reflects the relatively narrow scope of the assessment and a rigid application of study inclusion criteria (NICE, 2003; King et al., 2004a).

by once monthly medication visits[7]; Klein et al., 2004) were stable over two years, including effects on symptom improvement (Abikoff et al., 2004a), negative parental behaviors (Hechtman et al., 2004b), and social functioning (Abikoff et al., 2004b). Also short-term improvements of academic achievement and emotional status were maintained over two years, with no evidence of additional benefit from psychosocial interventions (Hechtman et al., 2004a). Furthermore, after 12 months children were switched to single-blind placebo, and methylphenidate was reinstituted when clinically indicated (as determined by an increase of 25% of the CTRS hyperactivity factor). All children relapsed when switched to placebo. These findings provide an important insight into the effects of treatment over time, although they are not mentioned in the Assessment Report. Most likely, this source of relevant information was not considered because the study did not exactly fit the search criteria defined in the assessment protocol (King et al., 2004a). However, the same is true for the NIMH MTA Study.

There has been no dispute among child and adolescent psychiatrists that the MTA Study, which involved 579 children with ADHD, represents the landmark study or "the mega trial"[8] in this field, that continues to provide crucial information about the relative efficacy of the major proven forms of treatment, i.e., high-quality medication management, intense behavioral interventions, and the combination of both – data that do not lend themselves to simplistic interpretations (cf. Taylor, 1999; Pelham, 1999; Jensen, 1999). It has been argued from a UK perspective that perhaps the clearest messages arising from the MTA Study are (a) that "intense and frequent monitoring [of medication management] ... is likely the key to improving results"[9] and (b) that "the challenge [is] to improve the focus and methods of psychological treatments" (Taylor, 1999).

For an interpretation of the key findings of the MTA Study, it is necessary to appreciate that it was an extensively standardized, highly manualized comparison of three treatment strategies and routine community care in the United States and Canada. All four approaches tested were highly effective and showed substantial improvement from baseline at 14 months (MTA Cooperative Group, 1999a). Two thirds of the children in the community comparison group received medication, principally methylphenidate (average daily dose at study completion 22.6 mg, administered, on average, as 2.3 divided daily doses). Emphasis on subject rapport, extensive use of manuals, and regular supervision of therapists by skilled clinician

---

[7] For cost-effectiveness evaluations of ADHD treatment strategies, another relevant aspect of this study is that its methylphenidate dose regimen corresponds closely to that used in the MTA medication management strategy (see main text, below). It was achieved without the administration of an MTA-style double-blind multiple-switch dose titration protocol (cf. Greenhill et al., 1999, 2001a).

[8] The term "mega trial" is used here with reference to Egger and Smith (1995).

[9] This suggestion by Eric Taylor (1999) also points – inter alia – to the importance of treatment compliance in the management of patients with ADHD. Eric Taylor has emphasized the importance of treatment compliance on various occasions, for example, in his recent contribution to the "Clinician's Handbook of Child and Adolescent Psychiatry" (Gillberg et al., 2006; Taylor, 2006). He also co-authored a "European treatment guideline" recommending availability and use of long-acting medications for ADHD, which noted the potential advantages associated with the omitted need of a midday dose, usually to be taken at school (Banaschewski et al., 2006).

investigators, together with robust monitoring measures, ensured a high degree of protocol adherence ("fidelity and compliance") for the active three treatment strategies investigated (MTA Cooperative Group, 1999a). Psychosocial interventions in the MTA Study involved three major integrated components, comprising parent training, school intervention, and summer treatment program, and was designed to maximize the opportunity to demonstrate treatment effects (Wells et al., 2000; Wells, 2001), not cost-effectiveness. Medication management in the MTA consisted of a structured set of algorithms (starting with a double-blind, daily-switch titration protocol for methylphenidate, followed sequentially by dextroamphetamine, pemoline, and imipramine, until a satisfactory response was obtained) rather than a single medication, which like the behavioral interventions were accompanied by extensive measures to ensure protocol fidelity. Of 289 children randomized to medication management, 256 adhered to and completed the full titration protocol. Of those 77% (198 out of 256) responded to one of the methylphenidate titration doses, and 88% (174 out of 198) were still taking methylphenidate at the end of maintenance at 14 months. Mean doses of methylphenidate at the end of 14 months were 31.1 mg per day for the combination management group and 38.1 mg per day for the medication management group (p<0.001); both groups received MPH-IR divided in three daily doses ("t.i.d."; cf. Greenhill et al., 1999, 2001a; Vitiello et al., 2001).

A wide range of outcome measures was assessed in the MTA Study, and complex relationships were observed between parameters (Owens et al., 2003). For instance, the presence of comorbidity was found to be an important variable influencing treatment response (Jensen et al., 2001a). One of these outcome analyses, that described response rates based on averaged parent and teacher ratings of ADHD and oppositional-defiant disorder symptoms on the SNAP-IV scale (Swanson et al., 2001), was used for economic analyses, including the present NICE assessment. So defined response rates were 25% for the community comparison group, 34% for behavioral management, 56% for medication management, and 68% for the combination of both (Swanson et al., 2001). At 10 months beyond the intensive treatment phase, the medication management strategy continued to show significant superiority over the behavioral management and community comparison groups for ADHD and oppositional-defiant symptoms, although effects were attenuated after the 14-months trial period. Continuing medication use was found to mediate, in part, the superiority of the medication management and combined strategies (MTA Cooperative Group, 2004).

Economic evaluations confirmed the value of intensive medication management also in terms of its relative cost-effectiveness; with incremental cost-effectiveness ratios (ICERs) for one additional patient with symptomatic normalization over a time frame of 12 months at around US-$ 350 for medication management (versus community care) and US-$ 2,500 for combination treatment versus behavioral treatment only (Jensen et al., 2004, 2005; Schlander et al., 2004a). For pure ADHD (i.e., ADHD according to DSM-IV diagnostic criteria, without co-existing anxiety, depression, conduct or oppositional defiant disorder), medication management dominated (i.e., it was more effective and less costly than) community care, and combination treatment versus behavioral treatment was associated with an ICER of US-$ 940 (Figure 6.1).

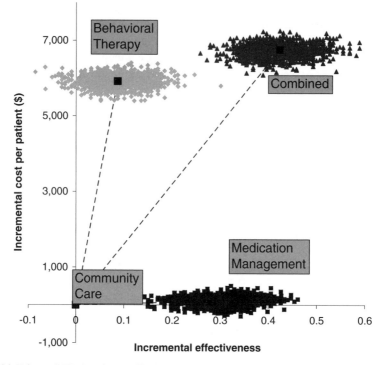

Fig. 6.1 Primary MTA-based cost-effectiveness analysis
Analysis of clinically proven treatment strategies for ADHD based on the NIMH MTA Study
(Jensen et al., 2004, 2005; Schlander et al., 2004a), compared to the community care group of
the study. Horizontal axis: incremental effectiveness, as determined by response rates according
to SNAP-IV symptom normalization (Swanson et al., 2001). Vertical axis: incremental cost per
patient from a US payers' perspective (US-$, 2000). Note that these data had been in the public
domain at the time of the NICE assessment

This translated into estimates of cost per QALY gained for medication management versus community care ranging between US-$ 3,000 and US-$ 5,500 for the
overall DSM-IV-defined study population; in patients with pure ADHD, medication
management dominated community care. Estimated costs per QALY for the comparison between combined treatment and behavioral management ranged between
US-$ 20,000 and US-$ 40,000 for the overall study population, and US-$ 8,000 to
US-$ 15,000 for pure ADHD (Jensen et al., 2005; Schlander et al., 2004a, 2005a).

A reanalysis for the patient sub-group that met ICD-10 diagnostic criteria for
hyperkinetic disorder (cf. Santosh et al., 2005) confirmed the cost-effectiveness
ranking of alternative strategies for the overall study population, further highlighting the economic attractiveness of intense medication management (Schlander
et al., 2005a).

In the meantime, European cost-effectiveness evaluations on the basis of the
NIMH MTA Study have become available (cf. Box 3). In order to address portability

Box 3 International relevance of the NIMH MTA study The NIMH-initiated Multimodal Treatment study ("MTA") currently represents the "mega-trial" in the field of clinical ADHD research, comparing three intense, "high-quality" treatment strategies (medication management, behavioral treatment, and the combination of both) with community care (MTA Cooperative Group, 1999a,1999b; for a brief description, see Chapter 6.1.1, *Insights from Clinical Long-Term studies*).

Patient-level data from the study were used to gain insights into the cost-effectiveness of the major clinically proven forms of ADHD treatment in the United States. Without exception, the MTA-based evaluations reported incremental cost-effectiveness ratios (ICERs), included both deterministic and probabilistic sensitivity analyses by nonparametric bootstrapping, and calculation of cost-effectiveness acceptability curves (CEACs). Direct medical costs were calculated using resource utilization data from the study, excluding its research component, in combination with unit costs determined from a payers' and from a societal perspective.

Primary analyses focused on symptomatic normalization rates (as determined using the SNAP-IV parent and teacher rating scale, which captures symptoms within the domains of inattention, hyperactivity/impulsivity and opposition/defiance, reflecting the definitions for ADHD and oppositional defiant disorder according to the DSM-IV and ICD-10 classifications; Swanson et al., 2001) and found an intense medication management strategy economically attractive (Jensen et al., 2004, 2005; Schlander et al., 2004a, 2005a).

Secondary extensions of these analyses looked at functional improvement as the therapeutic outcome of interest, using the Columbia Impairment Scale as a measure of clinical effectiveness (Foster et al., 2005, 2007). The Columbia Impairment Scale captures four domains of impairment, i.e., interpersonal relations, psychopathology (for example, depression, anxiety, or behavior problems), schoolwork, and use of leisure time. The questionnaire is completed by parents, and the scale has good internal consistency and construct validity (Bird, 2000; Bird et al., 1993, 1996). These secondary evaluations revealed a marked impact of comorbidity on the relative cost-effectiveness of MTA treatment strategies, indicating that – at higher levels of willingness-to-pay – for patients with internalizing comorbidity (i.e., anxiety or depression; 14% of the study population) behavioral treatment and for patients with both internalizing and externalizing comorbidity (i.e., conduct or oppositional defiant disorder; 25% of the study population) combined treatment may become cost-effective choices, too. At the same time, these extended evaluations confirmed the cost-effectiveness of medication management over the 12-months time horizon analyzed, also in terms of functional improvement.

Subsequent analyses addressed the portability of these findings from a European perspective (cf. Chapter 1, *Introduction*) by adopting an analytic strategy that additionally included (a) identifying and analyzing the study subpopulation meeting criteria for hyperkinetic (conduct) disorder (n=145; Santosh et al., 2005; Santosh, 2002), (b) modeling a hypothetical "Do Nothing" alternative to account for the context-specific community care arm, (c) calculating unit costs from a societal perspective and from a payers' perspective for Germany, The Netherlands, Sweden and the United Kingdom, and (d) a time horizon for analysis covering the full study period of 14 months (i.e., including the initial dose titration period).

The resulting cost-effectiveness estimates based on the NIMH MTA Study appeared robust across jurisdictions studied. For incremental costs per patient with symptomatic normalization from the perspective of the UK National Health Service (NHS), see Table 6.2.

These evaluations are not without limitations. Applying longer time horizons would likely improve cost-effectiveness estimates for all active treatment strategies. The measure of treatment costs was limited to the use of health services. In general, where there was uncertainty about assumptions, these were biased for analysis in favor of behavioral treatment. Finally, there remains a need for further studies assessing the cost-effectiveness of better-targeted psychosocial interventions. Source: Schlander et al., 2006a,b,c.

Table 6.2 Cost per patient with symptomatic normalization

UK	ADHD all	ADHD only	HKD/HKCD	HKD only
MedMgt vs CC	€ 3,720	€ 3,539	€ 3,998	€ 1,522
Comb vs MedMgt	€ 66,148	€ 57,605	€ 37,324	€ 26,459
Beh vs CC	€ 78,515	€ 63,811	€ 128,767	€ 26,872
Comb vs CC	€ 21,495	€ 22,029	€ 19,132	€ 14,540
Comb vs Beh	€ 6,731	€ 5,720	€ 6,052	€ 6,319
Beh vs MedMgt	inferior	inferior	inferior	inferior
CC vs DoNothing	€ 5,658	€ 5,030	€ 6,357	€ 7,975
Beh vs DoNothing	€ 24,263	€ 20,351	€ 27,393	€ 16,792
MedMgt vs DoNothing	€ 4,604	€ 4,356	€ 5,142	€ 4,676
Comb vs DoNothing	€ 15,558	€ 14,493	€ 14,797	€ 12,480

European cost-effectiveness evaluation based on the NIMH MTA Study (Schlander et al., 2006a; cf. Box 3). Costs expressed in € (2005; time horizon first 14 months of treatment), from the perspective of the UK National Health Service (NHS). "Symptomatic normalization" (response; time horizon 14 months) defined according to SNAP-IV summary scores ≤1, cf. Swanson et al., 2001.

Abbreviations: "ADHD all", total study population with ADHD according to DSM-IV criteria; "ADHD only", study subpopulation with "pure" ADHD, i.e., without coexisting psychiatric conditions; "HKD/HKCD", study subpopulation with hyperkinetic disorder (or hyperkinetic conduct disorder) according to ICD-10 criteria; "HKD only", study subpopulation with hyperkinetic disorder without coexisting psychiatric conditions (in particular, without concomitant conduct disorder); cf. Santosh et al., 2005. Treatment arms: MedMgt, medication management; Comb, combination treatment; Beh, behavioral treatment; CC, community care group; DoNothing, hypothetical "Do Nothing" alternative.

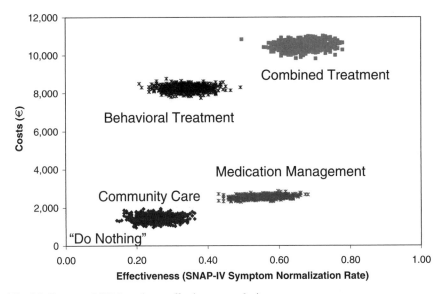

Fig. 6.2 European MTA-based cost-effectiveness analysis
Analysis of clinically proven treatment strategies for ADHD based on the NIMH MTA Study
(Schlander et al., 2006a), comparing the four MTA treatment strategies with a hypothetical "Do
Nothing" alternative. Horizontal axis: incremental effectiveness, as determined by response rates
according to SNAP-IV symptom normalization over 14 months (Swanson et al., 2001). Vertical
axis: incremental cost per patient from the UK NHS perspective (expressed in €, year 2005)

issues (cf. Drummond and Pang, 2001, and above, Chapter 1, *Introduction*), a number of assumptions had to be introduced to reflect international differences in care;
for instance, the model was extended by a hypothetical "Do Nothing" alternative
since North American routine community care was considered to not adequately
represent European treatment preferences (cf. Chapter 1, *Introduction*).

For the United Kingdom, these additional analyses yielded incremental cost-
effectiveness ratios in a range between € 1,500 and € 5,000 for medication management versus community care or the hypothetical "Do Nothing" alternative, respectively (time horizon 14 months, see Figure 6.2 and Table 6.2). The overall findings
from these analyses appeared robust across the five jurisdictions studied, namely
Germany, The Netherlands and Sweden, alongside the United States and United
Kingdom (Schlander et al., 2006a).

Further extensions of these analyses by Foster and colleagues (2005, 2007)
addressed the effects of the MTA treatment strategies on functional impairment,
and revealed profound differences between patient sub-groups by comorbidity: for
pure ADHD, high-quality MTA-style medication management was economically
superior to the studied alternatives at all levels of willingness-to-pay. For patients
with co-existing conditions and at relatively higher levels of willingness-to-pay,
(for the subgroup with internalizing comorbidity) psychosocial treatment and (for
the subgroups with externalizing or both comorbidities) the combined intervention
strategy were found likely to be cost-effective choices also (Foster et al., 2007).

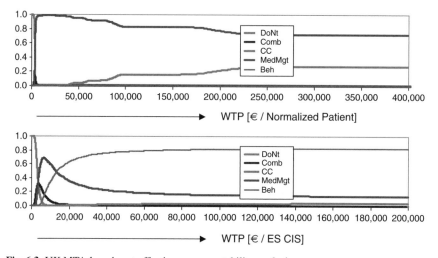

Fig. 6.3 UK MTA-based cost-effectiveness acceptability analysis
Analysis of clinically proven treatment strategies for ADHD by therapeutic objectives for patients with ADHD *and* internalizing psychiatric comorbidity based on the NIMH MTA Study (Schlander et al., 2006c), comparing the four MTA treatment strategies with a hypothetical "Do Nothing" alternative. Horizontal axis: willingness-to-pay (WTP) (a) per additional patient with symptomatic normalization (Swanson et al., 2001), (b) for functional improvement as defined as effect size (ES) on the Columbia Impairment Scale (CIS); time horizon: costs and effects over 14 months. Vertical axis: probability that treatment strategy is most cost-effective (as a function of WTP, expressed in €, year 2005). Abbreviations: DoNt, hypothetical "Do Nothing" alternative; Comb, combined treatment; CC, community comparison (US routine care); MedMgt, medication management; Beh, behavioral management (cf. Box 3)

These analyses were subsequently confirmed from the UK National Health Service (NHS) perspective as well, consistently showing for four European jurisdictions that more complex treatment may become relatively more cost-effective for more complex cases (in particular, behavioral interventions appeared relatively more attractive for patients with internalizing comorbidity, providing a therapeutic objective of functional improvement; cf. Box 3, see Figure 6.3), whereas an MTA-style intense medication management strategy remained the most cost-effectiveness choice for all patient subpopulations studied (Schlander et al., 2006b,c).

To reiterate, intense medication management in the MTA was a structured set of detailed strategies rather than a test of single medication (although most children received MPH-IR t.i.d., cf. above). It adhered to a psychopharmacology treatment manual including continuing treatment dosing algorithms, and was supported by monthly pharmacotherapy appointments and supportive sessions including counseling and parent guidance (Greenhill et al., 1999).

As mentioned earlier, it remains unclear from the Assessment Report exactly how the efficacy data from the MTA (on treatment strategies) were integrated in the economic model (of individual compounds) developed by the Assessment Group.

However, the assumption "that the medical management group in that trial represents treatment with MPH-IR" (AR, Ch. 6, p. 253) might well be subject to debate and controversy, and raises at least two questions:

First, do efficacy data for a highly controlled strategy relying on MPH-IR t.i.d. reflect *real-life effectiveness* of MPH-IR[10], or might the data better – and if so, to what extent – be interpreted as a proxy for the effectiveness of MPH-MR12 under routine care conditions?

Remarkably in this respect, mediator analyses revealed the important role of compliance for effectiveness of medication management and combined treatment (MTA Cooperative Group, 1999b). As-intended acceptance/attendance (defined as attendance for at least 80% of the monthly medication visits of the study protocol, with prescription written and delivered to family at those visits) was 78% in the medication management arm and 81% for the pharmacologic component of the combined treatment arm. As-intended acceptance/attendance was found to significantly enhance treatment response, "whereas in the below-intended sub-group, medication management was less effective, comparable to behavioral treatment" alone (MTA Cooperative Group, 1999b, p. 1092).

Second, would it have been more appropriate to interpret these data as direct evidence for one of the *treatment sequences* modeled?

Irrespective of the answer to these questions, not even having considered these aspects does constitute a critical omission of the assessment.

Even a more cautious interpretation of the North American data from the NIMH MTA Study would still support the cost-effectiveness of intense medication management (predominantly based on methylphenidate) and, thus, corroborate and extend key findings from previous technology assessments (Lord and Paisley, 2000; Miller et al., 1998). Importantly, the NIMH MTA Study now also provides insight into the impact of co-existing psychiatric conditions and therapeutic objectives on treatment cost-effectiveness.

6.1.2 Insights from Disease-Specific Effectiveness Measures

Once the economic acceptability of medication management strategies for ADHD has been established in principle, disease-specific measures may be useful to further differentiate between alternative approaches within this field (cf. Drummond et al., 2005, p. 103) on the grounds of their relative effectiveness and cost-effectiveness.

As previously described (cf. Chapter 5, *Outcome Measures*), the Conners' scales represent one such appropriate measure by virtue of their well-documented psychometric properties (Collett et al., 2003). These scales are widely used in ADHD

---

[10] One gap of the Assessment Report was noted before: it does not differentiate thoroughly between MPH doses and administration schedules used in clinical trials, despite evidence indicating, for instance, better efficacy of MPH-IR t.i.d. compared to MPH-IR b.i.d. (e.g., Stein et al., 1996). Individual variability in response to MPH dosages is another complicating factor (cf. Kimko et al., 1999).

studies and have been applied successfully in previous quantitative data synthe-
ses (Miller et al., 1998; Schachar et al., 2002). Since economic evaluations are
intended to ultimately translate into clinical decision-making – which they should
inform and support – usefulness of such measures from a clinical perspective should
imply usefulness from a "decision-making perspective" as well, notwithstanding
certain limitations[11]. This is particularly the case if and when alternative criteria such as QALYs – which are preferred by NICE and were used in the present
Technology Appraisal of ADHD treatments – are associated with substantial limitations, and when an exclusive reliance on QALYs may result in suboptimal use
of available evidence and missed opportunities to differentiate between treatments
(Schlander, 2007e).

Relevant to the present Technology Assessment, Kenneth Steinhoff and colleagues (2003) presented a comparative analysis of effects sizes achieved with three
once daily ADHD medications, namely Adderall[R] (mixed amphetamine salts), atomoxetine[12], and a modified-release preparation of methylphenidate with 12-hour
duration of action (MPH-MR12). These authors analyzed data from three phase III
trials (with study durations of three, four, and six weeks, respectively; Biederman
et al., 2002; Wolraich et al., 2001; Michelson et al., 2002) used by the manufacturers
of these products as part of their registration dossiers to obtain marketing authorization from the US Food and Drug Administration (FDA). All studies had enrolled a
respectable number of patients, were of parallel-group, double-blind, multi-center
design, and were placebo controlled. Likert-scale changes were examined on the
basis of Conners' ratings, and were compared using effect sizes. Effect sizes were
1.02 for MPH-MR12 and 0.62 for atomoxetine based on parent ratings, and 0.96 for
MPH-MR12 and 0.44 for atomoxetine based on teacher ratings. The authors concluded that these calculations suggested that non-stimulant (atomoxetine) treatment
"is less likely to be as effective a stimulant treatment and should be positioned for
trial after stimulant failure" (Steinhoff et al., 2003).

The results of Steinhoff and colleagues (2003) concurred with another analysis
indicating an effect size of long-acting stimulants in patients with ADHD of 0.95
as opposed to an effect size of non-stimulant medications of 0.62, which its authors
interpreted as "substantial and significant differences in efficacy between stimulant
and non-stimulant medications" (Faraone et al., 2003b, 2006; Faraone, 2003). For
comparison, in this meta-analysis the effect size for immediate-release stimulants
was estimated at 0.91 (Faraone, 2003). These analyses were controlled for confounding variables including study design and outcome measure. With regard to
the approach chosen by the Assessment Group, it seems noteworthy that Faraone
and colleagues (2006) explicitly noted that "comparing medication effect sizes in
different studies will lead to spurious conclusions without accounting for these
influences."

---

[11] The notion of outcomes criteria "useful from a clinical perspective," but less useful "from a
decision-making perspective," was introduced in the present context by the Assessment Group
(AR, Ch. 5, p. 179) to motivate its exclusive reliance on QALYs.

[12] As Steinhoff et al. (2003) note, all but one of the ATX studies submitted to the FDA were dosed
twice daily; these studies were excluded from their analysis of once-daily medications (Steinhoff
et al., 2003).

These findings also appear consistent with the results of two randomized head-to-head trials of MPH-MR12 versus atomoxetine (cf. above, Chapter 5, *Economic Model, Literature Review*, and Table 5.15), one of which had been overlooked by the Assessment Group. Taken together, these data strongly suggest the dominance of MPH-MR12 (and perhaps other methylphenidate formulations as well) over atomoxetine, as on the basis of best currently available evidence the stimulant product appears at least as or (most likely) more effective as ATX, whilst being less expensive (Table 1.2).

Two cost-effectiveness analyses (Annemans and Ingham, 2002; Schlander, 2004b) compared MPH-MR12 given once daily (o.a.d.) and MPH-IR divided in three daily doses (t.i.d.), using Conners' teacher and parent ratings as the clinical outcome measure. These analyses were extensions of the original CCOHTA model (Miller et al., 1998), adopted an explicit modeling approach to analyze the impact of non-compliance (as advocated by Hughes et al., 2001), and were informed by data and considerations discussed previously (see Box 4; cf. also Chapter 5, *Efficacy, Effectiveness, and Treatment Compliance*). Both analyses employed one- and two-way sensitivity analyses and found, from a Canadian third-party payer perspective (Annemans and Ingham, 2002) and from the perspective of the UK National Health Service (Schlander, 2004b; for details, see Box 4 and Figure 6.4), an extended dominance of MPH-MR12 over a wide range of model assumptions. Technically, extended dominance is defined as a state when one strategy under study (here MPH-IR t.i.d.) is both less effective and more costly than a linear combination of two other strategies (here, no drug treatment and MPH-MR12) with which it is mutually exclusive (Gold et al., 1996). In practical terms, extended dominance occurs when an alternative (MPH-MR12) is more effective and more costly, but provides better value for money.

Box 4 ADHD treatment compliance and cost-effectiveness In order to estimate the potential impact of noncompliance on the cost-effectiveness of a long-acting methylphenidate formulation from the perspective of the UK National Health Service (NHS), the economic model developed by the Canadian Coordinating Office for Health Technology Assessments (CCOHTA; Miller et al., 1998; Zupancic et al., 1998) for its appraisal of ADHD treatments was adapted to accommodate three alternatives, MPH-IR divided in three daily doses ("t.i.d."), MPH-MR12 given once daily ("o.a.d."), both combined with continuing nod-drug treatment, or non-drug treatment alone (Figure 6.4).

Efficacy data were derived from a meta-analysis of three double-blind, double-dummy, placebo-controlled randomized clinical trials comparing MPH-IR t.i.d. and MPH-MR12 o.a.d. in children with ADHD age 6 to 12 years (Swanson et al., 2003; Pelham et al., 2001; Wolraich et al., 2001), which assessed symptomatic improvement using IOWA Conners Ratings of inattention/overactivity as primary outcome measure.

These three trials were pooled to determine the combined point estimate for the standardized mean differences (SMDs) for teacher and parent/caregiver ratings using Cohen's d. The 95% confidence intervals around each estimate were also calculated (cf. Schlander et al., 2004b). Two models – a fixed effects model and a random effects model – were used to calculate those differences.

The economic model was populated with the results of the random effects model, and the primary economic analysis was based on teacher ratings. (These were conservative approaches, because the fixed effects model, but not the random effects model, had shown a statistically significant difference of parent ratings in favor of MPH-MR12, and because differences in favor of MPH-MR12 were greater for parent ratings than for teacher ratings).

Short-term symptomatic improvement was assumed to be maintained over the time horizon of the model (one year), providing patients adhered to therapy. This assumption was justified by clinical long-term data, indicating sustained symptomatic benefit from stimulant therapy over prolonged periods of time (e.g., Wilens et al., 2003; Abikoff et al., 2004a; and many others).

Data on resource utilization came from shared care protocols (NHS, 2001, 2003) and were combined with NHS unit costs (£, year 2003), which for drug treatment were taken from the British National Formulary, and for physician and psychosocial services (diagnosis, initial dose titration, monitoring visits during maintenance, and behavioral therapy) from the PSSRU compendium (Netten and Curtis, 2003). Model inputs for non-drug treatment were derived from the randomized clinical trial of cognitive behavioral therapy reported by Fehlings et al. (1991), which had been found useful by CCOHTA as well (Miller et al., 1998; Zupancic et al., 1998).

The initial modeling exercises (Schlander, 2004b; Schlander et al., 2004b) had been driven by the association between dose regimens and medication compliance described in the systematic review by Claxton et al. (2001) and rested on the plausible but unproven assumption of a direct relationship between short-term adherence and long-term treatment persistence. These analyses showed the potential of MPH-MR12 o.a.d. to be equivalent to MPH-IR t.i.d. in terms of cost-effectiveness and even indicated an extended dominance of MPH-MR12 under a broad range of conceivable assumptions, which were derived from the review of ADHD treatment compliance by Hack and Chow (2001). These initial estimates were supported by extensive sensitivity analyses.

In the meantime, observational studies have become available that provide real-world information on treatment-specific ADHD treatment persistence rates, (a) indicating relatively low long-term persistence rates and (b) consistently showing relatively higher persistence rates for patients receiving the long-acting medication with a simplified administration schedule. A replicate of the original model with empirical data from Sanchez et al. (2005) confirmed earlier results. – For a sensitivity analysis, see Figure 6.5. Source: Schlander, 2007d.

Such modeling is "an unavoidable fact of life" in economic evaluation (Buxton et al., 1997), with cost-effectiveness models intended to be aids guiding clinical and

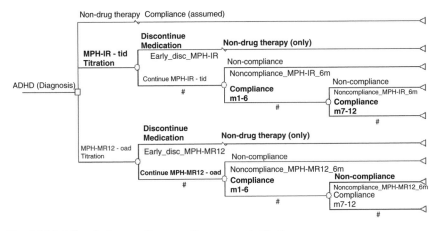

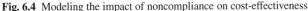

Fig. 6.4 Modeling the impact of noncompliance on cost-effectiveness
Adaptation of the CCOHTA model (Zupancic et al., 1998) used to estimate the impact of treatment noncompliance on the cost-effectiveness of methylphenidate treatment (cf. Box 4). Abbreviations: Early_disc_MPH-IR, early MPH-IR treatment discontinuation (due to tolerability problems; base case assumption, 6%); Early_disc_MPH-MR12, early MPH-MR12 treatment discontinuation (due to tolerability problems; base case assumption, 6%); Noncompliance_MPH-IR_6m, assumed treatment nonpersistence rate with MPH-IR over six months; Noncompliance_MPH-MR12_6m, assumed treatment nonpersistence rate with MPH-MR12 over six months; #, complementary probability

policy decisions; as such, they should not be misconceived as establishing "truth" (Weinstein et al., 2001). In fact, there is a broad consensus among health economists that failure to use models can lead to greater errors than the models themselves might introduce (Buxton et al., 1997; Gold et al., 1996). Importantly, the value of models lies not only in the results they generate, but also in their ability to reveal the logical connection between inputs (usually data *and* assumptions) and outputs (Weinstein et al., 2003).

The initial versions of the model had been limited by a paucity of data on treatment persistence with different formulations of methylphenidate. Therefore, assumptions had to be made on the relation between adherence rates under different administration schedules and long-term treatment persistence (cf. Box 4). Since the earlier review by Hack and Chow (2001; see Table 5.6), administrative database analyses have been published, providing further information on treatment-specific persistence rates in children and adolescents with ADHD (Table 6.3).

One of the typical difficulties with administrative data is the absence of reliable means to distinguish clinically appropriate discontinuation from premature treatment termination. Another issue relates to the control for confounding variables and sources of bias. The analyses based on the Integrated Health Care Information Services (IHCIS) National Managed Care Benchmark Database (covering 17 million managed care lives in the United States; Table 6.4; Kemner and Lage, 2006a,b; Lage and Hwang, 2003, 2004) are of particular interest, because they were controlled for demographic characteristics, patient general health status, comorbid diagnoses, and medication use. Patients receiving modified-release methylphenidate

Table 6.3 Administrative data on ADHD treatment persistence

Study	Origin of data	Patient population	Key findings of interest	Comments
Schirm et al. (2001): Pharmacy dispensing data from InterAction database analysis, University of Groningen and community pharmacies, northern part of The Netherlands	Netherlands 1997–1999 (and 1995–1997, n=98)	Age 0–19 years; *de novo* stimulant prescriptions between 1997 and 1999 (n=271)	Stimulant prescriptions,12-months persistence rate (n=271) approximately 58%	Data presented in graphical form only
Cox et al. (2003): Nationwide random sample from Express Scripts, Inc (ESI) members, who were commercially insured with pharmacy benefit management (PBM)	USA 1999	Age 5–14 years; at least one stimulant prescription during 1999 (n=7,510)	Median number of 30-day equivalent prescriptions among stimulant users was 4	Study objective different from treatment persistence analysis; no correction for data edge effects in sample
Miller et al. (2004): Linked prescription and health database analysis, British Columbia	Canada 1990–1996	Age 0–19 years; *de novo* MPH prescriptions (n=18,081)	4-months persistence rate 50%; 12-months persistence rate 15%	Average therapy duration 19 months
Sanchez et al. (2005): Texas Medicaid prescriptions claims database analysis	USA 2001–2002	Age 5–18 years; ADHD diagnosis (n=9,549)	6-months persistence rates: MAS, 42% (n=3,425); MPH-IR, 37% (n=3,343); MPH-MR12, 50% (n=2,781); extrapolated to 12-months: 18%, 14%, 25%, resp.	All differences statistically significant

Marcus et al. (2005): California Medicaid claims database analysis	USA 2000–2003	Age 6–17 years; *de novo* MPH prescriptions for ADHD (n=11,537)	Mean duration of MPH treatment episodes: MPH-IR, 103.4d (n=8,093); MPH-ER, 140.3d (n=3,444); hereof: MPH-MR08*, 101.1d and 113.0d, resp. (n= 586); MPH-MR12, 147.2d (n=2,858); 12-months persistence rates reported only in graphical form: MPH-IR, ~8%; MPH-MR08*, ~8% and ~10%, resp.; MPH-MR12, ~20%	All differences statistically significant; study also reports total number of treatment days during 12-months period: MPH-ER, 193.5 days (n=3,444); MPH-IR, 171.2 days (n=8,093)
Kenner and Lage (2006a,b): National Managed Care Benchmark Database analyses	USA 2000–2002	Age 6-65 years; ADHD diagnosis; *de novo* MPH-IR (t.i.d.) or MPH-MR12 prescriptions (n=5,939)	Number of days on ITT medication over 365d period: MPH-IR, 108d (n=1,154); MPH-MR12, 199d (n=4,785)	Analysis controlled for demographic characteristics, health status, comorbidity; patients receiving MPH-MR12 were less likely to be hospitalized and experienced less emergency room visits

(continued)

Table 6.3 (continued)

Study	Originof data	Patient population	Key findings of interest	Comments
Lage and Hwang (2003, 2004): National Managed Care Benchmark Database analyses	USA 1999–2002	Age 6-12 years; *de novo* MPH-IR (t.i.d.) or MPH-MR12 prescriptions (n= 1,775)	Medication supply during 12-months follow-up period, number of days: MPH-IR (t.i.d.), 127d (n=344); MPH-MR12, 186d (n=1,431); Discontinuation rate (incl. switches of medication): MPH-IR (t.i.d.), 72% (n=344); MPH-MR12, 47% (n=1,431), during 12 months	Analysis controlled for covariates; patients receiving MPH-MR12 were less likely to experience injuries and accidents and had fewer emergency room visits; all differences statistically significant

Since the review by Hack and Chow (2001; cf. Table 5.6), a number of claims database analyses reporting treatment persistence rates have become available. These analyses consistently describe longer treatment episodes with extended-release formulations. Abbreviations: MAS, mixed amphetamine salts; ITT, intent-to-treat; d, day(s); n, size of sample; resp., respectively; *in the study of Marcus et al. (2005), data on two MPH-MR08 formulations (Metadate[R] CD and Ritalin[R] LA) were reported

were treated for 199 days on average, compared to 108 days for patients receiving immediate-release methylphenidate (Kemner and Lage, 2006b; cf. also Chapter 5, *Treatment Compliance of Patients with ADHD*).

In some of the other database studies, observed differences in treatment persistence were less pronounced between immediate-release and modified-release formulations of methylphenidate (Table 6.3). Thus it should represent a conservative modeling approach to replicate the earlier cost-effectiveness analyses based on the CCOHTA model with the low persistence rates derived from the Texas Medicaid study by Sanchez and colleagues (2005). This analysis translates into ICER estimates of £1,617 for MPH-IR t.i.d. per additional effect size (ES) improvement on the Conners' Teacher Rating Scale (CTRS) maintained over one year of treatment, and £1,501 for MPHR-MR12 o.a.d., both versus non-drug treatment, and £ 1,179 (per ES over 1 year) for MPH-MR12 o.a.d. versus MPH-IR t.i.d. (cf. Figures 6.4 and 6.5).

For comparison, for the original analysis (Box 4; Schlander, 2004b; Schlander et al., 2004b) higher one-year persistence rates had been assumed (for MPH-IR t.i.d., 65%, and for MPH-MR12 o.a.d., 79%; following the meta-analysis by Claxton et al., 2001), and base case results had indicated ICERs of £1,120 (MPH-IR t.i.d. versus no treatment), £1,161 (MPH-MR12 o.a.d. versus no treatment) and £1,345 (MPH-MR12 o.a.d. versus MPH-IR t.i.d.), each per effect size (ES) CTRS improvement maintained over one year. Further analyses based on parent ratings (CPRS scores) had shown extended dominance of MPH-MR12 o.a.d. over MPH-IR t.i.d. (Schlander et al., 2004b).

Overall, adaptations of the economic evaluation model developed by CCOHTA (Miller et al., 1998; Zupancic et al., 1998) consistently indicate an acceptable to attractive cost-effectiveness of modified-release methylphenidate compared to immediate-release formulations.

Given the uncertainty surrounding both the empirical data as well as the assumptions entering models, it is an essential component of good modeling practice to thoroughly assess the sensitivity of model outputs to critical data inputs and assumptions (e.g., Philips et al., 2004, 2006; Akehurst et al., 2000; Brennan and Akehurst, 2000; Buxton et al., 1997). Figure 6.5 depicts the sensitivity of incremental cost-effectiveness ratios for MPH-IR t.i.d. and MPH-MR12 o.a.d. to the assumed non-compliance rates associated with MPH-IR t.i.d. treatment over a time horizon of 12 months (cf. Box 4), on the basis of the described replicate of the initial model using a one-year treatment persistence rate of 50% with MPH-MR12 o.a.d., as reported in the database analysis by Sanchez et al. (2005). This sensitivity analysis further indicates a threshold one-year compliance rate with MPH-IR t.i.d. of 20%, below which extended dominance of MPH-MR12 o.a.d. will occur.

Comparable data on ADHD treatment persistence with non-stimulants, especially atomoxetine, which is usually administered once daily, have not (yet) been made available (cf. Waxmonsky, 2005; Stein, 2004; Banaschewski et al., 2004). Accordingly, the submission to NICE by its manufacturer apparently did not consider issues related to treatment compliance, which should be better for atomoxetine compared to immediate-release methylphenidate products (cf. King et al., 2004b).

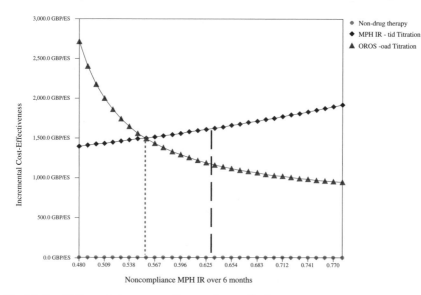

Fig. 6.5 Sensitivity analysis: noncompliance and cost-effectiveness

Replicate of the original UK cost-effectiveness model (Figure 6.4) using empirical data from Sanchez et al. (2005), illustrating the sensitivity of incremental cost-effectiveness ratios (ICERs) for MPH-IR and MPH-MR12 to varying treatment persistence rates with MPH-IR (cf. Box 4).

Vertical axis: ICERs, incremental cost (GBP = £) for one additional patient with symptomatic improvement by one effect size (ES) on the inattention/overactivity IOWA Conners teacher scale, maintained over 12 months.

Horizontal axis: Varying persistence rates on MPH-IR. Numbers on axis give six-months-attrition (nonpersistence) rates, cf. model structure, Figure 6.4. Note that a 63% (or 55% or 50%) nonpersistence rate at six months corresponds to a 12-months persistence rate of 14% (or 20%, or 25%, respectively).

Dashed vertical line: Base case according to prescription claims data analysis by Sanchez et al. (2005).

Dotted vertical line: Threshold analysis – *ceteris paribus* (assuming a constant 12-months-persistence rate of 25% with MPH-MR12), MPH-MR12 will exhibit no longer extended dominance over MPH-IR when six-months nonpersistence rates with MPH-IR are below 55% (i.e., when 12-months-persistence rates with MPH-IR exceed 20%)

In contrast, both manufacturers of modified-release methylphenidate products (Table 1.2) had submitted evaluation models that included consideration of treatment compliance (King et al., 2004b). As described earlier, the Assessment Group had reasoned that assumptions required for modeling the impact of noncompliance "would not be reasonable given the lack of available data, which would render the results of *any* sensitivity analysis around compliance uninformative to decision-makers"[13] (AR, Ch. 6, p. 233; italics added), although the extensive literature on the

---

[13] Interestingly, the senior author of the Assessment Report stated elsewhere: "Given the weaknesses in trial-based economic evaluation for purposes of decision-making, the appropriate vehicle is evidence synthesis and decision modeling. This provides a framework for bringing together all sources of evidence and explicit assumptions to inform decisions, given existing knowledge," and "To inform decision-making, a clear principle is that economic evaluations should include all relevant evidence" (Sculpher and Drummond, 2006, p. 1090f.).

role of treatment compliance in ADHD had not been addressed in the assessment (cf. also *Appendix*).

Meanwhile, a number of further cost-effectiveness analyses have become available. To date, many of these have been published as conference presentations only, and their key findings are summarized in Table 6.4.

Collectively, these data provide strong support for the economic value of pharmacological treatment for ADHD in children and adolescents. They further suggest the possibility of a ranking of treatment options in terms of their cost-effectiveness, with MPH-IR and MPH-MR12 essentially equivalent to one another, and each likely to dominate atomoxetine (which is more expensive and most likely less effective, cf. above). Dexamphetamine (the option identified as "clearly optimal" by the Assessment Group) has not been addressed here in light of the paucity of high-quality clinical data and its more restricted license as "an adjunct in the management of refractory hyperkinetic states in children" (NICE, 2005c; Joint Formulary Committee, 2005). Likewise, mixed amphetamine salts (Adderall^R) are currently not available in the UK.

The foregoing brief review of currently available evidence does not intend to represent (or substitute for) a more systematic evaluation; this is beyond the scope of this critical review of the present NICE Appraisal and would need to consider also safety profiles and adverse events in greater depth. Further research in this area seems warranted.

It is notable, however, that organizations other than NICE that perform health technology assessments have reached conclusions concordant with this critique. The Scottish Medicines Consortium, for instance, initially did not recommend atomoxetine in February 2005, apparently on grounds of the same evidence base as NICE, reasoning that the economic case for atomoxetine had not been demonstrated (Scottish Medicines Consortium, 2005a). Following a resubmission, it accepted atomoxetine for restricted use within the NHS Scotland only in June 2005, limiting its use to children and adolescents with ADHD "who do not respond to stimulants or in whom stimulants are contraindicated or not tolerated." Essentially this placed atomoxetine as a *second line option after stimulants* (Scottish Medicines Consortium, 2005b).

Also, in a different environment, in November 2005 the Australian Pharmaceutical Benefits Advisory Committee (PBAC) rejected a submission by the manufacturer of atomoxetine, who had applied for listing of atomoxetine on the Pharmaceutical Benefits Scheme (PBS) of the Australian government, "because of unacceptable and uncertain cost-effectiveness," even as a second line option after treatment failure with or contraindications to stimulants (Australian Government, 2005a,b).

Finally, a group of European clinical experts reviewed the use of long-acting medications for ADHD and proposed a treatment guideline placing both dexamphetamine and atomoxetine as second line options for patients who did not respond to or suffered adverse effects on methylphenidate (Banaschewski et al., 2006), although this group had been aware of the technology assessment done on behalf of NICE.

These NICE-independent decisions, therefore, support the suspicion that the present Assessment Report, Appraisal and subsequent Guidance by NICE do not adequately reflect the current status of knowledge in this field. Moreover, the in-depth case analysis suggests that the observed anomalies of the assessment

Table 6.4 Overview of cost-effectiveness evaluations of attention-deficit/hyperactivity disorder (ADHD) treatment options

	Jurisdiction	Comparison	Effectiveness measure	Key conclusions (and/or ICERs reported)
Gilmore et al., 1998 (Wessex DEC Report 1998); Gilmore and Milne, 2001	UK	MPH-IR t.i.d. vs. "Do Nothing" alternative	QALYs (utilities based on expert estimates)	MPH-IR (t.i.d.) £7,446 – £9,177/QALY (vs. "Do Nothing" alternative)
Miller et al., 1998; Zupancic et al., 1998 (CCOHTA Assessment 1998)	CAN	MPH-IR (b.i.d.) vs. DEX vs. Pemoline vs. "NDT", vs. Combination Therapies vs. "Do Nothing" alternative	Conners Teacher Rating Scale (CTRS), six point improvement (or ~1 standard deviation); compliance modeled	MPH-IR (b.i.d.) dominates DEX, NDT and Combination; MPH-IR (b.i.d.) vs. "Do Nothing" $384 - $498 / six-point CTRS gain over 12 months
Lord and Paisley, 2000 (NICE Assessment 2000)	UK	MPH-IR vs. "Do Nothing" alternative	QALYs (utilities based on EQ5D expert estimates); CTRS; SNAP-IV	MPH-IR £9,200 – £14,600/QALY (vs. "Do Nothing" alternative) or £958 / six-point CTRS gain, or £1,600 for 1 standard deviation SNAP-IV gain, over 12 months
Annemans and Ingham, 2002	CAN	MPH-MR12 (o.a.d.) vs. MPH-IR (t.i.d.)	IOWA Conners parent ratings; compliance modeled	Extended dominance MPH-MR12 (o.a.d.) over MPH-IR (t.i.d.)
Iskedjian et al., 2003	CAN	ATX vs. MPH-IR	"symptom free days" (SFDs)	ATX vs. MPH-IR $8.83 / additional SFD (government perspective), or $2.00 / additional SFD (societal perspective); sensitivity analyses: range $1.12 – $20.34/SFD

Donnelly et al., 2004	AUS	DEX vs. MPH-IR	DALYs averted (utilities estimated on the basis of effect sizes, which were derived from meta-analysis)	Both DEX and MPH-IR are cost-effective; ICERs (government perspective) $4,100 / DALY saved for DEX, and $15,000 / DALY saved for MPH-IR; "If MPH[-IR] were listed at a similar price to DEX, ... MPH[-IR] would become as cost-effective as DEX"
Schlander, 2004b; Schlander et al., 2004b	UK	MPH-MR12 (o.a.d.) vs. MPH-IR (t.i.d.)	IOWA Conners (parent and teacher ratings; effect sizes based on metaanalysis); compliance modeled	Extended dominance MPH-MR12 (o.a.d.) over MPH-IR (t.i.d.) "over a wide range of assumptions"
Jensen et al., 2004, 2005; Schlander et al., 2004	USA	Medication management (mostly MPH-IR t.i.d.) vs. psychosocial treatment vs. combined treatment vs. community comparison (many MPH-IR b.i.d.)	SNAP-IV symptomatic normalization; QALYs (utilities based on expert and parent estimates); data from NIMH MTA Study	Medication management most cost-effective, $360 per additional patient symptomatically "normalized"; ~$3,000/QALY gained (expert estimates) or ~$5,500/QALY gained (parent estimates) vs. community comparison group, with some differences for comorbid subgroups

(continued)

Table 6.4 (continued)

	Jurisdiction	Comparison	Effectiveness measure	Key conclusions(and/or ICERs reported)
King et al., 2004b, 2006 (NICE Assessment 2004)	UK	37 alternative treatment sequences (drug treatment only: DEX, MPH, ATX)	QALYs (utilities based on parent estimates); data from mixed treatment comparison (MTC) primarily based on CGI-I subscale	"Clearly defined optimal strategy: 1st line DEX, 2nd line MPH-IR, 3rd line ATX" (dominant in model); "results largely driven by drug cost"
Narayan and Hay, 2004	USA	Adderall[R] (mixed amphetamine salts) vs. MPH-IR	QALYs (utilities based on Index of Health-Related Quality of Life (IHRQOL) scale; response rates from literature; compliance modeled	"MPH-IR dominated" by MAS (Adderall)[R], with an ICER of $21,957/QALY versus no treatment; findings "difficult to generalize"
Laing et al., 2005	NL	ATX vs. "current practice"	QALYs (utilities based on "a survey of 83 parents of ADHD children")	ICERs estimated at €18,800 to €22,800 versus MPH-IR and MPH-ER, respectively; model description not transparent
Tilden et al., 2005	Norway	ATX vs. stimulants and "no medication"	QALYs (source of utilities not given in abstract)	ICERs estimated at NOK 149,900 to NOK 199,200 compared to stimulants; model description not transparent
Foster et al., 2005, 2007	USA	Medication management (mostly MPH-IR t.i.d.) vs. psychosocial treatment vs. combined treatment vs. community comparison (many MPH-IR b.i.d.)	Columbia Impairment Scale (CIS) scores reflecting functional improvement; data from NIMH MTA Study	Medication management more cost-effective than intensive behavioral treatment; behavioral interventions relatively more cost-effective in comorbid patient subgroups

Sandberg, 2005	USA	Threshold analysis: "what QALY gains are needed for psychosocial treatment strategies to become cost-effective?	Analysis based on cost calculations using resource utilization estimates derived from the NIMH MTA Study	Conclusions essentially consistent with Jensen et al. (2004, 2005) but research question inadequate for behavioral management, since the NIMH MTA Study was designed to maximize its effectiveness: the relevant question is whether better targeted, lower cost behavioral interventions might achieve similar outcomes (cf. also Taylor, 1999)
Schlander et al., 2005a	USA	Medication management (mostly MPH-IR t.i.d.) vs. psychosocial treatment vs. combined treatment vs. community comparison (many MPH-IR b.i.d.)	SNAP-IV symptomatic normalization; QALYs (utilities based on expert and parent estimates); data from NIMH MTA Study	Extension of MTA-based cost-effectiveness results (Jensen et al. 2005) for patients with an ADHD diagnosis according to ICD-10 criteria
Schlander et al., 2006a,b,c	D, NL, UK, S, USA	Medication management (mostly MPH-IR t.i.d.) vs. psychosocial treatment vs. combined treatment vs. community comparison (many MPH-IR b.i.d.) vs. a hypothetical "Do Nothing" alternative	SNAP-IV symptomatic normalization; functional impairment (Columbia Impairment Scale); subgroup analyses by diagnostic criteria and coexisting conditions	Medication management "acceptable to attractive", dominating psychosocial treatment; psychosocial interventions my become relatively more acceptable in comorbid subgroups when functional improvement is sought; findings "robust across jurisdictions"

resulted not only in an incomplete appraisal of available information. It seems likely that the identified gaps of the assessment constituted a source of distorted, potentially biased conclusions. Given the intended far-reaching consequences of NICE guidelines on the level of care available to patients within the framework of the National Health Service (NHS) in England and Wales, as well as its implications for the efficient use of limited resources available to the NHS, this is more than an academic issue.

6.2 Case Analysis: Symptoms and Underlying Problems

The late Alan Williams certainly spoke for many health economists when he described NICE as "the closest anyone has yet come to fulfilling the economist's dream of how priority-setting in health care should be conducted. It is transparent, evidence-based, seeks to balance efficiency with equity, and uses a cost-per-QALY benchmark as the focus for its decision-making" (Williams, 2004, p. 3). His following question, "What more could anyone ask for?" perhaps epitomizes the broadly conceived notion of NICE as a role model.

Paradoxically, Alan Williams was well aware that "it is not uncommon for an economist's-dream-come-true to be seen as a nightmare by everyone else." The medical profession, notably specialists involved in health care provision for children with attention-deficit/hyperactivity disorder (ADHD), might feel justified in agreeing with that observation, and it is less than certain that all health economists would feel comfortable with the actual implementation of such a concept in real life assessments[14]. This is evident from the current NICE appraisal of ADHD treatment strategies, which falls short of its stated objectives.

In the most general terms, in the context of NICE the expected role of technology appraisals is to provide the basis for NICE to issue guidance about the optimal use of health technologies (NICE, 2004b, p. 1). This guidance, referred to as "appraisal recommendations" in the information by NICE to "National Collaborating Centres and Guideline Developers," "should be reproduced unchanged ... within a guideline" (NICE, 2004a, section 10.1.3). It should be given the highest rating for strength of evidence (NICE, 2004a, section 11.3), implying the assumption that highest quality standards will be attained consistently. Arguably this expectation has not been met in the present case.

Interestingly, in contrast to the reference case defined for technology assessments (NICE, 2004c, section 5[15]), for the process of clinical guideline development the

---

[14] As to the normative premises underpinning the prioritization framework adopted by the NHS and NICE, see next sections of main text (Chapter 6.5 *Implications for International Health Care Policy-Makers*, and Chapter 7, *Which Way Forward?*).

[15] It should be added here that the NICE Guide to the Methods of Technology Appraisal (in section 5.3.4.2) at least in principle gives some flexibility to deviate from or amend the "reference case" evaluation, if justifiable: "Despite the role of cost per QALY in the reference case, the Institute recognises that other forms of cost-effectiveness analysis ... may have a role to play, as

use cost-effectiveness analyses is encouraged as "there are two general approaches to modeling that may be considered: cost utility analysis (CUA) using QALYs, and cost-effectiveness analysis (CEA) using alternative measures of effectiveness" (NICE, 2004a, section 8.2). It is explicitly acknowledged that "where there are no good-quality data to estimate QALY gains, an alternative measure of effectiveness might be considered (such as ... some more disease-specific outcome)" (NICE, 2004a, section 8.2). This remains remarkable, even though the preference for QALYs has been somewhat strengthened with the April 2006 update of the NICE guidelines manual (NICE, 2006g).

The frequent occurrence of substantial gaps between the scopes of NICE clinical guidelines and technology appraisals, which are expected to inform clinical guideline development, has been identified earlier (NICE, 2004a, section 10; Williams, 2004[16]). In the present case, this gap related to the management of ADHD in adults, the place of non-drug treatment (especially psychosocial interventions), the influence of illness sub-types including hyperkinetic disorder (the bulk of clinical data came from studies applying DSM-IV-based diagnostic criteria), and the management of comorbidities (NICE, 2003, 2006a). This gap seems attributable to the overall approach adopted by NICE, which allowed two very different streams of work (i.e., technology appraisal and clinical guideline development) to develop. It appears that NICE has not yet succeeded integrating clinically driven guideline development and economically driven technology-related guidance development (Williams, 2004).

Although the scope of the technology appraisal was narrower than that of the clinical guideline, however, the assessment did not accomplish to address important aspects specified in advance in its scope (NICE, 2003) and in its assessment protocol (King et al., 2004a), notably outcome measures related to core symptoms (regarding the economic model; for effectiveness review, hyperactivity – but not inattention and impulsivity – was included), co-existent problems, and treatment in the presence of comorbid disorders. In summary, then, the Assessment Report fell short of the objectives defined by its scope as well as those outlined in the reference case.

The Assessment Report also did not adhere to "technical" criteria defined by NICE for reference case analysis, beyond not covering the issues specified in its defined scope. For instance, discount rates used did not reflect NICE guidance, the sources of preference data used were stated incorrectly (alongside some confusion apparent in the respective discussion), and data synthesis did not meet criteria specified by NICE regarding assessment of heterogeneity (cf. NICE, 2004c, section 5.4.2.2, and interestingly also NICE, 2004a, section 7.3.2), specifically relating to

---

non-reference case analyses in specific situations" (NICE, 2004c). There are reasons to doubt the practical relevance of this statement for the Technology Appraisal process, as Anthony J. Culyer (at the time non-executive director and Deputy Chair of NICE) said to this author in Stockholm on June 06, 2002, with reference to manufacturer submissions to NICE: "If you do not provide us with QALYs, we will do them for you." (Source: personal communication.)

[16] For a further discussion of the need to better integrate clinical and economic perspectives in the process of clinical guideline development, cf. Wailoo et al., 2004, and Littlejohns et al., 2004.

"different study circumstances" (in the present case, randomized controlled efficacy versus real-life effectiveness studies) as a potential source of heterogeneity.

In addition, the pooling of different effect measures without controlling for possible confounding effects, protocol deviations regarding study inclusion and exclusion criteria, including, but not limited to, the idiosyncratic interpretation of the three-week-duration criterion, as well as certain problems associated with its internal consistency (such as the double-counting of non-responders, owing to the basic structure of the economic evaluation model combined with data inputs chosen), may be regarded as erroneous.

The alarming proportions of the anomalies identified with Technology Appraisal No. 98 (Table 6.1) raise the intriguing question of whether a causal relationship may exist between these observations and structural characteristics of the specific NICE approach to health technology assessments (HTAs). Keeping in mind the limitations of case study research, and those of qualitative research in general, the following exploration of potential underlying problems should be interpreted as an invitation to further debate and inquiry, not as presentation of definitive conclusions.

6.2.1 Separation of Clinical and Economic Perspectives

One candid reason is the separation of clinical and economical guidance (or "guideline," for that purpose) development at NICE that had been noted before with respect to differing scopes (cf. Williams, 2004; NICE, 2004a). This separation might also account, at least in part, for a range of specific observations related to the present case study, including: (a) the complete absence of a discussion of the literature on clinical effect measures (and their psychometric properties) used in ADHD treatment studies (Chapter 5, *Outcome Measures Considered* and *Appendix*); (b) the almost complete absence of consideration of the role of treatment compliance for clinical effectiveness in general, and its particular importance in ADHD[17]; (c) the rationale given for the three-week minimum duration criterion for study inclusion[18], combined with the absence of a discussion of carryover effects in crossover studies included in the review (cf. Chapter 5, *Data Selection for Assessment*). It seems conceivable that the economists involved in the NICE assessment may have felt compromised, and possibly overstrained, by expectations of them

---

[17] For instance, child psychiatrist Kenneth Steinhoff from the University of California (at Irvine) Medical Center, emphasized in July 2004, at the time when the assessment was begun, that ADHD-specific symptoms, such as forgetfulness, inability to complete tasks, lack of follow-through, and easy distractibility make it difficult for patients to adhere to ≥ 3-times-daily dosing schedules (Steinhoff, 2004).

[18] This criterion was introduced because "the literature suggests that three weeks is the minimum length of treatment chosen by investigators who are examining clinical outcome," though it was recognized "that even three weeks is a short period in which to examine the effect of a drug intended to modify a chronic condition" (AR, Ch. 3, p. 44f.). The three-weeks cut-off was neither justified by empirical evidence nor correctly applied.

Table 6.5 Symptoms and suggested underlying issues (1)

Symptoms that may be explained in part
by the separation of clinical and economic perspectives

- *Differences in scope*
  between technology appraisal and clinical guideline development (impairing relevance of technology appraisal for guideline development)
- *Selection of clinical studies*
  (including inappropriate interpretation of 3-weeks-duration criterion and absence of consideration of carry-over effects in crossover trials)
- *Dissociation between effectiveness review and cost-effectiveness evaluation*
  of technology assessment, the latter not using findings of the systematic review (i.e., use of hyperactivity scores versus CGI-I subscale scores)
- *Disorder-specific outcome measures not (or inappropriately*) included in economic evaluation,*
  contributing to the exclusion from analysis of clinical long-term evidence (including absence of literature review on clinical measurement instruments)
- *Distinction between efficacy and effectiveness not taken into account*
  (including absence of compliance literature review)
- *Patients (children with ADHD) as a source of utility values*
  considered relevant to the review (AR, p. 182), and, for secondary model extensions, confusing narrow-band symptom scales with quality of life measures, raising doubt whether the clinical problem was understood properly by analysts

*For secondary model extensions, results from narrow-band symptom scales were pooled with clinical global impressions - see last item on list above. AR: Assessment Report; CGI-I: clinical global impressions, improvement subscale

to unravel a complex set of clinical problems under serious resource (time) constraints. It seems likely that injection of a stronger dose of clinical expertise at the stage of the assessment process might have served to ameliorate, if not prevent, these issues (Table 6.5). Except for one clinical specialist, who provided input and comments, the Assessment Group was exclusively composed of staff from the Centre for Reviews and Dissemination (CRD) and the Centre for Health Economics (CHE), both within the University of York (AR, pp. 1–3). Thus expertise of the assessment team could be expected predominantly in the fields of review methodology and health economics, whereas the clinical subject area of interest was underrepresented.

6.2.2 High Level of Standardization

A second candid reason to explain a number of problematic issues observed is the high level of standardization of technology assessments by NICE (cf. NICE, 2004b,d,h,i,j,k), which was achieved at the expense of flexibility to adapt the solution to the problem faced. A key element of standardization applied by NICE is the definition of the "reference case" by NICE, which prescribes – *inter alia* – systematic reviews and the use of meta-analyses for synthesizing evidence on treatment outcomes and the use of QALYs (using preferences elicited by a choice-based method as opposed to a rating scale) for valuation of health effects (Table 3.1; NICE, 2004c).

Interestingly, as was noted above (Chapter 6, *Symptoms and Underlying Problems*), the clinical guideline development process is more flexible (compared to technology appraisals) to accommodate "alternative measures of effectiveness" (NICE, 2004a, 2006g). At least in principle, NICE also permits a non-quantitative overview of evidence "where sufficient relevant and valid data are not available" (NICE, 2004c).

This extensive standardization of technology assessments, and the appraisal process in general, has been driven by a desire to achieve consistency between submissions and evaluations, to ensure that health-related benefits are comparable across evaluations, and perhaps to serve as a substitute for knowledge of the analysts (NICE, 2004c; CRD, 2001; Kanavos et al., 2000; Rennie and Luft, 2000; Paltiel and Neumann, 1997; Siegel et al., 1997; Gold et al., 1996; Rovira, 1994; Drummond et al., 1993a).

It has been asserted that government and industry interests "have ensured that [health] economic evaluation is a heavily regulated environment," and it has been argued that "under-education and over-regulation" may not only be detrimental to the further evolution of the discipline but also place junior health economists at risk of "becoming the 'worker bees' of a heavily regulated industry" (Bridges, 2005). From a welfare theoretic perspective it has been further remarked that "one key advantage of taking an artificially determined objective function, such as cost per QALY, is that many … (real-world) complications are avoided" (Bridges, 2005). While others have taken alternative positions relating to the extrawelfarist logic of cost-effectiveness (cf. below, Chapter 6, *Objectives*, and Chapter 7, *Which Way Forward?*), in the present context it is probably most important to acknowledge that the fundamental idea underpinning cost per QALY evaluations, as the standard form of "cost-utility analyses," has been the application of QALYs as a universal and comprehensive measure of health benefits.

In the ADHD assessment a very rich clinical evidence base was reduced to a limited number of short-term studies reporting clinical global impression improvements on a sub-scale with dubious psychometric properties (cf. Figure 5.1 and Tables 5.1, 5.2, 5.7, and 6.6), which was motivated to use "the most common definition of response in the included studies" (AR, Ch. 6, p. 225), enabling cost per QALY calculations. Adhering by the book to the reference case prescribed by NICE, the assessment did not adequately address the substantial caveats surrounding the use of QALYs, in particular in pediatric (De Civita et al., 2005) and psychiatric populations (Centre for Reviews and Dissemination (CRD), 2003; Gilbody et al., 2003). A critical review of the subject by a group of researchers from the University of Bristol, UK, also concluded that "comparisons of the relative cost-effectiveness reported as cost per QALY gained across interventions for different diseases and populations should be treated with extreme caution" (Griebsch et al., 2005). As a consequence it became impossible to differentiate between treatments on the grounds of clinical effectiveness, and the resulting economic model was ultimately driven by drug cost differentials (King et al., 2004b, 2006).

While there is virtue in process standardization as a means to achieve procedural justice (Gibson et al., 2002), over-restrictive use of available evidence and

Table 6.6 Symptoms and suggested underlying issues (2)

Symptoms that may be explained in part by the high level of standardization ("reference case analysis")

Exclusive focus on cost-utility analyses

- At the expense of insights from cost-effectiveness evaluations
- Reliance on utility estimates of questionable validity
- For calculation of quality-adjusted life years (QALYs), linking utility estimates based on complex health state descriptions with response estimates based on clinical global impressions subscales
- Inability to identify differences between treatments

Highly restrictive use of clinical evidence for economic evaluation

- Clinical long-term studies (largely) excluded from analysis (enigmatic inclusion of data from the NIMH MTA study)
- Commonly used effectiveness measures excluded from analysis
- Mathematical precision of quantitative meta-analysis not in tune with imprecision of binomial input data ("response rates") from small-scale short-term clinical studies and CGI-I ratings
- Need to use data from clinical studies that had been excluded from effectiveness review for quality concerns

reliance on small-scale short-term studies may be a cause of bias and misleading results of data synthesis. For example, even for the extended economic model, evidence on dexamphetamine – recommended as a first-line option by the Assessment Group – was limited to two small crossover trials with three-week treatment periods each, and one of these had not passed criteria for effectiveness review and studied girls only (Sharp et al., 1999), while the other one used different diagnostic criteria and endpoint definitions (Elia et al., 1991; Castellanos et al., 1997; cf. Tables 5.7 and 5.8).

In view of reported discrepancies between meta-analyses and subsequent large randomized controlled trials, most researchers agree that direct comparisons of treatments should be sought whenever possible (Song et al., 2003; Bucher et al., 1997; LeLorier et al., 1997). The problematic issues are exaggerated if other sources of heterogeneity, such as the pooling of efficacy and effectiveness studies, are not addressed. It has therefore been recommended that a formal meta-analysis should be conducted only after it has been determined "whether quantitative synthesis is at all possible and if so whether it would be appropriate" (CRD, 2001). Other scholars have observed that, even the most advanced, sophisticated "statistical tests cannot compensate for lack of common sense, clinical acumen, and biological plausibility in the design and protocol of a meta-analysis" (Lau et al., 1997). According to a paper accompanying a recent consensus statement on "decision analytic modeling in the economic evaluation of health technologies" (Brennan and Akehurst, 2000), the structural quality of a model should be judged by two attributes: (a) it should be consistent with the stated decision problem, and (b) its "structure should be dictated by a theory of disease, not by data availability" (Sculpher et al., 2000).

Accordingly, any representation of stochastic uncertainty based on such calculations may be misleading, as it does not reflect sources of uncertainty related to the underlying assumptions of the analysis, such as the double-counting of non-responders or those related to the impact of treatment compliance. For recipients of an analysis, mathematical precision, like utility differences extending to the third decimal place, might be suggestive of levels of reliability that cannot reflect the quality of data accrued from one seven-point "clinical global impressions" sub-scale (consisting of one question only), which was reported as a secondary endpoint of a small sub-set of clinical trials only.

In conclusion, therefore, one effect of standardization apparently was that the problem was redefined to fit a predetermined approach to solve it, as opposed to seeking the most suitable solution based on the decision problem and the available evidence.

6.2.3 Technical Quality of Assessment

A third candid reason relates to the apparent absence of an effective quality assurance system for assessments that can be inferred from the limited technical quality of the Assessment Report (Table 6.7; for a summary of consistency issues, cf. *Appendix*). While reviews of the quality of economic evaluations have suggested a high prevalence of serious methodological flaws (Drummond and Sculpher, 2005; Neumann et al., 2000, 2005b; Jefferson et al., 2002; Hill et al., 2000; Gerard et al., 1999), this is surprising here given (a) the efforts of NICE to standardize assessments (see above), which, at least in the present case, apparently failed to ensure consistent quality, and (b) the fact that NICE assessment teams are recruited from some of the leading and most reputable health economics research centers worldwide.

It should be emphasized at this point that these issues are not simply attributable to a failure of the Assessment Group. For example, some technical issues might be attributable, at least in part, to the Assessment Group's insufficient access to clinical expertise (a problem for which structural reasons can be identified at NICE). As discussed earlier, limited use or availability of clinical expertise may be reflected by the inappropriate treatment of compliance, the use of the less-than-optimal three-week study duration cut-off for as a study selection criterion, the exclusion of effects on impulsivity and inattention in the effectiveness review, the absence of a sound discussion of the relative merits of the various effectiveness measures used in ADHD, and/or the absence of any meaningful consideration of the substantial long-term sequelae associated with the disorder.

As one would expect, the Assessment Group offered justifications and *caveats* for many of its assumptions and assertions. A closer inspection of these reveals a number of problems related to the internal and external consistency of the assessment (listed in the *Appendix*). Further anomalies of a predominantly technical nature do fall under the responsibility of the review team, such as the departure from search criteria pre-specified in the assessment protocol, discount rates deviating from NICE reference case recommendations, heterogeneity of trials and endpoints pooled, and lack of preparedness to incorporate into the evaluation model the well-established distinction between clinical efficacy and effectiveness.

Also for these problems, however, obvious contradictions – for instance between the Assessment Report and (a) statements made elsewhere by its senior author or (b) existing economic expert consensus – indicate the possible role of process-related constraints. One might speculate that, perhaps, another contributing factor was insufficient resources available to the Assessment Group, for instance in terms of time (given the complexity of the task at hand) and/or in terms of funding (given the need to attract sufficient involvement of senior economists).

6.2.4 Process-Related Issues

The highly structured processes, from scoping to assessment and appraisal, were followed through by NICE in a highly predictable manner (cf. Chapter 4, *NICE Appraisal of ADHD Treatments*). This provided manufacturers of the products under review as well as other consultees with predictable opportunities to contribute throughout the assessment and appraisal process. Insofar it might seem that criteria of procedural fairness were met. Not only the content of technology assessments (cf. the "reference case" definition, Table 3.1), but also the appraisal process adopted by NICE is highly standardized. This high level of standardization certainly contributes to the predictability and reliability of appraisal time schedules (cf. Figure 1.5 and Table 3.2) and, thus, facilitates stakeholder participation and minimizes surprises.

Table 6.7 Symptoms and suggested underlying issues (3)

Symptoms that may be explained in part
by the absence of effective quality assurance

Deviation of assessment from NICE guidance

- Discount rates used for long-term economic model
- Discussion of appropriate sources of utility estimates

Issues related to technical quality of assessment

- Multiple violations of search criteria specified in assessment protocol
  e.g., concerning relevant effectiveness studies;
  e.g., concerning relevant economic evaluations;
  e.g., inclusion of studies rejected for quality concerns
- Pooling of heterogeneous studies for quantitative synthesis
  e.g., efficacy vs. effectiveness; clinical effectiveness measures
- Not controlling for potential confounding effects
  e.g., effectiveness measures used and treatment strategies
- Mismatch between clinical global impressions
  (and other response criteria used)
  and health state descriptions used for utility estimates
- Economic model structure
  e.g., double-counting of non-responders as a source of distortion

See also *Appendix, Consistency Issues*

Yet, the standardized approach of NICE reminds of a "one size fits all" philosophy, not only in terms of analytic procedures ("content"), but also in terms of time and resources allotted to review teams. It appears conceivable that an unintended effect of this standardization is the loss of flexibility to adapt the process (e.g., resources and time) to the level of the complexity of the assessment at hand. Resource constraints had already been identified by the WHO review (WHO, 2003; cf. Chapter 1, *Introduction*); in particular it was noted that "the late deadline for stakeholder submissions puts unreasonable time pressure on the Technology Assessment Groups" and that "the quality of reports may be compromised by late arrival of stakeholder submissions" (WHO, 2003). The detrimental effect of such pressures may be exacerbated when the clinical problem is as complex and challenging as ADHD. In this case, the three months remaining for completion of the technology assessment after receipt of company submissions were in stark contrast to the 33 months it took from initial scoping to the issuance of guidance (Table 3.2).

6.3 NICE Accountability for Reasonableness

Norman Daniels and James Sabin (1997, 1998, 2002; Daniels, 2000) have developed an ethical framework of accountability for reasonableness ("A4R") which "fair-minded people" should accept based on the idea that there exists a core set of reasons, that all center on fairness, on which there will be no disagreement. A4R is strongly focused on a fair institutional process and, according to Daniels and Sabin, comprises four conditions: publicity, relevance, appeals, and enforcement (cf. Chapter 2, *A Note on Objectives and Methods*). Based on justice theories of democratic deliberation, fulfillment of these conditions, which accentuate fairness and openness, has been proposed to give legitimacy to resource allocation decisions.

As mentioned earlier (Chapter 2, *A Note on Objectives and Methods*), NICE has explicitly adopted the principles of procedural justice – A4R – espoused by Daniels and Sabin (2002), at the same time confirming its commitment to "ensure that NHS resources are used in a manner that takes both clinical and cost-effectiveness into account; but that also embodies equity" (Rawlins and Dillon, 2005b).

In light of the findings of the case study of Technology Appraisal No. 98, the technology appraisal process adopted by NICE can be compared to the conditions for A4R developed by Daniels and Sabin (Tables 2.1 and 6.8).

6.3.1 Publicity

Overall, the condition of *publicity* was met to a great extent. Key documents were continuously posted on the NICE website, enabling tracking the progress and providing stakeholders with well-defined opportunities to participate. A timetable was also published and continuously updated on the NICE website, creating a high level

Table 6.8 NICE accountability for reasonableness (A4R)

A4R condition	Key features	Key limitations
Publicity	**Overall process** well-defined structure; detailed timelines, key documents continuously published; predictable opportunities for stakeholders to provide input	Selection of topics for appraisal (sometimes)
	Assessment Phase Assessment Protocol and Assessment Report published	"Commercial-in-confidence" data withheld. Economic model not released ("intellectual property")
	Appraisal Phase Appraisal Committee meeting agendas published meeting minutes published ACD, FAD published	Uninformative Appraisal Committee meeting minutes Criteria beyond cost -effectiveness neither codified nor transparent
	Appeal Phase (optional) Appeal Panel holding public hearings; detailed meeting minutes	
Relevance	**Fairness Condition** High level of procedural fairness within NICE framework; NICE seeking input from Citizens Council on social value judgments	No codified criteria for fairness; "efficiency-first" approach
	Integration of clinical and economic perspectives	Poor alignment of scopes (for technology appraisals and clinical guideline development). Sometimes (?) poor integration of both perspectives
Revisions and appeal	**NICE definition of "appeal"** differs from that of A4R; appeals may be lodged by consultees only	Conditions for appeal more restrictive than A4R recommendations; this appears unlikely to be fully compensated for by opportunities for stakeholder participation
Enforcement	**Consistency of technical quality of assessment reports**	Absence of effective quality assurance system for technology assessments
	Implementation	Mixed record of guidance implementation in the NHS

of predictability for stakeholders wishing to submit information. NICE also demonstrated a high degree of flexibility in adjusting its process in response to changes in the environment, notably related to atomoxetine (cf. Table 3.2). Reasons for any changes were provided by NICE. At the same time, except for sensible adaptation to a changing environment, NICE consistently kept published deadlines. This appears especially remarkable given the substantial complexity of the clinical problem under consideration (cf. Chapter 1, *Introduction*). Thus, at first glance there remain relatively few concerns related to transparency. These concerns are primarily related to the treatment of "commercial-in-confidence" data and economic models developed by assessment groups.

First, transparency of the appraisal process was limited as a consequence of commercial-in-confidence data submitted, which were not available for review and comment. In fact, four trials included in the economic model had been designated "commercial-in-confidence," of which three could nevertheless be identified with presentations at congresses or full publications in peer-reviewed journals. This treatment of clinical data is arguably outdated at a time when clinical trial registries are established to make unbiased information available to health care professionals and patients in a timely manner.

In the meantime, NICE have addressed the debate about use of confidential information in technology assessments (Mauskopf and Drummond, 2004), and NICE have reached an agreement with the pharmaceutical industry defining the circumstances under which non-publication of data would be acceptable (NICE, 2004g). This agreement between NICE and the Association of the British Pharmaceutical Industry (ABPI) was made on October 27, 2004, i.e., after the September 17, 2004 deadline set for submissions by consultees for the ADHD appraisal reviewed here (Table 3.2). A more restrictive use of the "commercial-in-confidence" provision should serve to further increase transparency. It would also enhance the existing opportunities for stakeholders to contribute to the appraisal process. In particular, unreferenced sources of "commercial-in-confidence" data may impede stakeholder participation quite substantially, given the limited time periods allowed to prepare and submit comments.

Second, NICE Appraisal Committee meeting minutes (cf. Chapter 4, *NICE Appraisal of ADHD Treatments*; e.g., NICE, 2005b,d) are hardly informative and do not enhance transparency of arguments and decision-making. This practice does not conform with reasonable expectations created by NICE's own process description related to the operation of the appraisal committees, stating that "the minutes [...] provide [...] an accurate record of its proceedings and discussions and also inform the public of the matters discussed at the meeting" (NICE, 2004b).

Third, economic models used by the assessment groups remain confidential (NICE, 2004b), with the effect of insulating an essential part of the assessment groups' work from public scrutiny. While transfer of intellectual property rights to academic assessment groups for work commissioned by NICE may be primarily a concern relevant to British taxpayers, there remain at least three further issues with the current practice:

First, at the time of writing this book it seemed possible that it might soon be tested whether this practice is in compliance with the British Freedom of Information Act (Scrip, 2006). Meanwhile, two pharmaceutical companies have taken NICE to court after their appeal against an appraisal determination was dismissed. Apparently, part of the dispute revolves around the transparency (or the lack hereof) of the economic model underlying the controversial assessment (cf. below; Scrip, 2007; Childs, 2006).

Second, secrecy prevents public academic debate about the relative merits of modeling approaches and may impede advances of methodological standards in the discipline of cost-effectiveness evaluations, to the potential detriment of its various stakeholders.

Third, the review of the ADHD technology assessment may serve to under-score the importance of transparency of economic models, as at present there is no opportunity for observers to uncover important elements of the model – in the present case, for instance, it is not even clear which clinical trials were actually included. Restrictions placed by NICE on the transparency of economic models include that, if the model has been provided to consultees and com-mentators (upon their request in writing), "the model must not be re-run with alternative assumptions or inputs," and that "the consultees and commentators will not publish the model wholly or in part, or use it to inform the develop-ment of other economic models" (NICE, 2004b, section 4.4.1.9, p. 14). Insofar not only the publicity condition of A4R is not met for an essential part of the NICE appraisal process, but also a key characteristic of good modeling practice is missed (Philips et al., 2004; Drummond, 2003; Brennan and Akehurst, 2000). Publicity and the resulting exposure of models to scrutiny by third parties might also assist effective quality assurance (cf. below, *Enforcement*). This observation corresponds to the conclusion of Jefferson and colleagues (2002) who "believe that urgent action should be taken to address the problem of poor methods in eco-nomic evaluations. [. . .] Economic models used in evaluations should be readily accessible to reviewers and readers. [. . .] Editorial teams, regulatory institutions, and researchers should implement and assess quality assurance" (Jefferson et al., 2002).

Next, the importance of the issues above is related to the observation that the appraisal phase of the process relies heavily on the initial technology assess-ment. Despite softening of certain conclusions proposed by the group of health economists, the ADHD assessment seemed to largely predetermine the range of possible outcomes of the subsequent appraisal. This last observation, however, is somewhat speculative since the contributions and comments that NICE received from the various stakeholders are not transparent.

Finally, there are distinct transparency issues related to the criteria other than cost-effectiveness, which are used for decision-making on guidance by the appraisal committees. These will be examined in more detail below (cf. sections on *Relevance, Objectives of Health Care Provision*, and *Objectives, Reconsidered*).

6.3.2 Relevance

The *relevance* of the present NICE ADHD technology appraisal is less clear. First, its scope is narrow compared to clinical guidelines in development, nec-

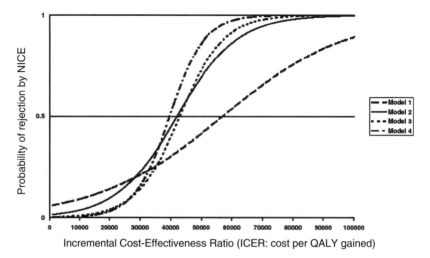

Incremental Cost-Effectiveness Ratio (ICER: cost per QALY gained)

Fig. 6.6 Probabilistic NICE cost-effectiveness thresholds
NICE has officially rejected the use of an absolute threshold for cost-effectiveness, as "there may be circumstances in which NICE would want to ignore a threshold" (Rawlins and Culyer, 2004). NICE is using a "benchmark" in the range of £20,000 to £30,000 per QALY gained to determine acceptability of a technology in the NHS (NICE, 2004b). The "probabilistic approach" adopted by NICE (Devlin and Parkin, 2004) creates issues related to the transparency of the other factors it is using to inform its decisions.
Source: "Does NICE have a cost-effectiveness threshold and what other factors influence its decisions? A binary choice analysis" by Nancy Devlin and David Parkin (2004), published in *Health Economics* 13 (5), pp. 437–452. © John Wiley & Sons Limited, Chichester. Reproduced with kind permission.

essarily reducing its relevance in this respect. Second, quality-adjusted life-years (QALYs) are understood to represent an intrinsically problematic instrument to measure clinical outcomes in children (De Civita et al., 2005; Griebsch et al., 2005). Third, the QALY aggregation rule implicitly underlying cost per QALY rankings (viz., "league tables"; cf. Mauskopf et al., 2003; Drummond et al., 1993b), even though relaxed by NICE (Figure 6.6; NICE, 2004c; Dakin et al., 2006; Devlin and Parkin, 2004; Towse et al., 2002), carries with it some morally controversial (if not unacceptable) assumptions (Schlander, 2005a,b; Daniels and Sabin, 2002; Dolan, 2001; Nord, 1999), which have been found to be empirically flawed (Dolan et al., 2005; cf. below, section on *Objectives of Health Care Provision*). Finally, an economically meaningful evaluation of allocative efficiency would have required a complete assessment of alternative treatment options, including psychosocial interventions.

In this context, it should be kept in mind that emphasis on due process and democratic deliberation does not necessarily provide an indication of the exact *content* of the process (Hasman and Holm, 2005; Daniels, 2000). While NICE has officially rejected the use of an absolute threshold for cost-effectiveness, as "there may be circumstances in which NICE would want to ignore a threshold" (Rawlins and Culyer, 2004), it has remained somewhat unclear what these circumstances could be, and "their relative importance and trade-offs between them are not made explicit" (Dakin et al., 2006). This is a major issue related to the *publicity* condition of A4R that also was subject to critique by the WHO review team (WHO, 2003). For example, independent analyses did suggest that budgetary constraints may be taken into account, despite explicit statements by NICE representatives to the contrary (e.g., Rawlins and Culyer, 2004). Multinomial modeling of NICE decision-making revealed that "interventions recommended for restricted use [within the NHS] had a significantly higher potential budget impact than those recommended routinely and the addition of this variable to the cost-effectiveness ratio and number of RCTs [available for a technology assessment] explained a greater proportion of the variance than any other variable" (Dakin et al., 2006).

Next, there is a real possibility that the requirement to be evidence-based (Daniels and Sabin, 1998) might have been missed during assessment, since the economic model was built exclusively on a highly restrictive selection of short-term clinical data as described earlier. Although the Appraisal Committee moderated the clear conclusions brought forward by the Assessment Group, the critique above strongly suggests that the limited focus on a small subset of randomized clinical trials was an important source of distortion and potential bias; the gaps of the assessment resulting from the exclusion of relevant information on the clinical and cost-effectiveness of treatments considered could not be compensated for by the subsequent appraisal. Also Health Technology Assessments by other agencies, such as the Scottish Medicines Consortium or the Australian Pharmaceutical Benefits Advisory Committee (PBAC), have reached different results (Scottish Medicines Consortium, 2005a,b; Australian Government, 2005a,b).

6.3.3 Appeal

NICE provisions for *appeal* appear to be markedly more restrictive than those proposed for A4R by Daniels and Sabin (1997, 1998, 2002). Appeals are limited to specific grounds and do not allow to reopen debate, which differs from A4R recommendations.

On the other hand NICE offers, beyond A4R requirements, ample opportunities for stakeholder participation (or more precisely, for input from invited consultees and commentators) during the process. In practice, however, these opportunities may be hampered by tight timelines – consultees and commentators are given four weeks to submit comments on the ACD and three weeks to lodge an appeal against the FAD – in combination with limited transparency of commercial-in-confidence information and economic models. This difficulty may be exacerbated when the Technology Assessment Report (a document comprising 605 pages in the case of the ADHD assessment) is made publicly available simultaneously with the ACD (Table 3.2).

Nevertheless, NICE's appeal system may have improved consistency and, until recently, prevented appellants from proceeding to legal challenge (Scrip, 2007; Childs, 2006; Raftery, 2006).

6.3.4 Enforcement

Finally, under A4R provisions are required to ascertain that the three other components are maintained. This is referred to as the *enforcement* condition. However, there is no indication that NICE has implemented an effective quality assurance system for health technology assessments. Design of effective provisions would have to appreciate that conventional peer-review processes are unlikely to be up to this task (Brennan and Akehurst, 2000; Hill et al., 2000).

Given the technical anomalies and inconsistencies identified with the ADHD technology assessment (cf. Table 6.7 and *Appendix*), there appears to be a need for NICE to reconsider arrangements with its review teams in that respect (WHO, 2003), as they apparently stand in the way of full publication of models (NICE, 2006k). The current NICE policy constitutes a peculiar contrast with broadly accepted quality criteria for economic models (Philips et al., 2004; Brennan and Akehurst, 2000).

Following Hasman and Holm (2005), proper enforcement of decisions may also be expected to result in implementation of guidance. Implementation of NICE guidance is subject to debate in England, and the record of NICE (and the NHS) in this respect has not been convincing to date (e.g., Freemantle, 2004; Sheldon et al., 2004; Howard and Harrison, 2004; but also Rawlins and Dillon, 2005a). Further exploration of this aspect is beyond the scope of the present analysis, but it should be noted that NICE now provides on its website an impressive number of generic and guidance-specific tools to assist the implementation of guidance. These tools include a "forward planner" summarizing published and forthcoming NICE guidance, slide sets highlighting key messages and likely implementation issues, audit criteria designed to assist monitoring actual implementation, and costing tools helping to determine the financial impact of guidance implementation (cf. NICE, 2006l).

Summing up, using the A4R framework as a benchmark for the NICE technology appraisal process paints a mixed picture. This might well be considered slightly disappointing given the explicit commitment by NICE to adhere to the principles of A4R (Rawlins and Dillon, 2005b).

The specific NICE approach appears well-structured, highly predictable, and to provide well-defined opportunities for (invited) stakeholders to participate. Transparency is generally good but far from perfect, and issues remain as to the relevance of NICE technology assessments, concerning the restrictive provisions for appeal, and the apparent absence of effective quality assurance as well as the implementation of guidance (enforcement). These observations suggest substantial room for further improvement.

6.4 NICE Technology Appraisal No. 98 – A Unique Outlier?

At first glance it might seem tempting to relegate the qualitative study of NICE Technology Appraisal No. 98, "Methylphenidate, atomoxetine and dexamfetamine for attention–deficit/hyperactivity disorder (ADHD) in children and adolescents. Review of Technology Appraisal 13" (NICE, 2006b), to the growing inventory of controversial criticisms that a priority-setting body has to expect (Rennie, 2001; Rennie and Luft, 2000). Why bother with an obvious outlier when there is so much praise for the approach adopted by NICE? After all, isn't the feasibility of the case study testimonial enough of a transparent appraisal process?

There are a number of reasons, however, why its findings should not be so quickly dismissed. First, agencies like NICE are most likely to draw fire from interested parties when their recommendations imply restrictions of use or denial of reimbursement (cf. Chapter 1, *Introduction*), which does not apply to the present case. Others however have questioned NICE's ability to say "no," except in obvious cases (Cookson et al., 2001; Raftery, 2001; Smith, 2000), or even the appropriateness of cost-effectiveness analysis since it does not capture the opportunity cost of adopting programs (Birch and Gafni, 2006a; Gafni and Birch, 1993; 2003a,b; 2006; Donaldson et al., 2002) or, from a policy-maker's perspective, the notion of "affordability" (cf. also below). Second, even if the case study dealt with an exceptional outlier, its findings were still relevant, as they would indicate an unsatisfactory robustness, suggesting difficulties when dealing with a complex clinical decision problem. These may have potentially far-reaching implications for the comparability of appraisals across a wide range of indications and interventions, which are intended to form the basis of decisions affecting large numbers of patients. Third, as emphasized earlier, qualitative methods in health and health services research can "reach the parts other methods cannot reach," and as such can complement quantitative studies: Case study research has been recognized to be especially useful to explore contemporary phenomena not amenable to quantitative analysis, for instance where complex interrelated issues are involved (cf. Chapter 1, *Introduction*; Pope and Mays, 1995).

Clearly, then, there remains the undeniable risk of implicit or explicit overgeneralization of observations largely based on one case study only. International observers, including this author, have been suitably impressed by the attempts by NICE to ensure rigorous systematic reviews, objective economic evaluation, stakeholder participation and transparency of process as well as value judgments (e.g., Schlander, 2007a; Neumann et al., 2005a; WHO, 2003).

This notwithstanding, even a single outlier must cast doubt on the attained robustness of its technology assessment process, which is an important requirement for its sustained widespread acceptance. It appears impossible to rule out that certain problems identified with the ADHD technology appraisal might be less unique than one would hope.

There is little if any dispute about the need to integrate clinical and economic evidence for health technology assessments to be meaningful in the context of a priority-setting body like NICE. Apart from the emergence of two streams of work – technology appraisals and clinical guideline development – that have developed very differently (Williams, 2004), others have observed that there are some difficulties "in ensuring that all academic centers [which provide the assessment groups] have the appropriate combination of clinical and economic expertise" (WHO, 2003).

Within the realm of technology assessments, problems seem to be more common in reconciling clinical data availability for systematic effectiveness review and the perspective of cost-utility analysis requiring units of outcome that facilitate the calculation of QALYs. For instance, for the recent economic evaluation of newer drugs for epilepsy in adults, effectiveness data – usually reported in terms of the reduction of seizures over a defined time period – were transformed into the categories of full (seizure-free) or partial (>50% reduction in seizure frequency) responders, which were subsequently combined with utility estimates for each state. This approach did not enable incorporation of side effect profiles (Wilby et al., 2003) – incorporation of which has generally proven difficult (cf. Chapter 2, *Methods*; Fletcher, 2000) – and no significant effectiveness differences could be confirmed in the systematic review prepared for NICE (Wilby et al., 2003). A meta-analysis performed on this basis, in order to produce economic model inputs, showed a difference in expected QALYs of only 0.025 between the drugs studied (Wilby et al., 2003). Different from the conclusions of NICE (NICE, 2004l), clinical guidelines developed at the same time by the Scottish Intercollegiate Guidelines Network (SIGN) – without formal consideration of cost-effectiveness – included two of the newer compounds (lamotrigine and oxcarbamazepine) for first-line treatment of partial and secondary generalized seizures SIGN (2003), and the American Epilepsy Society even recommended four of the newer compounds for newly diagnosed epilepsy (French et al., 2004).

Although *post-hoc* departures from pre-defined search strategies for data on the clinical or cost-effectiveness of interventions (cf. above, Chapter 5, *A Critique*) should be a rare occurrence, it is clear that abstracts and conference proceedings represent a challenge to review teams. While the critique of the ADHD assessment illustrates their importance in HTAs of rapidly evolving technologies, this is a time- and resource-consuming endeavor that often requires efforts to obtain further information from the authors. In this respect, there have been "variations in policy and practice" of assessment groups (Dundar et al., 2006).

Next, the health economics literature (Drummond et al., 2005; Brennan and Akehurst, 2000; Gold et al., 1996; Rittenhouse, 1996) suggests a broad consensus about the fundamental distinction between efficacy, effectiveness, and cost-effectiveness. Dealing with results of randomized clinical trials, the question for the economic analyst is "what does this mean in practice?" (Buxton et al., 1997). It is less evident how this insight has translated into real-life decision-making, since pragmatic open-label trials are frequently considered of lower quality than well-controlled, double-blind studies (NICE, 2006g; Busse et al., 2002; CRD, 2001), seen to provide evidence of a lower hierarchy level, "and so should be interpreted with caution" (NICE, 2005c). Specifically concerning treatment compliance, which may differ greatly between settings, analysts and decision-makers face pertinent issues related to the appropriate criteria to distinguish between mere convenience and clinical relevance. Challenges include what type of evidence to expect and how to weight it, from models driven by assumptions or expert consensus, over randomized pragmatic clinical trials (usually open-label!), to observational studies and retrospective database analyses.

Finally, transparency of economic models appears to be an issue far exceeding the ADHD technology assessment. Lack of transparency may not only impede effective stakeholder participation, but might even violate legal provisions. Two pharmaceutical companies, whose appeal against a recent NICE appraisal determination had been dismissed (NICE, 2006k), have taken NICE to court on grounds that its conclusions were "irrational" and "not supported legally," and that NICE "refused to disclose a fully-working version of the cost-effectiveness model used" (Scrip, 2007; Childs, 2006).

Combined with the ADHD case analysis, this brief collection of random observations does justify a further exploration of potential issues and underlying problems.

6.5 Implications for International Health Care Policy-Makers

There are compelling reasons to formally evaluate the trade-offs between alternative allocations of limited resources in any given health care system. Economic analyses, using concepts such as opportunity cost and incremental analysis (of costs and benefits, i.e., outcomes in the broadest sense), may inform such decisions and assist increasing their transparency and consistency. NICE has been heralded as a role model to achieve this goal in a reasonable way (Williams, 2004). As a result, international health care policy-makers will be interested not only in the performance of the NICE approach in relation to this expectation, but also what might be learned from NICE. A number of key issues that deserve careful consideration will be offered below.

6.5.1 Objectives of Health Care Provision

NICE has adopted the "extrawelfarist" proposition that the principal (although, as Anthony Culyer was keen to point out, "this does not mean 'only'") objective of the health care systems (or, more specifically, the National Health Service in England and Wales) "ought to be to maximize the aggregate improvement in the health status of the whole community"[19] (Culyer, 1997). The fundamental equity position of

---

[19] 20 years earlier, Weinstein and Stason (1977) had written: "The underlying premise of CEA [cost-effectiveness analysis using QALYs as outcome measures] in health problems is that for any given level of resources available, society (or the decision-making jurisdiction involved) wishes to maximize the *total aggregate* health benefit conferred" [italics added]. George Torrance, in a brief historical account of the early evolution of the conceptual underpinnings of cost-utility analysis, simply states "There was consensus in the literature that the objective of health care was to maximize health [...], i.e. to maximize both the quantity and quality of life" (without providing references) – from this it is evident that the development of the fundamental approach was charac-

NICE has been the assumption that "a QALY is a QALY is a QALY" resulting from the decision to (a) adopt QALYs as a universal outcome measure and (b) to give no differential weight to QALYs on the premise that "an additional adjusted life year is of equal importance for each person" (Rawlins and Culyer, 2004; NICE Citizens Council, 2003).

The social value judgments of NICE are not shared universally. In fact, the extrawelfarist proposition has come under attack via two different lines of thought. On the one hand, some economists assert, "that, for economists (as economists) wishing to influence policy, welfare economics is the only real game in town" (Pauly, 2003a). From this perspective it has been argued that the approach currently adopted by NICE[20], i.e. cost-utility analysis using arbitrary (e.g., Eichler et al., 2004) benchmarks for acceptable incremental costs per QALY gained, may in fact be expected to result in increased inefficiency (Birch and Gafni, 1993, 2006a; Gafni and Birch, 1993; 2003a,b; 2006; Bridges, 2005; Donaldson et al., 2002). However, the conventional view that QALY-based measurements are intrinsically inferior to willingness-to-pay-based cost-benefit analysis, as a proxy for overall social welfare composed of some aggregate of "lifetime welfare units," has been challenged (Adler, 2005).

On the other hand, empirical studies provided evidence that the simple (linear) QALY maximization assumption "is empirically flawed" (Dolan et al., 2005), as it does not reflect public preferences; technically, there seems to be a diminishing marginal social value associated with changes in both quality and length of life (Dolan et al., 2005). It has been proposed that "we find strong reasons to fear that to rank projects in terms of costs-per-QALY as often as not will tend to distort resource allocation decisions rather than to inform and aid them" (Nord, 1999). One consequence of this is that economic evaluations of medical interventions might be "answering questions people are unwilling to ask" (Schlander, 2005b). There are also important normative concerns, which include the implied valuation of human life as a function of health status, as opposed to viewing the value of life as a dimension distinct from health (cf. Arnesen and Nord, 1999).

As Daniels and Sabin (2002, p. 37) state, "It may well matter morally to us that someone who is much more seriously ill gets the extra benefit rather than someone less ill, or we may not be willing to aggregate minor benefits across large populations and outweigh, in the aggregate, major benefits, such as saving lives, for a few."[21] This issue will be addressed in more depth below, see Chapter 7, *Which Way Forward?*

---

terized by the application of decision analytic concepts without any empirical exploration of social values (Torrance, 2006; cf. also Nord, 1999).

[20] NICE initially had denied using a benchmark.

[21] There is extensive literature devoted to this issue, e.g., Dolan et al., 2005; Schlander, 2005a; Daniels and Sabin, 2002; Sen, 2002; Dolan, 2001; Ubel, 2000; Nord, 1999; Williams, 1997; and many others. See also later, Chapter 7, *Objectives, Reconsidered.*

6.5.2 (Almost) Exclusive Reliance on QALYs as Outcome Measure?

A key motive for the widespread use of QALYs has been the wish to make comparisons across a wide range of morbidities supported by a universal and comprehensive measure of health outcomes with interval scale properties. Any relaxation of, or deviation from, the extrawelfarist approach would immediately alleviate the restrictions associated with an (almost) exclusive reliance on QALYs as an outcome measure of interest. As has been seen in the ADHD case study, this narrow analytical focus was a prime reason contributing to the highly selective use of clinical evidence[22] and the resulting exclusion of an existing relevant, rich clinical (and cost-effectiveness) evidence base (Schlander, 2007e).

Even if acceptability on grounds of "efficiency" (cf. below, Chapter 7, *Objectives, Reconsidered*) was established by some cost per (weighted or unweighted) QALY ratio, current limitations of the methods used to derive utility estimates (see Bleichrodt and Pinto, 2006; Schlander, 2005a; Dolan, 2000; Kahneman et al., 1997; and many others), including the availability (or lack) of suitable clinical data, might still encourage policy-makers to have such evaluations *complemented* by appropriate examinations using other techniques, for instance, cost-effectiveness analysis. Instead of relying on restricted data sets, this might enable utilization of the best available clinical evidence and would imply greater flexibility in use of analytic approaches compared to the NICE reference case[23].

6.5.3 Technology Appraisal Processes

In particular the processes of NICE have been understood by observers to set a new standard internationally (e.g., Schlander, 2007a; Buxton, 2006; WHO, 2003). The technology appraisal process adopted by NICE is highly predictable and transparent in relation to timelines and methods used (and expectations for submissions) by NICE. In this respect it may indeed serve as an admirable role model, offering well-structured opportunities for stakeholders to participate throughout all phases, from scoping through assessment up to appraisal, with an Appraisal Consultation Document preceding Final Appraisal Determination and the issuance of

---

[22] It is clear, though, that an incomplete search for relevant evidence by the Assessment Group aggravated the problem.

[23] While it is clear that additions ("where one or more aspects of the methods differ") to the reference case are explicitly permitted by NICE (NICE, 2004c, section 5.3, pp. 20ff.), the Assessment Group did not make use of this option in the present case. Reasons might be related to (a) resource constraints (e.g., time, funding, access to clinical expertise and senior economic experts) and/or (b) insufficient encouragement to utilize methods different from those specified in the reference case.

guidance. Finally, consultees are given the chance to lodge an appeal against the Final Appraisal Determination.

Using the accountability for reasonableness (A4R) framework inaugurated by Daniels and Sabin as a benchmark, a number of differences between conditions for A4R and NICE processes were nevertheless identified, including the highly acclaimed transparency of the NICE approach. Thus, international policy-makers may wish to consider alternatives that ensure that stakeholders and third-party observers will be put in a position to replicate approaches chosen for modeling (including the impact of modified assumptions). Models developed with taxpayers' funding might be put in the public domain to foster academic debate about the relative merits of modeling approaches, to support further advances of methodological standards in the science of health economic evaluation (which would be to the advantage of all stakeholders), and not least as a tool enabling external quality assurance.

The process-related accomplishments of NICE have been supported by a high level of standardization, which in turn has contributed to a certain lack of flexibility to adapt the analytic process to the complexity of the specific decision situation. It would appear more appropriate if the assessment strategies pursued were better adapted to the problems at hand. Solving a number of decision problems may be fairly straight-forward, not requiring application of the full arsenal of analytic methods, such as probabilistic sensitivity analyses, and, hence, be less resource-consuming (cf. also Buxton, 2006; Fendrick, 2006). On the other hand, there may be challenging evaluation problems (such as a meaningful ADHD technology assessment) that can be met only if sufficient resources (time, manpower, budget, access to expertise) are available and that demand a problem-solving strategy different from the currently prescribed standard.

A more flexible, less schematic evaluation process could also allow for more than one stage of assessment, contingent on the problem. A meaningful approach could be to invite assessment groups to submit proposals; this could be organized as a competitive process among a selected group of academic centers with established excellence. Within the pre-defined scope, such proposals would usefully present "convincing arguments that the objectives of the review have been understood (and refined if necessary)," demonstrate the necessary range of expertise of the assessment group, describe an appropriate and feasible methodology for undertaking the review, and cover the resources (funds and timescales) required (CRD, 2001). If and when a process consisting of more than one stage was considered adequate, the principle objective of a first phase could be to determine the social desirability of funding a technology; this would sensibly include, but not be limited to, consideration of *allocative efficiency* (cf. Chapter 7, *Objectives, Reconsidered*). These criteria would need to be codified (WHO, 2003). A subsequent phase of evaluation then might address in more detail issues of *technical efficiency*, which would offer an opportunity for a more complete review of available evidence, including a more cautious use of quantitative meta-analysis, and cost-effectiveness analysis using clinical endpoints considered meaningful.

6.5.4 Timing of Technology Appraisals

It is well understood that the cost-effectiveness of technologies does change over time (Remak et al., 2003; Buxton, 1987). The rapid evolution of our understanding of the economic implications of ADHD (which was briefly delineated earlier, see Chapter 6, *Insights from Clinical Long-Term Data and from Disease-Specific Effectiveness Measures*) underscores the relevance of this observation, illustrating the inherent dynamics of the evidence of effectiveness and cost-effectiveness.

There is no ideal solution to the resulting dilemma, for which the term Buxton's law has been coined: "*It's always too early [to evaluate] until, unfortunately, it's suddenly too late*" (Buxton, 1987). If anything, this dilemma is aggravated by the possibility that sound economic evaluations of complex clinical problems require substantial resources – including time – especially when they are embedded in truly participatory processes. In the ADHD case it took 33 months from initial scoping to the issuance of NICE guidance (Table 3.2), and it seems quite possible that the six-months assessment period was too short to successfully mount the task.

In an attempt to better address the problem described by Martin Buxton, NICE itself recently announced the introduction of a revised process allowing more rapid appraisal of important new technologies (NICE, 2005g, 2006i). It will be interesting to see how NICE is going to deal with the challenging task to assure sufficiently broad scope and high quality of such rapid reviews (cf. Buxton and Akehurst, 2006).

Two further consequences seem worth mentioning here.

First, there is a need to use decision analytic modeling to extrapolate beyond the data observed in clinical trials (e.g., Philips et al., 2004, 2006; Brennan and Akehurst, 2000; Buxton et al., 1997). This will often include inferring final outcomes from intermediate clinical endpoints, if and when a relationship between both has been shown to exist (Buxton et al., 1997; Rittenhouse, 1996). The need for modeling has been recognized by NICE (2004b,c), and NICE has played an important and laudable role in methods development in this area, in particular regarding the consideration of decision uncertainty associated with the use of models (e.g., Ades et al., 2006; Griffin et al., 2006; Ginnelly, 2005; Claxton et al., 2005).

Second, in order to use the best evidence available at the time of an assessment, it appears necessary to include conference abstracts and presentations of new data that have not yet been published in peer-reviewed journals. This creates challenges regarding complete search strategies, access to relevant data, and evaluation of quality of findings presented (cf. Dundar et al., 2006).

The critique of the ADHD assessment indicates that even NICE may not (yet) have succeeded to consistently implement these consequences (see Chapter 5, above).

6.5.5 Multidisciplinary Assessment Teams

Technology appraisals need to address clinical problems, some of which may be extremely complex, and are expected to derive meaningful conclusions that will exert direct and/or indirect influence on clinical decision-making (viz., "resource allocation"). The ADHD case study lends support to the conjecture that it is unlikely that complex problems can be handled successfully by either discipline – the medical profession or economists – working in isolation.

It seems likely on the basis of this case study that NICE has not (yet) sufficiently accomplished the desirable (if not necessary) integration. The implications are potentially far-reaching and transcend the issue of how to relate clinical guideline development to the technology appraisals. Beyond sharing expertise, a higher level of integration of the key disciplines involved in technology assessments and clinical guideline development could also assist addressing the challenging differences between the professions in terms of attitudes, values, and beliefs relevant to prioritization problems in health care (cf. again Chapter 7, *Objectives, Reconsidered*).

6.5.6 Quality Assurance

High levels of standardization do not suffice to assure consistent quality of technology assessments. There seems to be a need for some kind of *enforcement* as postulated by Daniels and Sabin (1998) as part of their "accountability for reasonableness" framework. This would extend to the technical quality of reviews.

Beyond disclosure of potential conflicts of interest, transparency of methods used for modeling might be useful[24]. Further precautions might be built into the appraisal process to achieve the important requirement of effective quality assurance. It is not sufficient to rely on conventional peer review processes, which cannot be expected to be up to this task (cf. Hill et al., 2000; Reinhardt, 1997).

6.5.7 Implementation

Economic evaluations are useless unless their results can be applied in clinical practice. However, the implementation of NICE guidance within the UK National Health Service to date has been mixed (e.g., Sheldon et al., 2004; Howard and Harrison, 2004), and NICE has responded by launching an implementation support strategy (NICE, 2004m, 2006l; cf. also Rawlins and Dillon, 2005a). In principle, there are several possible approaches to improve implementation, in-depth discussion of which is beyond the scope of the present study.

One straightforward way to implement economic evaluation results is to tie them directly to pricing or indirectly to reimbursement decisions, such as coverage and payment policies or formulary listings. This approach, which is commonly referred to as "fourth hurdle" regulation (in addition to the three traditional "hur-

---

[24] This corresponds to the conclusion of Jefferson and colleagues (2002, p. 2811); see Chapter 6, *NICE Accountability for Reasonableness: Publicity.*

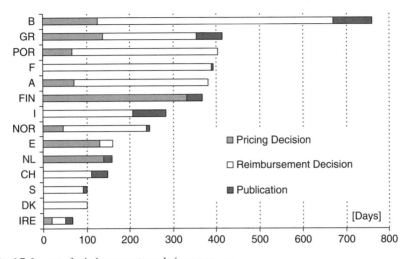

Fig. 6.7 Impact of reimbursement regulation on access
Delayed access to new medicines: average time from pricing and/or reimbursement application to actual reimbursement for new pharmaceutical products in European markets; data source: analysis by Cambridge Pharma Consultancy (2002) for the Commission of the European Communities, 2003; from Schlander, 2004c.
Abbreviations: B, Belgium; GR, Greece; POR, Portugal; F, France; A, Austria; FIN, Finland; I, Italy; NOR, Norway; E, Spain; NL, Netherlands; CH, Switzerland; S, Sweden; DK, Denmark; IRE, Ireland

dles," efficacy/effectiveness, safety, and product quality, that need to be taken by new pharmaceutical products prior to market authorization), does exist in a number of jurisdictions (with or without the use of economic evaluations). One of its key disadvantages is delayed access (a) to new medicines from the perspective of patients and (b) to markets from the perspective of pharmaceutical innovators.

For example, mean times to listing on the Australian Pharmaceutical Benefits Scheme (PBS) of new products or new indications were found in a range between 22 and 30 weeks during the years 1999 to 2003, according to a recent review (Wonder et al., 2006). A study commissioned by the G10 working group of the European Commission found the delays of market access for new pharmaceutical products to vary greatly by country (Figure 6.7; Commission of the European Communities, 2003).

In contrast, (abstracting from the Pharmaceutical Price Regulation Scheme, PPRS, in the United Kingdom) NICE operates in a free-pricing environment for pharmaceutical products[25]. Nevertheless, it has been argued that NICE technology assessments also lead to held-back prescribing especially of innovative, costly new medicines (Redwood, 2006). The phenomenon – sometimes called "NICE Blight" – describes the reluctance of physicians to prescribe a new treatment before it is

---

[25] In February 2007, the Office of Fair Trading (OFT) suggested to replace the current system of profit and price controls under the PPRS with a value-based approach to pricing (OFT, 2007)

known whether NICE guidance will be prepared, and if so, whether NICE will actually recommend its use within the NHS.

A separate implementation issue may emerge after issuance of a positive recommendation by NICE, because NICE has no control over the resources of the NHS and their deployment, and budget constraints faced by NHS bodies such as Regional Health Authorities and Primary Care Trusts may either stand in the way of guidance implementation or require displacement of other technologies, cost-effectiveness of which may be unknown (e.g., Williams, 2004; Towse and Pritchard, 2002). This problem has also been recognized by the UK Audit Commission (2005), and recommendations have been put forward to improve the situation.

Specifically in the context of the ADHD case study it is interesting that it has been observed that guidance seems "more likely to be adopted when there is strong professional support, a stable and convincing evidence base, ... Guidance needs to be clear and reflect the clinical context" (Sheldon et al., 2004).

In order to gain the respect of the medical profession, health economists wishing to influence clinical resource allocation decisions should be prepared to meet the expectation that they do adhere to quality standards no less than those expected to be met routinely in medical decision-making. As John Maynard Keynes once wrote, "if economists could manage to get themselves thought of as humble, competent people, on a level with dentists, that would be splendid.[26]"

---

[26] J.M. Keynes, *Collected Works* (1971–1989), Vol. IX, p. 332.

Which Way Forward?

Chapter 7
Which Way Forward?

Apparently there is no universally correct – possibly not even a universally applicable – answer to this key question; any reasonable way forward will necessarily depend on the respective *starting point* and on the *objectives* ultimately pursued, as well as the specific *institutional context*.

7.1 Starting Points

While the number of organizations involved in health technology assessments (HTAs) has grown in recent years, the approaches adopted internationally differ, perhaps most markedly with respect to the use of economic evaluation as a part of HTAs (cf. Hutton et al., 2006; Henry et al., 2005; Hjelmgren et al., 2001). Some organizations, including the Centers for Medicare and Medicaid Services (CMS) and the Veterans Administration (VA Technology Assessment Program, VATAP) in the United States, the German Institute for Quality and Efficiency in Health Care (Institut für Qualität und Wirtschaftlichkeit im Gesundheitswesen, IQWiG), and the Spanish Agency for Health Technology Evaluation (Agencia de Evaluación de Tecnologías Sanitarias, AETS), do not (yet) use formal economic analyses (cf. IQWiG, 2005, 2006; García-Altés et al., 2004; Tunis, 2004). The German IQWiG, for example, evaluates whether or not medical technologies offer "therapeutically relevant" advantages over existing options, without considering cost. Owing to the resulting difficulties to link effectiveness and cost, important opportunities to increase quality and efficiency of health care may be missed (Schlander, 2003). With this constraint being increasingly realized, interest has been growing in NICE as a role model for the implementation of economic evaluations, which have the potential to add important information on the trade-offs associated with prioritization decisions.

First and foremost, expectations for cost-effectiveness analyses should be realistic. A rigid application of the logic of cost-effectiveness has not been unequivocally successful, neither in Oregon, nor in New Zealand or elsewhere, though it is seen by many analysts as an essential ingredient into rational resource allocation processes (Maynard and Bloor, 1995). In particular, international experience – including Australia and Canada – indicates that implementation of cost-effectiveness analyses

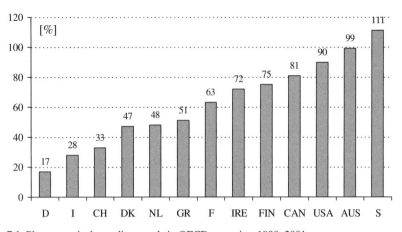

Fig. 7.1 Pharmaceutical spending trends in OECD countries, 1990–2001
Australia and Canada were the first jurisdiction implementing cost-effectiveness analyses to inform
reimbursement decisions. At the same time, Australia and Canada were among the OECD markets
recording the highest per-capita growth of total pharmaceutical expenditures, 1990–2001 (Aus-
tralia and Switzerland, 1990–2000; Germany, 1992–2001; no UK data available). Source: OECD
Health Data, 2003; Schlander, 2004c.
Abbreviations: D, Germany; I, Italy; CH, Switzerland; DK, Denmark; NL, Netherlands;
GR, Greece; F, France; IRE, Ireland; FIN, Finland; CAN, Canada; Aus, Australia; S, Sweden.

tends to increase spending (cf. Figure 7.1), as – according to one interpretation – it
tends to reveal relatively more undertreatment than overtreatment (Neumann, 2004;
Schlander, 2004c; Mitchell, 2002). A prevailing focus on the evaluation of new
technologies rather than existing ones may be another important factor contributing
to inflationary pressures created by the current use of cost-effectiveness analyses
(Maynard et al., 2004).

In England, prescription drug spending increased from £5.58bn in 2000 to
£7.94bn in 2005, i.e., by a compound annual growth rate of 7.4%, and NICE
guidance has been seen by many analysts as one important underlying reason
(e.g., Maynard et al., 2004; Macdonald, 2003; Taylor, 2002; Cookson et al., 2001).
According to recent internal estimates from NICE, full implementation of NICE
guidance from 1999 through 2004 would have had a cumulated budgetary impact
on the NHS of £ 800 million, equivalent to 1% of total NHS spending (Audit
Commission, 2005).

It has also been pointed out by health economists that ranking interventions on
the basis of incremental cost-effectiveness ratios (ICERs) does not provide information about the opportunity costs associated with the adoption of a new program (e.g.,
Birch and Gafni, 2006a; Gafni and Birch, 1993; 2003a,b; 2006; Donaldson et al.,
2002). As a pragmatic solution attempt, it has been suggested to complement cost-
effectiveness evaluations with budgetary impact analyses (Trueman et al., 2001).
This approach implies the introduction of a fifth criterion[1] and thus a departure from

---

[1] It is a fifth criterion (or "*fifth hurdle*") following common parlance, which refers to the cost-
effectiveness criterion as a *fourth hurdle* from the perspective of manufacturers to gain reim-

the simple decision rules of the logic of cost-effectiveness – although in practice both types of analysis can be conducted using a common technical framework (cf. Nuijten and Rutten, 2002). Besides the economic concept of opportunity costs, budgetary impact analysis is related to the notion of affordability, and the computation of "affordability curves" has been suggested, reflecting the probability that a technology is affordable for a range of "threshold budgets" (Sendi and Briggs, 2001).

7.1.1 Affordability

In many publicly financed health care systems, whether they are organized according to the National Health Service model or as (mandatory) insurance systems, resource availability or "affordability" is predetermined by some kind of global budget. In these cases, limits to available resources are most obvious. Albeit economic (cost-benefit) evaluation may contribute to determining appropriate limits, ultimately these resource constraints are the result of public or political trade-off processes. Ideally, these are the consequence of democratic deliberation about competing social goods, such as education and child care, but also social benefits (e.g., unemployment benefits and pension funds) and broader economic objectives, for instance job creation, and even military defense and police to protect law and order – all of which contribute to protecting basic liberties, individual opportunities and relevant capabilities (cf. Rawls, 1971; Sen 1985).

In other words, public spending on health care will be constrained by the demand for public non-health spending and the limits to society's willingness to be taxed. As such, a key issue about global limits to health care spending will be democratic deliberation. Following Daniels and Sabin (2002), accountability for reasonableness should begin with transparency about limits and their implications. As a consequence, transparency should be expected as to the difference between "affordability" or ability-to-pay, and willingness-to-pay on the societal level. *Per se*, the notion of affordability, often discussed in relation to a growing share of health care expenditures of gross national product (GDP), represents an ill-defined, highly subjective concept (see Box 5).

There is no feasible scientific way to determine an optimal share of health care spending (e.g., Aaron, 2003; Pauly, 2003b; Reinhardt et al., 2002). More than that, as it turns out, the future affordability of health care spending growing faster than GDP is highly sensitive to real per-capita economic growth rates, particularly those falling below 1% per year (Figure 7.2). If and when sufficient economic growth rates (above about 1% per year) can be realized, ability-to-pay for health care expenditures rising faster than GDP would exist, even under reasonably conservative assumptions (Box 5), for several decades (Figure 7.2). Thus, at the societal or macro

---

bursement and hence market access for a given technology; the first three criteria are efficacy/effectiveness, safety, and product quality, which are evaluated during the traditional new product approval process.

Box 5 On the notion of "affordability" Without exception, OECD countries have experienced dramatic increases of their health care expenditure. Expressed as a share of gross domestic product (GDP), health care spending in the United States climbed from 5.0 percent in 1960 to 13.9 percent in 2001. Health care's share of the US economy has been predicted to reach 18 percent by 2012 (Heffler et al., 2003). Long-range forecasts for the United States indicate health care expenditures might well consume 38 percent of GDP by 2075 (Chernew et al., 2003).

A Medicare Technical Review Panel (2000) defined affordable growth of health care spending in terms of non-health spending, postulating that maximum affordability be reached at a level of spending when non-health expenditures would no longer rise – i.e., when the increase of GDP would be consumed entirely by growing health expenditures. One advantage of this approach is that its definition of minimum acceptable non-health spending relies on observed consumption patterns instead of some more theoretical construct. This simple idea implies that, with increasing GDP, a society can afford to spend a greater share of income on health care – a suggestion not only in line with observations from studies at the macro level of nations but, likewise, with the "dictionary definition" of affordability (cf. Reinhardt et al., 2004).

Chernew et al. (2003) provided an extrapolation under an assumed real GDP growth rate of 1.2 percent per year. Allowing for a separate demographic adjustment of health care spending of 0.43 percentage points per year, real health care spending rising one percentage point faster than real GDP would then be "affordable" beyond 2075. Under the same set of assumptions a two-percentage point gap between the annual growth rates would still be affordable until 2039. However, future economic growth rates are uncertain.

The time period of future "affordable" health care cost growth can be estimated as a function of the combined effects of health care cost and real GDP growth rates on non-health care spending, allowing for an investment share of 18 percent of GDP required to support rising GDP. Then real non-health expenditures start to decrease after t years if the rise of health expenditure exceeds the rise of investment adjusted GDP. (Note that the mathematical formulas do not show the adjustment made for the assumed investment share.)

$$(GDP_t - GDP_{t-1}) - (HE_t - HE_{t-1}) < 0 \qquad (7.1)$$

where GDP_t = gross domestic product per capita (adjusted for an 18% investment share) in year t, and HE_t = total health expenditures per capita in year t

Transformation of (7.1) with real growth rates for health expenditure g_{HE} and GDP g_{GDP} results in:

$$\left[GDP_0 \cdot (1 + g_{GDP})^t - GDP_0 \cdot (1 + g_{GDP})^{t-1} \right]$$
$$- \left[HE_0 \cdot (1 + g_{HE})^t - HE_0 \cdot (1 + g_{HE})^{t-1} \right] < 0 \qquad (7.2)$$

Equation (7.2) may be rewritten:

$$GDP_0 \cdot (1 + g_{GDP})^{t-1} \cdot g_{GDP} - HE_0 \cdot (1 + g_{HE})^{t-1} \cdot g_{HE} < 0 \qquad (7.3)$$

After derivation with respect to t the number of years with rising non-health care expenditures despite positive health expenditure growth rate is:

$$t = \frac{\ln(HE_0 \cdot g_{HE}) - \ln(GDP_0 \cdot g_{GDP})}{\ln(1 + g_{GDP}) - \ln(1 + g_{HE})} + 1 \qquad (7.4)$$

Hence, total non-health expenditures start to decrease after t years. Technically, this corresponds to the time when the slope of the curve of health care spending equals the slope of the curve of gross domestic product. On this basis the time span t can be calculated until rising health spending will completely consume the increase of GDP under different combinations of assumed growth rates of health spending and GDP (per capita in real terms). The resulting number of years can then be interpreted as an upper limit of the future "affordability" of escalating health care expenditures, according to the definition adopted by the Technical Review Panel.
Source: Schlander et al., 2004c,d; Schlander and Schwarz, 2005b.

level, the relevant issue is not "affordability" – in the sense of whether the economy can sustain increasing spending on health care – but actual willingness-to-pay – or, in the context of collectively financed health care, willingness to be taxed.

Of course, this observation does in no way abolish the social choice problems associated with health care resource allocation decisions. On the contrary, it may serve to highlight the extent to which there are indeed critical choices to be made at all levels of decision-making. Also pointing to the abstract existence of affordability should not be misinterpreted as an attempt to invalidate the ethical imperative to strive for "efficient" use of resources, in particular, to eliminate wasteful spending (cf. Anderson et al., 2003; Maynard, 2001a).

7.1.2 Institutional Context

Institutional context will have to be taken into account in various ways. One aspect relates to specific features of health care systems, such as centralization (National

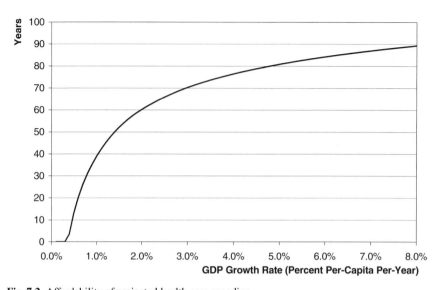

Fig. 7.2 Affordability of projected health care spending
Affordability of projected US health care spending according to a definition proposed by the
Medicare Technical Review Panel (2000): number of years of rising non-health expenditures as
a function of the future (real per-capita) GDP growth rate, assuming a two-percentage point gap
between the growth rates of health expenditures and GDP. See also Box 5. GDP is gross domestic
product. Source: Schlander et al., 2004d

Health Service model) versus decentralization (e.g., competition in the United States
system), which will influence the optimal way of implementation of economic
evaluations, obviously without invalidating the principal usefulness of the discipline
(cf. Siegel, 2005; Berger and Teutsch, 2005).

   Also the level of decision-making will matter. At the central or macro level,
usually an agency is entrusted with the task of making decisions for the whole
health care system. At the local or micro level (sometimes referred to as "meso"
level, as opposed to the "micro" level of bedside decisions), for instance Regional
Health Authorities, Primary Care Trusts or hospitals, various constraints (e.g., budget pressures, limited available health economic expertise, etc.) may dictate different approaches. Moreover, local implementation of central guidance rests – among
other factors – on alignment between recommendations and funding (e.g., Audit
Commission, 2005; Sheldon et al., 2004).

   More importantly, legal environments will impose constraints on prioritization
decisions. A well-known incident in the United States was the revisions of the Oregon Health Plan required by the Health Care Financing Administration (HCFA)
to comply with the Federal Americans with Disabilities Act (ADA). QALYs value
life as a function of health status (e.g., Nord et al., 1999; Savulescu, 1999; Menzel,
1990; Harris, 1987; cf. also the recent dispute between Harris, 2005a,b, and Rawlins
and Dillon, 2005b). However, any discrimination of (groups of) patients on grounds
of their reduced capacity to gain "quality of life," for instance the disabled or the
chronically ill (people in so-called "double-jeopardy;" cf. Richardson and McKie,
2005; Singer et al., 1995; Harris, 1995), would still have to stand the test of the

declaration of human rights, stating that "recognition of the inherent dignity and of the equal and inalienable rights of all members of the human family is the foundation" (United Nations, 1948). In many jurisdictions there exist constitutional provisions that set limits to a utilitarian or quasi-utilitarian approach that is exclusively or primarily concerned with maximizing the distribution-independent sum of individual utilities, as "distribution indifference does not take the distinction between persons adequately seriously" (Sen, 2002; Rawls, 1971).

7.2 Objectives, Reconsidered

Keeping specific legal context in mind as a constraint, it is a fundamental principle of decision analysis that "the identification and structuring of objectives essentially frames the decision being addressed. It sets the stage for all that follows" (Keeney and Raiffa, 1993). To be relevant, thus, analytic decision support relies on prior clarification of values and objectives to be pursued (Keeney, 1992). For this reason Uwe Reinhardt has emphasized repeatedly that there is no point in discussing "efficiency" (invariably an instrumental or secondary objective) unless effectiveness criteria (i.e., primary objectives) have been agreed on (Reinhardt, 1992, 1998).

7.2.1 Efficiency

Cost-effectiveness analysis has been conceptualized as a tool to maximize "value for money" (i.e., not to minimize spending), which immediately raises the issue of identifying and valuing the appropriate outcomes (Gold et al., 1996). If limited to issues of *technical efficiency*, i.e., the evaluation of alternative ways to achieve a given clinical outcome (such as peptic ulcer healing, eradication of Helicobacter pylori, life years gained by implementation of a specific type of screening program, or, related to the present case study, symptomatic and/or functional improvement of patients), cost-effectiveness analysis clearly can provide useful information.

The situation is more complicated when issues of *allocative efficiency* need to be addressed, which inevitably arise in an environment of scarce resources, i.e., when group decisions must consider a broad range of consequences across multiple decisions. For example[2], should limited resources better be used to fund the provision of sildenafil (Viagra[R]) for patients with erectile dysfunction, pharmacological or behavioral treatment for children and adolescents with ADHD, or beta-interferon and glatiramer for patients with multiple sclerosis (...)? Cost-utility analysis using QALYs as the universal (and comprehensive) measure of (health-related) outcomes

---

[2] Of course, this would have to be further specified according to different patient subgroups (e.g., by disease severity – the "*clinical margin*") and varying intensity of interventions (the "*intensity margin*"), as the real choices are not about blanket in- or exclusions, but about addressing incremental costs and effectiveness at the margin (e.g., Briggs, 2000; Briggs and Gray, 2000).

purports to solve the inherent problem of comparing outcomes that are different in kind[3] (Drummond et al., 2005, 1997; Gold et al., 1996). The relative desirability of a given medical intervention then rests on its incremental cost per QALY ratio. Some implications of this logic were briefly discussed earlier (see Chapter 6, *Objectives of Health Care Provision*). Ultimately, there are fundamental ethical choices to be made, detailed discussion of which exceeds the scope of this case study.

For instance, policy-makers might wonder about the validity of rankings derived from cost-effectiveness ratios (viz., "*league tables*"), the meaning of which is based on a quasi-utilitarian aggregation rule[4]. As there is no gold standard against which to judge criterion validity, an alternative may be to use the so-called reflective equilibrium approach (Nord, 1992; Daniels, 1979; Rawls, 1971). Empirically, this would imply to examine to what extent rankings derived from health state valuations (quality weights) used for QALY computations are in accordance with directly elicited preferences for resource allocation. In other words, assuming the cost per QALY gained was, for example, ∼£3,600 for sildenafil in erectile dysfunction (Stolk et al., 2000), ∼£7,000 for medication in ADHD (NICE, 2006b), and >£120,000 for beta-interferons and glatiramer in multiple sclerosis (NICE, 2002), would this ranking reflect the comparative social desirability of these interventions (cf. McGregor, 2003)?

For health economic analyses it is usually assumed that, because health care produces health, the objective of collectively-financed health care should be to maximize either (a) the aggregate of ordinally measured individual utilities, with health being one out of many arguments of the utility function (cf. Pauly, 1995, 2003a; Breyer et al., 2003; Hurley, 2000), or (b) cardinally measured health gains, i.e., treating health as an independent argument of the utility function (cf. Schlander, 2005a; Rawlins and Culyer, 2004; Culyer, 1971, 1989, 1997). In its pure form, this view results in an "*efficiency-only*" approach, with efficiency being defined either (a) based on the welfare theoretic principles of Pareto and Kaldor-Hicks (cf. Ng, 2004; Boadway and Bruce, 1984) or (b) their extrawelfarist variant seeking to produce the maximum amount of QALYs (or a comparable construct) for a given budget (cf. Weinstein, 2006; Schlander, 2005a; Rawlins and Culyer, 2004; Weinstein and Zeckhauser, 1973). Then, the tools to determine efficiency are cost-benefit or cost-utility analysis, respectively. While the debate between the proponents of either approach continues (Birch and Gafni, 2006a,b; Birch and Donaldson, 2003; Gafni and Birch, 2003a,b; Donaldson et al., 2002; Blaug, 1998), it is noteworthy here that both approaches are "mean-based" (cf. Vanness and Mullahy, 2006), i.e., they represent attempts to maximize an average expected consequence irrespective of its actual distribution across individuals, and have been criticized for overlooking the frequent impossibility of compensating "losers" for foregone health benefits (Schlander, 2005a,b; Ng, 2004; Reinhardt, 1998; Boadway and Bruce,

---

[3] For instance: "Cost-utility analysis should be used … when the programs being compared have a wide range of different kinds of outcomes and you wish to have a common unit of output for comparison" (Drummond et al., 1997, p. 141f.).

[4] Cf. above, Chapter 6, see also Culyer, 1997, and Weinstein and Stason, 1977. For recent reviews, cf. Dolan et al., 2005, and Schlander, 2005a.

1984; Mishan, 1971). Apart from normative concerns, the quasi-utilitarian QALY aggregation rule has been shown to be empirically flawed, i.e., there is a wealth of evidence that it does not adequately reflect prevailing social value judgments (Richardson and McKie, 2005; Schlander, 2005a; Dolan et al., 2005; McKie and Richardson, 2003).

The approach adopted by NICE may be characterized as *"efficiency-first"* (Buxton, 2006; Pearson and Rawlins, 2005; Rawlins and Culyer, 2004), following the extrawelfarist proposition and using a cost-effectiveness benchmark of "a most plausible" £20,000 to £30,000 per QALY gained (NICE, 2004c) while rejecting an absolute threshold (Pearson and Rawlins, 2005; Rawlins and Culyer, 2004), specifying that it would also consider other factors including "the particular features of the condition and population receiving the technology" (NICE, 2004c), which may include social value judgments such as "special considerations of equity" (Rawlins and Culyer, 2004). NICE established a Citizens Council to provide input "on the topics it wants the council to discuss," in order "to ensure that these values resonate broadly with the public" (Rawlins and Culyer, 2004), while maintaining that guidance "is based on clinical and cost-effectiveness evidence" (NICE, 2007).

The Citizens Council (NICE, 2006c,d,e) has shown some concern for these issues[5] but endorsed NICE's approach, concluding that "cost-utility analysis is necessary, but should not be the sole basis for decisions on cost-effectiveness" (NICE, 2005f,k). It is unclear whether the Citizens Council was confronted with the issue of cost-per-QALY rankings such as those cited above. Neither is it clear whether implications of the logic of cost-utility analysis were exposed in such a way as Jeff Richardson and John McKie suggested, namely "When a health state is rated as having a utility score of 0.8 it may be inferred that curing five people in this health state and returning them to normal health for the rest of their lives is equivalent to saving the life of a single person," because $5 \times (1.0-0.8) = 1$, which is also the utility obtained from saving one person's life (Richardson and McKie, 2005, p. 272).

A related concern found by the WHO review team has been the lack of transparency regarding considerations other than cost-effectiveness (WHO, 2003), which has led to second-guessing and scientific inquiry by academic researchers (cf. Chapter 6, *Discussion and Implications*; Figure 6.6; Dakin et al., 2006; Devlin and Parkin, 2004; Towse and Pritchard, 2002). NICE has denied speculation that it considers the budgetary impact of technologies (Pearson and Rawlins, 2005; Rawlins and Culyer, 2004) despite some indications to the contrary (Dakin et al., 2006), which has caused critique from a theoretic perspective as well as for its practical consequences (cf. above; e.g., Cookson et al., 2001; Gafni and Birch, 1993). The WHO team recommended that "NICE codifies and justifies the specific criteria used in decision-making" (WHO, 2003). Other observers analyzed NICE's positive appraisal of riluzole for motor neuron disease on the basis of an ICER of a cost per

---

[5] In particular, the published meeting minutes of the NICE Citizens Council provide for instructive reading material – for instance, NICE, 2006e.

QALY of £34,000 to £43,500 (NICE, 2001), which had initially been estimated at £58,000 (Stewart et al., 2000) and had later been brought down to £16,500 to £20,000 (Bryan et al., 2001). Independent analyses demonstrated substantial uncertainty surrounding these estimates (Ginsberg and Lowe, 2002), and it was argued by observers that NICE "should not need to fabricate an efficiency criterion to support the reimbursement of riluzole" because it "tried to resolve two impossible statements," (a) "uncertainty on effectiveness" and (b) "a cost per QALY in a tightly circumscribed range" (Freemantle et al., 2002). They concluded that it might "be better to accept that resources are more reasonably and appropriately allocated on the basis of the rule of rescue or fair innings rather than a strict efficacy [note added: *efficiency*?] criterion" (Freemantle et al., 2002).

The "rule of rescue" refers to "the imperative people feel to rescue identifiable individuals facing avoidable death" (Jonsen, 1986). Whereas being "identifiable" has been described as morally irrelevant, the preference for lifesaving over non-lifesaving measures – which the rule entails – may be justifiable from a utilitarian perspective but is not captured by standard techniques of utility measurement for cost-effectiveness analysis (McKie and Richardson, 2003). The "fair innings" argument as proposed by Alan Williams (1997) reflects the notion that "everyone is entitled to some 'normal' span of health (usually expressed in life years)." These concepts represent just two examples of "values" which may be considered relevant to health care resource allocation decisions that standard cost-utility evaluation does not encompass adequately.

A concern has been raised that the NICE approach in practice may result in "the marginalization of factors other than clinical and cost-effectiveness as outside NICE's terms of reference" (Redwood, 2006; cf. Berg et al., 2001), and one might indeed expect this effect to occur as a consequence of NICE's focus on cost-effectiveness benchmarks as the primary proxy of "social desirability" within the context of the NHS. Unfortunately, there is no simple way to measure community values for direct use in setting health care priorities (Nord, 1995, 1999), and a Canadian qualitative analysis of health reform documents revealed a "Tower of Babel" that is contemporary "values talk," concluding that the capacity of any one scholarly theory of values was limited to encompass the diversity of "policy values" (Giacomini et al., 2004).

7.2.2 Fairness

Despite some undeniable difficulty in deriving workable alternative solutions to the health care resource allocation problem, it has been argued that the primary objective of a collectively financed health scheme (and, therefore, the relevant unit of analysis) is *not* the maximization of an *aggregate* of utility or construct of population health, but includes prominently to give *individuals* the *chance* to achieve a "decent basic minimum" of health (Daniels, 1985) or the "capability" of achieving good health (Anand, 2005; Sen, 1985, 2002), in order to gain "a normal range of opportunities" to pursue their individual conceptions of the "good" (Daniels,

1985; cf. Rawls, 1971). This would imply an explicit *"fairness-first"* approach to health care resource allocation decisions, which would make treatment of motor neuron disease or reimbursement coverage for expensive drugs for rare diseases ("orphan drugs," the development of which is encouraged by European policy: Aronson, 2006) not *necessarily* (!) "a small extravagance" (McGregor, 2006), which is (still) tolerated owing to its limited budgetary impact (*sic!*) but not justifiable on the grounds of cost-effectiveness (Table 7.1; McCabe et al., 2005, 2006; Hughes, 2006; Connock et al., 2006; Hughes et al., 2005; Marshall, 2005; Sheehan, 2005; NICE, 2004n; McKie and Richardson, 2003; but also, Anonymous, 2002). Assigning a higher priority to the objective of fairness compared to efficiency may have both normative and empirical support (e.g., Richardson and McKie, 2005; Dolan et al., 2005; Schlander, 2005a,b; McKie and Richardson, 2003; Nord, 1993, 1999; Nord et al., 1999; Savulescu, 1999; Menzel, 1990; Harris, 1987; Daniels, 1985), but it would absolutely not abolish the need for economic analysis to moderate fairness-driven reasoning. Importantly, however, it has been argued that current standards of health economic evaluation might need reinterpretation, concerning both the appropriate valuation of benefits (e.g., Mortimer, 2006; Pinto-Prades and Abellan-Perpinan, 2005; Schlander, 2005a; Nord, 1993, 1999; McGregor, 2003; but also Chong, 2003) and the determination of relevant costs (Richardson and McKie, 2006). This represents an equally intriguing and important area for further scientific endeavor and debate.

At the extreme end of the spectrum would be a *"fairness-only"* approach, but this is not considered here since it would appear too naïve to pretend that clinical decision-making has nothing to do with cost.

Some implications should be obvious from the ADHD case and the discussion above. If, for instance, the overarching objectives of collectively financed health care prominently included to protect (to maintain, to restore, or to compensate for

Table 7.1 Cost-effectiveness ratios for orphan treatments
Cost-effectiveness ratios for orphan treatments Cost-effectiveness ratios for many orphan treatments (sometimes referred to as "expensive treatments for rare diseases"; cf. Laupacis, 2006) will not meet the benchmark adopted by NICE (£20,000 to £30,000 per QALY gained; NICE, 2004c). Should these treatments be excluded from reimbursement, with the consequence of depriving patients afflicted with these rare disorders from any *chance* of effective treatment? ICER, incremental cost-effectiveness ratio; MPS, mucopolysaccharidosis. Estimates by NICE. Data source: www.nice.org.uk/download.aspx?o=296850.

Condition	Prevalence	Product	ICER ("preliminary estimated £ per QALY")
M. Gaucher (Type I and III)	270	Imiglucerase (Ceredase[R])	391,200
MPS Type 1	130	Laronidase (Aldurazyme[R])	334,900
M. Fabry	200	Agalsidase beta (Fabrazyme[R])	203,000
Hemophilia B	350	Nonacog alpha (BeneFIX[R])	172,500
M. Gaucher (Type I)	270	Miglustat	116,800

the loss of) normal functioning and, thereby, [strive to] guarantee that individuals have a fair range of opportunities to pursue their personal life plans, as proposed by Norman Daniels (1985, 2001; cf. also Harris, 1997), then current standards of health economic evaluation would not (yet) be aligned with this goal. In this case, instead of relying (almost) exclusively on QALYs as an instrument to measure health-related outcomes, other approaches to economic evaluation might be pursued by policy-makers, either as complements to or as substitutes for cost-utility analysis. Explicit criteria to determine acceptability and desirability of medical interventions might be specified, which could be used in combination with formal economic evaluation. Scorecards might be developed to consider distributional issues and to balance quantitative and qualitative information in an explicit and transparent manner. Formal economic evaluation would continue to provide key quantitative input. However, once the claim of the alleged superiority of extrawelfarist cost-utility analyses over cost-benefit evaluation has been given up (or is no longer necessary), allocation decisions might be informed by cost-benefit analyses, which have the advantage that they are firmly grounded in economic theory (cf. Birch and Donaldson, 2003). To make optimal use of the available clinical evidence base, any type of analysis might be appropriately supported by supplementary cost-effectiveness evaluations, which would enable better differentiation of alternative medical intervention strategies, i.e., serve to address issues related to technical efficiency.

Assuming the Department of Health (DoH), the National Health Service (NHS), and NICE were not prepared to modify their currently prevailing social value judgments[6], they would still have an option to use cost-effectiveness analyses in addition to cost-utility estimates. Again, once desirability at the level of resource allocation has been established, additional cost-effectiveness analyses would be useful to maximize technical efficiency.

7.3 Research Agenda

A number of important areas for further research can be identified. NICE itself has initiated research in fields such as implementation of guidance, further development of its methods, or the societal value of a QALY[7].

---

[6] The NICE Citizens Council, in its January 26–28, 2006, meeting (for minutes, see NICE, 2006e), considered the "rule of rescue," which was broadly understood to pertain to "exceptional cases" where someone's life was in immediate or imminent danger. Many of its members felt that "allowing 'exceptional case treatment' was the mark of a civilised and humane society" (NICE, 2006e, p. 14). The Citizens Council noted that NICE apparently had implicitly – without transparent criteria – applied a "rule of rescue" in previous appraisals, citing the cases of (a) temozolomide (for treatment of certain brain tumors, at an estimated cost per QALY (ICER) of ~£35,000); (b) riluzole (motor neuron disease, ~£34,000 to ~£43,500); (c) imatinib (advanced leukemia, ~£48,000). It will be interesting to see whether NICE will respond by defining a set of explicit criteria, which might imply moving to a variant of the "scorecard approach" proposed above.

[7] For a review of some related issues, see Gyrd-Hansen, 2005.

The simple linear (quasi-utilitarian) QALY aggregation rule implies a maximization principle[8] rather than a methodology of fairness (cf. Ubel et al., 2000; Menzel et al., 1999), and in cost-utility analysis, there is some obvious confusion between social values and preferences or utilities (Nord et al., 1995). This raises the challenge to construct an ethically sensitive framework for cost-effectiveness analysis (Daniels, 2004). One such approach would be to systematically determine community values relevant to health care resource allocation decisions (Richardson and McKie, 2006; Ubel, 1999b). Research in this field should be pursued with high priority.

Another promising approach was proposed by Erik Nord (1995, 1999) but is not without its own problems (cf. Osterdal, 2003). The basic idea is to establish a person trade-off methodology as a basis for "cost-value analysis" that reflects the trade-offs society wishes to make between competing programs. Cost-value analysis certainly requires further research, which seems justified as it promises to enable public policy following the public's values.

It has been further proposed that there is a need to reconsider current practice as to the inclusion or exclusion of various types of cost in meaningful economic evaluations, i.e., those reflecting the real world situation of social transfer payments resulting from the decisions evaluated, instead of solving an artificially defined decision analytic problem in isolation, as has been briefly mentioned earlier. It might appear more appropriate to fully consider existing alternatives and their consequences, an observation which creates an intriguing field for further debate about relevant economic support of medical resource allocation problems (see Richardson and McKie, 2006).

Yet another path forward might be to reexamine the potential of cost-benefit analysis in health care (Birch and Donaldson, 2003; Johannesson and Jönsson, 1991; and some others). In environmental economics, for example, cost-benefit analysis has been a standard method for decades now. Research into ways of how best to address distributional concerns associated with cost-benefit analysis (with or without additional qualitative criteria) would seem a good investment (cf. various contributions in Barer et al., 1998).

Finally, projects have been initiated in Canada and Europe to define a health benefit basket, i.e., "the totality of services, activities, and goods covered by publicly funded insurance schemes or National Health Services" (Schreyögg et al., 2005; Flood et al., 2004). Beyond description of the status quo (jurisdictions, including the United Kingdom [Mason, 2005] do not usually have explicit benefit catalogs), a major research avenue needs to address which services *should* be publicly covered, and what should be the criteria for such decisions, recognizing that priority-setting decisions involve competing goals and multiple stakeholder relationships, and are not amenable to simplistic solutions. The optimal role of economic evaluation might be better defined by explicit reference to its context (cf., for instance, Mitton and Donaldson, 2004).

---

[8] As was briefly discussed earlier, this aggregation rule is empirically flawed (e.g., Dolan et al., 2005; Schlander, 2005a).

7.4 Final Note

This critical case analysis needs to be seen in the context of the evolving achievements and the pioneering role of NICE. Although "still in its infancy" (Williams, 2004), NICE has changed the way of thinking about resource allocation far beyond its area of remit in England and Wales. Its processes have been hailed for their predictability, transparency, and participatory nature. The level of sophistication and rigor that NICE has been striving for in its innovating role is admirable from an international viewpoint. New standards have been set, for instance, with the adoption of probabilistic sensitivity analyses (though on occasion one might wonder about other sources of uncertainty hidden in critical assumptions).

Yet, even NICE is not perfect. Given its high international profile, health care policy-makers elsewhere, who are contemplating making better use of economic analyses, need to be aware of strengths and weaknesses of the NICE approach to enable the distinction to be made between copying NICE and learning from NICE. This case analysis, it is hoped, may contribute insights into the real-life application of NICE processes, so to speak, "when the rubber hits the road." Its findings do not exactly confirm "NICE's use of cost effectiveness as an exemplar of a deliberative process" (as claimed by Culyer, 2006).

Even strong conceptual face-validity – which in any event should not be confused with criterion validity – would have to be confirmed by impeccable quality of realization. If and when that cannot be accomplished consistently, health economists might find that they are indeed "just kidding themselves" about the full potential of their discipline (cf. Drummond, 2004). When it comes to health care resource allocation decisions affecting large numbers of patients, consistent attainment of the highest standards in terms of validity, objectivity, and reliability of the underlying evaluations should be expected. International policy-makers would seem well advised not to settle for anything less.

Appendices

Appendix A
Abbreviations and Use of Terminology

A4R	"Accountability for reasonableness," a framework for fair processes to reach priority setting decisions (Daniels and Sabin, 1997, 1998, 2002)
AC	NICE Appraisal Committee
ACD	Appraisal Consultation Document
Adderall[R]	A combination of DEX and amphetamine salts, not licensed for use in the UK
ADHD–RS	A narrow band ADHD symptom scale, in its version IV updated for and directly derived from DSM–IV symptom criteria (Collett et al., 2003)
AG	Assessment Group
AR	Assessment Report
ATX	Atomoxetine hydrochloride (Strattera[R]), a non-stimulant drug for treatment of ADHD; cf. Table 1.2
Beh	Behavioral treatment arm of the NIMH MTA Study
b.i.d.	Administration divided in two daily doses
CC	Community comparison arm of the NIMH MTA Study
CD	Conduct disorder
CEA	Cost-effectiveness analysis
CEAC	Cost-effectiveness acceptability curve (cf. Fenwick et al., 2004)
CGI	Clinical Global Impressions Scale, a global outcome measure widely used in clinical psychopharmacology trials, consisting of three "sub–scales" (one question each); easy to administer, but controversial psychometric properties (cf. Guy, 2000)
Ch.	Chapter
CI	Confidence interval
CIC	Commercial-in-confidence

CIS | Columbia Impairment Scale, a fully structure questionnaire to assess functioning in four domains, interpersonal relations, psychopathology, job or schoolwork, and leisure time (cf. Bird, 2000)

Comb | Combination treatment arm of the NIMH MTA Study

Commentators | Organizations involved in the NICE appraisal process; without right of appeal

Consultees | Organizations involved in the NICE appraisal process asked to submit information; with right of appeal (typically manufacturers, professional and patient/caregiver groups)

CPRS(-H) | Conners' Parents' Rating Scale (-H: hyperactivity sub-scale)

CRS | Conners' Rating Scales, a family of related narrow band scales; most widely used in the assessment and treatment of ADHD

CTRS(-H) | Conners' Teachers Rating Scale(-H: hyperactivity subscale)

CUA | Cost-utility analysis

DALY | Disability-adjusted life year

DoH | Department of Health

DEX | Dexamphetamine sulphate (e.g., Dexedrine^R); cf. Table 1.2

DSM-IV | Diagnostic criteria of the American Psychiatric Association; for ADHD, specifying three subtypes: primarily inattention, primarily hyperactivity and impulsivity, and a combined type of ADHD; DSM-IV criteria are commonly used in North America

EQ–5D | A generic instrument for measuring health–related quality of life (HRQoL), formerly known as "EuroQoL"

ER | Extended release (used by AG to collectively describe modified release formulations of MPH)

FAD | Final Appraisal Determination

HRQoL | Health-related quality of life

HTA | Health technology assessment

ICD–10 | Diagnostic criteria of the World Health Organization; for ADHD (hyperkinetic disorder, HKD), requiring the presence of symptoms of inattention and hyperactivity/impulsivity, resulting in a narrower definition of "ADHD" compared to DSM-IV; ICD-10 criteria are frequently used in Europe

ICER | Incremental cost-effectiveness ratio

IHRQL | Index of health-related quality of life

MAS | Mixed amphetamine salts; see Adderall^R

MedMgt	Medication management treatment arm of the NIMH MTA Study
MPH	Methylphenidate hydrochloride
MPH–IR	Methylphenidate hydrochloride, immediate-release formulation (Ritalin[R], Equasym[R], generics); cf. Table 1.2
MPH–MR08	Methylphenidate hydrochloride, modified-release formulation with a duration of action of $\sim$8h (Equasym[R] XL); cf. Table 1.2
MPH–MR12	Methylphenidate hydrochloride, modified-release formulation with a duration of action of $\sim$12h (methylphenidate-OROS; Concerta[R] XL); cf. Table 1.2
MR	Modified-release (preparation)
MTA	(1) "Multimodal Treatment Study," a landmark study in clinical ADHD research initiated by the US National Institute for Mental Health (NIMH)
	(2) "Multiple technology appraisal," the standard process adopted by NICE for health technology appraisals (cf. NICE, 2004b,c)
MTC	Mixed treatment comparison
NDT	Non-drug treatment (primarily psychosocial interventions, such as cognitive behavioral therapy)
NIMH	National Institute of Mental Health, Bethesda, MD
o.a.d.	Administration as one dose per day
ODD	Oppositional-defiant disorder
PD	Pharmacodynamic(s)
PK	Pharmacokinetic(s)
QALY	Quality-adjusted life year
q.i.d.	Administration divided in four daily doses
RCT	Randomized controlled trial
Reference Case	As "reference case," NICE specifies methods it considers most appropriate for the Appraisal Committee's purpose (cf. Table 3.1; NICE, 2004c) – not to be confused with the "reference case" defined by the Washington Panel (Gold et al., 1996)
SNAP–IV	Swanson, Nolan and Pelham-IV Questionnaire, a narrow band ADHD symptom scale reflecting core symptoms defined by DSM-IV, essentially similar to (most of) the Conners' Rating Scales (cf. Collett et al., 2003)

STA	"Single technology appraisal," a new process complementing standard "multiple technology appraisals" (MTAs), adopted by NICE in November 2005 to provide faster guidance on new technologies (cf. NICE, 2006i)
t.i.d.	Administration divided in three daily doses
WAG	Welsh Assembly Government
WHO	World Health Organization

Appendix B
Critical Gaps of Assessment

According to the list of references quoted in the Assessment Report, which comprises a total 320 items, a number of essential sources were not tapped.

In particular, literature review is missing on some areas critical to the assessment. Note that all references listed below had been available at the time the technology assessment was undertaken.

Clinical Effect Measures in ADHD

The extensive literature related to clinical measurement instruments and their psychometric properties was not addressed in the Assessment Report.

For instance, the following references were not reviewed:

APA, 2000;
Beneke and Rasmus, 1992;
Bird et al., 1996;
Bird et al., 1993;
Conners, 2000;
Conners, 1997;
Dahlke et al., 1992;
Danckaerts et al., 1999;
DuPaul, 1991;
DuPaul et al., 1998;
Gilbody et al., 2003;
Guy, 2000;
Guy, 1976;
Kashani et al., 1985;
Loney and Milich, 1982;
Swanson, 1992.

As a consequence, another important aspect also was not addressed in the Assessment Report: There is currently no conclusive evidence available on the long-term effects of short-term symptomatic or functional improvements. (In principle, this knowledge gap is of equal importance for any of the clinical outcome measures considered in the present case analysis.) This, however, is one of the most pressing issues in ADHD treatment research, as important long-term sequelae have been linked to the disorder (cf. main text and, for instance, Wilens and Dodson, 2004; Mannuzza and Klein, 2000)

Impact of Treatment Non-Compliance in ADHD

The extensive literature on treatment compliance was largely missed in the Assessment Report.

For instance, the following references were not reviewed:

Andrade et al., 1995;
Brown et al., 1987;
Brown et al., 1985;
Caro et al., 1999a;
Caro et al., 1999b;
Coghill, 2003;
Cramer et al., 1990;
DiMatteo et al., 2000;
Feinstein, 1990;
Firestone, 1982;
Hack and Chow, 2001;
Hughes et al., 2001;
Hwang et al., 2003
Johnston and Fine, 1993;
Kass et al., 1986;
Kauffman et al., 1981;
Lage and Hwang, 2003;
Lage and Hwang, 2004;
Meredith, 1999;
Métry, 1999;
Miller et al., 2004;
Peck, 1999;
Pelham et al., 2000;
Revicki and Frank, 1999;
Sleator et al.,1982;
Swanson, 2003;
Urquhart, 1999;
Wasson et al., 1992;
Weinstein et al., 2003;
Wilens and Dodson, 2004.

Pharmacokinetic and Pharmacodynamic Properties of Stimulants

Among others, the following references were not discussed in the Assessment Report:

Cox, 1990;
Greenhill, 1992;
Greenhill et al., 2001b;
Kimko et al., 1999;
Patrick et al., 1987;
Pelham et al., 2000;
Swanson et al., 1978;
Vitiello and Burke, 1998.

The gaps above are interpreted here to underscore the need for better integration of clinical and economic perspectives.

Data Synthesis (Meta-Analysis and Mixed Treatment Comparisons)

The following references related to issues encountered in quantitative meta-analyses were not addressed in the Assessment Report:

Borzak and Ridker, 1995;
Bucher et al., 1997;
Chalmers et al., 1987a;
Chalmers et al., 1987b;
Egger and Smith, 1995;
Eysenck, 1978;
Faraone et al., 2003b;
Higgins and Whitehead, 1996;
Hunter and Schmidt, 1990;
Lau et al., 1997;
LeLorier et al., 1997;
Lu and Ades, 2004;
Petitti, 2000;
Peto et al., 1995;
Song et al., 2003.

Comparative Effectiveness and Cost-Effectiveness Analyses

The following economic evaluations of ADHD treatment strategies were not addressed in the Assessment Report:

Annemans and Ingham, 2002;
Donnelly et al., 2004;
Faraone, 2003;
Faraone et al., 2003b;
Iskedjian et al., 2003;
Jensen et al., 2004;
Michelson et al., 2001;
Newcorn et al., 2004 (and 2005);
Schachar et al., 2002 (review);
Schlander, 2004b;
Schlander et al., 2004a,b;
Steinhoff, 2004 (review);
Steinhoff et al., 2003.

Appendix C
Consistency Issues Associated with NICE Assessment

Subject	Statements and Rationales	Consistency Issue
Search criteria	"Economic evaluations reported as conference proceedings or abstracts were excluded since the data may not be complete" (AR, p. 178)	Departure from assessment protocol (King et al., 2004a), which had promised to include "abstracts, conference proceedings, gray literature, ..."
		Violations of predefined search strategy, e.g., overlooked RCTs and CEAs in the public domain.
		The incomplete search did not prevent from claiming that "the review highlighted a number of potential limitations in the existing literature ... in particular ... in estimating treatment effectiveness ..., [which] may stem from a lack of available data" (AR, p. 266).
		Inclusion of (at least) one study in economic model that had been excluded from the effectiveness review and not listed in appendix.
	"This review presents a comprehensive overview of existing *economic* evaluations of MPH, ATX and DEX for children and adolescents with ADHD" (AR, p. 266).	Cost-effectiveness analyses in the public domain (see Table 6.4 and *Appendix, Critical Gaps of Assessment*) were excluded from consideration owing to the illicit change of search criteria (cf. above).
Study inclusion criteria	Minimum study duration was chosen because "the literature suggests that three weeks is the minimum duration for therapeutic trials" assessing "the impact	More than one third of studies included in the effectiveness review were short-term crossover studies with *treatment duration* of one week or less, and some of

on the social adjustment of the child" (AR, pp. 44ff.)

them had been conducted without washout phases between treatment periods (cf. Chapter 5, footnote 9).

There was no review of "the literature" supporting the assertion; except for one reference to the DSM-IV diagnostic manual (AR, p. 45).

If social adjustment of a child is the clinical outcome of interest, then (a) a clinical effect measure capturing functional impairment (which was discarded: AR, p. 46) would have been more appropriate than CGI ratings, which were used as a proxy for health-related quality-of-life (for instance: AR, pp. 16, 17, 46, 48), and (b) crossover designs will be problematic due to frequent violation of the requirement that "a similar baseline condition must be present at the start of each of the treatment periods, ... and there must not be any carryover (i.e. residual) effects (even psychological ones) after either treatment" (Spilker, 1991).

Outcome measures

A "plethora of instruments" was noted (AR, p. 178) and it was recognized that "the choice of an outcome measure is a critical design issue" (AR, p. 178)

These observations were not followed up by an exploration of the extensive literature on this subject area (cf. CRD, 2003; Collett et al., 2003; APA, 2000).

Conners Rating Scales

Rejected for economic modeling...

... although representing the most widely used effect measure in ADHD research to date, and the only one enabling quantitative synthesis in previous reviews.

... on the basis of a critique of the "implicit assumption that a small gain in CTRS score for many children is assumed to be the same as the cost and desirability of achieving a large gain in CTRS score for few children" (AR, p. 186). Further it was argued that, "if this measure is used, a gain of 1 point on the scale is valued the same, regard

A remarkably similar critique has been put forward (and been supported by a large body of empirical evidence showing that identical QALY differences will not be attached equal social value across the scale – Mortimer, 2006; Richardson and McKie, 2005; Dolan et al., 2005; Nord et al., 1999) against QALYs, the

less of where you begin on that scale, so the relative value of different effect sizes is not readily interpretable" (AR, p. 224).

... on the basis of a critique of the "implicit assumption ... that efficacy is constant across baseline levels of ADHD severity. ... However, the efficacy of stimulants [or medication in general] *may* depend on the quality and severity of symptoms" (AR, p. 186).

outcome measure used for economic evaluation following NICE reference case guidance.

The advantage of the CGI-I scores selected for primary evaluation remains unclear, as this score consists of only one item, reading "Rate total improvement ... compared to the patient's condition and admission to the project" (Guy, 1976) – hardly constituting a measure independent from baseline severity or commanding interval-scale properties.

QALY calculation

For utility estimates it was explicitly recognized that "the validity of these measures depends on the content and style of the vignette used to describe each health state" (AR, p. 181).

Health state utilities derived from a company submission were used for extended sensitivity analyses (AR, p. 235, pp. 240ff.), ...

Utility data for the primary economic evaluation came from "values obtained using a *standard gamble* technique from parents of children with ADHD, providing proxy ratings for their children" (AR, p. 235).

Utility "values *obtained directly from patients*, using standard gamble methodology, may be [more] relevant to this review" (AR, p. 182).

Health state descriptions for utility measurement (responders and non-responders) did not match the CGI Criteria (as well as other criteria synthesized) criteria (cf. AR, pp. 359ff.).

... although inconsistencies of these values had been identified (AR, p. 217), and inspection of health state descriptions (e.g., AR, pp. 359ff.) reveals "double-counting" of side effects for MPH-IR and MPH-MR.

In fact, these utilities were derived from *EQ-5D questionnaires* completed by parents or caregivers (Coghill et al., 2004).

NICE guidance asks for a representative sample of the public as the source of utility data. Further, there are specific concerns about the reliability of self-reports of children with ADHD.

Quantitative synthesis (meta-analysis using mixed-treatment comparison technique)

For the base case economic model (primary evaluation), CGI-I based "response rates" were synthesized and combined with utility estimates for responders and non-responders.

Primary analysis resulted in *inconsistent rankings* of strategies (Table 6.7 of AR, p. 237), which were not even mentioned in the body of the text, except for the remark that "the difference in QALY gains between the alternative treatments strategies was very small" (AR, p. 236).

Full text:

For secondary extensions of the model, response rates, which had been derived from heterogeneous criteria, were synthesized. Scales included (besides CGI-I and CGI-S) the ADHD-RS and the SNAP-IV (AR, p. 254), which were described as "disease specific instruments" measuring "health-related quality of life in children" (AR, p. 176).

The ADHD-RS and the SNAP-IV are typical narrow-band symptom scales.

The assessment protocol had stated that "relative risks will only be pooled when this is statistically and clinically meaningful."

Heterogeneity of parameters such as patient populations (age, sex, comorbidity, etc.), study designs (efficacy, effectiveness), treatments (intensity, combination with non-drug treatment), and effect measures was mentioned repeatedly.

Despite heterogeneity of effect measures across treatments and studies, there is no evidence that potential confounding effects between treatment strategies and effect measures were assessed.

Effectiveness versus efficacy distinction

The distinction between efficacy and effectiveness was not addressed in the assessment report; both terms were apparently used interchangeably, without discrimination.

In his authoritative textbook, the senior author of the Assessment Report explained the fundamental importance of this differentiation for a meaningful economic analysis. He stated that "clinical trials are artificial environments, and do not provide all the economic information needed by decision-makers" (Drummond et al., 1997), and "for economic evaluations to be relevant, they need to reflect the real-world conditions faced by the decision-maker" (Buxton et al., 1997).

Discussion of the MTA study in the AR ran over five pages in the clinical effectiveness review (AR, pp. 164ff.).

However, the extensive measures to ensure fidelity and adherence were not described (MTA, 1999a,b), and the mediator analyses clearly showing the impact of treatment adherence on treatment response were missed; cf. AR, pp. 167ff.

"The effect of compliance on response rates to MPH-IR and MPH-MR is reflected in the model" (AR, p. 250).

This approach ignored the difference between efficacy and effectiveness trials and the AR did not discuss the extensive literature on non-compliance in general and in ADHD specifically.

Non-compliance was assumed to be a subset of non-response in RCTs (AR, p. 232: implying that "double-blind, double-dummy trials" ... "capture the effects of compliance").

In contrast, the senior author of the assessment stated elsewhere, "great efforts are typically made in the conduct of a clinical trial to ensure that patients consume their prescribed medications" and, referring to the situation outside trials, "to the extent that patients do not comply with the prescribed therapy, there may be a dilution of the treatment effect originally observed in the trial" (Drummond et al., 2005). He explicitly recommended the review of Hughes et al (2001) who concluded "that *sensitivity analysis* should be applied appropriately to ascertain the impact of non-compliance on the cost-effectiveness of drug therapies".

"The exploration of the effects of non-compliance would involve a number of assumptions ... it was felt that these modeling assumptions would not be reasonable given the lack of appropriate data, which would render the results of any *sensitivity analysis* around compliance uninformative to decision-makers" (AR, p. 233).

Any assumption was felt unjustified concerning "the distribution of reduced compliance between morning, lunchtime, and evening doses of medication" (AR, p. 232f.).

A study from Canada had been in the public domain that indicated that MPH doses were frequently missed, with the second and, in particular, the third daily doses most affected (Hwang et al., 2003). This study was not discussed in the AR.

"Health outcomes [...] in an economic analysis [...] should also consider overall treatment effectiveness as observed in real-world settings. Effectiveness can include outcomes such as loss of efficacy [...], compliance with therapy..." (Drummond, 2003).

Economic model

Stochastic analysis: "The model is probabilistic, meaning that relevant input parameters are entered as probabilistic distributions rather than point estimates in order to *represent the uncertainty* around each point estimate" (AR, p. 220). "The output from the model incorporates the uncertainty around the estimated response rates..." (AR, p. 229). As to the MTA subgroup analyses, it was stated that these evaluations "should

This is inconsistent with the use of CGI-I scores as a primary efficacy parameter, because these were not the primary outcome parameters of the underlying RCTs. While it is quite legitimate to carry out secondary analyses, these should not be presented as main results *assumed to capture the uncertainty*.

be seen as 'exploratory', because of the danger of *repeated statistical testing* with a sample not designed for this purpose" (AR, p. 167).

Although double-counting of non-responders in the economic model was recognized (AR, p. 230) ...

... there was no further exploration of the resulting distortion, because it was (erroneously) reasoned that "none of the ... trials calculated response in an intent-to-treat analysis" (AR, p. 230). Data on withdrawal rates indicate that not all treatments assessed were affected equally (cf. AR, Table 6.3, p. 231, and AR, Table 6.6, p. 236).

"The nature of the treatment received in the community comparison arm of the MTA trial is still unclear, and as a result this data is omitted from the analysis" (AR, p. 254).

A table in the Assessment Report, however, states that three of its four arms were included: "results for behavioral treatment were omitted as not relevant to this review" (AR, Table 6.17, p. 254). Thus it remains enigmatic which arm of the MTA was actually omitted from analysis.

For secondary analyses, "we can also incorporate the results of the MTA trial, but only by assuming that the medical management group in that trial represents treatment with MPH-IR" (AR, p. 253).

It was noted in the effectiveness review (AR, p. 165) that "most of the children in the community care group (97/146) received stimulant medication." Using the medication management arm of the MTA study as a proxy for MPH-IR contradicts the importance of treatment adherence found in that study (see above; MTA Cooperative Group, 1999b) as well as the extensive measures to ensure treatment fidelity and adherence in this trial (MTA Cooperative Group, 1999a).

"A number of studies excluded from the effectiveness review, for reasons of data presentations, were nevertheless ... included in the calculation of response rate for the cost-effectiveness analysis. Further details of these excluded studies are given in appendix 3" (AR, pp. 225ff.)

Appendix 3 of the AR lists all studies excluded and does *not* provide any information about which studies might have been included in the economic model in addition to five studies of the clinical effectiveness review and Sharp et al. 1999; (cf. AR, pp. 333ff.).

Extrapolation over 12 years

"In this extended analysis, costs are discounted at an annual rate

NICE guidance specifies that costs and health benefits should

	of 6%, and health benefits are discounted at an annual rate of 1.5%, in accordance with NICE guidance" (AR, p. 233).	be discounted at an annual rate of 3.5% (see Table 3.1).
	"There is little data on long-term efficacy [...] associated with medical management of ADHD" (AR, p. 19).	Inclusion of 14-months data from the MTA study remained enigmatic (see above, *Economic Model*), and other long-term studies were excluded from the review.
	Long-term sequelae of the disorder briefly mentioned as potential "long-term benefits of treatment" (AR, p. 247).	Long-term sequelae of ADHD were neither mentioned in Executive Summary nor in Conclusions of the Assessment Report, and were not explored by literature search. Long-term extrapolation model did include a discussion of mid- to long-term effects ("sensitivity to time horizon": AR, pp. 245ff.).
Limitations	"Clear conclusions," stated repeatedly (cf. below, Executive Summary): AR, pp.19, 261, 266).	*Caveats* scattered throughout the report (e.g., AR, pp. 45, 224, 261ff.). Porzsolt et al. (2005) identified "a serious problem" in "HTA reports which ... express limitations in the discussions (read by many scientists) but not in the conclusions (read mainly by policy-makers)."
Executive Summary on Cost-Effectiveness (AR, pp. 18ff.)	"For a decision taken now, with current available data, the results of the economic evaluation clearly identified an optimal treatment strategy. That is, ..."	Limitations of the model described incompletely, suggesting limited available information without indicating impact of study selection criteria chosen (e.g., regarding long-term studies excluded from review and economic model – see above).
	Caveats: "The model is not without limitations. As identified in the clinical effectiveness review, the reporting of studies was poor, there is little data to discriminate between the drugs in efficacy or adverse events and there is little data on long-term efficacy and adverse events associated with medical management of ADHD. The data do not allow discrimination between patients with ADHD in terms of ADHD subtype, age, gender or previous treatment."	Model, however, was limited to response rates based on CGI-I ratings, which were subsequently pooled for secondary "sensitivity" analysis with various (heterogeneous) "response rates".

Irrespective of their interpretation, each of the inconsistencies identified constitutes a gap of the assessment, i.e., important aspects were not adequately considered. AR, Assessment Report.

References

References

Aaron, H.J. (2003) Should public policy seek to control the growth of health care spending? *Health Affairs*, Web Exclusives January 2003: W3-28-W3-36.

Abikoff, H.G., Hechtman, L., Klein, R.G., et al. (2004a) Symptomatic improvement in children with ADHD treated with long-term methylphenidate and multimodal psychosocial treatment. *Journal of the American Academy of Child and Adolescent Psychiatry* 43 (7): 802–811.

Abikoff, H., Hechtman, L., Klein, R.G., et al. (2004b) Social functioning in children with ADHD treated with long-term methylphenidate and multimodal psychosocial treatment. *Journal of the American Academy of Child & Adolescent Psychiatry* 43 (7): 820–829.

Abikoff, H., Jensen, P., Arnold, L.E., et al. (2002) Observed classroom behavior of children with ADHD: relationship to gender and comorbidity. *Journal of Abnormal Child Psychology* 30: 349–359.

Achenbach, T.M., Edelbrock, C.S. (1987) *Manual for the Youth Self-Report and Profile*. Burlington, VT: Department of Psychiatry, University of Vermont.

Adler, M.D. (2005) *QALYs and policy evaluation: a new perspective*. University of Pennsylvania Law School, Paper 59. Available online at http://lsr.nellco.org/upenn/wps/papers/59.

Ades, A.E., Lu, G. (2003) Correlations between parameters in risk models: estimation and propagation of uncertainty by Markov chain Monte Carlo. *Risk Analysis* 6: 1165–1172.

Ades, A.E., Claxton, K., Sculpher M. (2006) Evidence synthesis, parameter correlation and probabilistic sensitivity analysis. *Health Economics* 15 (4): 373–381.

Ahmann, P.A., Waltonen, S.J., Olson, K.A., et al. (1993) Placebo-controlled evaluation of Ritalin side effects. *Pediatrics* 91: 1101–1106.

Akehurst, R., Anderson, P., Brazier, J., et al. (2000) Decision analytic modelling in the economic evaluation of health technologies: a consensus statement. *Pharmacoeconomics* 17 (5): 443–444.

American Academy of Child and Adolescent Psychiatry [AACAP] (2002) Practice parameter for the use of stimulant medications in the treatment of children, adolescents, and adults. *Journal of the American Academy of Child & Adolescent Psychiatry* 41 (2 Supplement): 26S–49S.

American Academy of Pediatrics [AAP] (2001) Subcommittee on Attention-Deficit / Hyperactivity Disorder and Committee on Quality Improvement. Clinical practice guideline: treatment of the school-aged child with attention-deficit/hyperactivity disorder. *Pediatrics* 108 (4): 1033–1044.

American Psychiatric Association [APA] (2000) *Handbook of Psychiatric Measures*. Washington, DC: APA.

American Psychiatric Association [APA] (1994) *Diagnostic and statistical manual of mental disorders (DSM-IV)*. Washington, DC: American Psychiatric Association, 4th edn.

Anand, P. (2005) Capabilities and health. *Journal of Medical Ethics* 31: 299–303.

Andersen, S.L., Teicher, M.H. (2000) Sex differences in dopamine receptors and their relevance to ADHD. *Neuroscience & Biobehavioral Reviews* 24 (1): 137–141.

Anderson, G.F., Reinhardt, U.E., Hussey, P.S., Petrosyan, V. (2003) It's the prices, stupid: why the United States is so different from other countries. *Health Affairs* 22 (3): 89–105.

Andrade, S.E., Walker, A.M., Gottlieb, LK, et al. (1995) Discontinuation of antihyperlipidemic drugs – do rates reported in clinical trials reflect rates in primary care settings? *New England Journal of Medicine* 332 (17): 1125–1131.

Annemans, L., Ingham, M. (2002) Estimating cost-effectiveness of Concerta OROS in attention-deficit/hyperactivity disorder (ADHD) – adapting the Canadian Coordinating Office for Health Technology Assessment's (CCOHTA) economic model of methylphenidate immediate release versus behavioural interventions from a parent's perspective. *Value in Health* 5 (6): 517.

Anonymous (2002) When rules about 'orphan drugs' go wrong, costs rise. *Annals of Oncology* 13: 1327.

Arcia, E., Conners, C.K. (1998) Gender differences in ADHD? *Journal of Developmental and Behavioral Pediatrics* 19 (2): 77–83.

Arnesen, T., Nord, E. (1999) The value of DALY life: problems with ethics and validity of disability adjusted life years. *British Medical Journal* 319: 1423–1425.

Arnold L.E. (2001) Alternative treatments for adults with attention-deficit hyperactivity disorder (ADHD). *Annals of the New York Academy of Sciences* 931: 310–341.

Arnold, L.E. (1996) Sex differences in ADHD: conference summary. *Journal of Abnormal Child Psychology* 24 (5): 555–569.

Arnold, L.E., Molina, B., Swanson, J., et al. (2005) *New ADHD insights from MTA data through 36 months*. Presented at the 52nd Annual Meeting of the American Academy of Child & Adolescent Psychiatry (AACAP), Toronto, Ontario, October 18-23, Scientific Proceedings, C69, p. 150.

Aronson, J.K. (2006) Editor's view: Rare diseases and orphan drugs. *British Journal of Clinical Pharmacology* 61 (3): 243–245.

Asherson, P., and the IMAGE Consortium (2004) Attention-deficit hyperactivity disorder in the post-genomic era. *European Child & Adolescent Psychiatry* 13 (Suppl. 1): 50–70.

Audit Commission (2005) *Managing the financial implications of NICE guidance.* (September 08, 2005) Available online at: http://www.audit-commission.gov.uk/reports/national-report.asp?categoryid=&prodid=cc53ddfe-42c8-49c7-bb53-9f6485262718&from reportsanddata=national-report&page=index.asp&area=hplink.Last accessed December 20, 2005

Australian Government, Department of Health and Ageing (2005a) *November 2005 PBAC Outcomes – Subsequent decisions not to recommend.* Available online at: http://www.health.gov.au/internet/wcms/publishing.nsf/Content/pbacrecnov05-subsequent_rejections.Last accessed February 15, 2006.

Australian Government, Department of Health and Ageing (2005b) *Atomoxetine hydrochloride, capsules, 10mg, 18mg, 25mg, 40mg and 60mg, Strattera^R, November 2005.* Available online at http://www.health.gov.au/internet/wcms/publishing.nsf/content/pbac-psd-atomoxetine-nov05. November 2005. Last accessed September 01, 2006.

Avorn, J. (2006) Part "D" for "defective" – the Medicare drug-benefit chaos. *New England Journal of Medicine* 354 (13): 1339–1341.

Baltussen, R., Leidl, R., Ament, A. (1999) Real world designs in economic evaluation: bridging the gap between clinical research and policy-making. *Pharmacoeconomics* 16 (5): 449–458.

Banaschewski, T., Coghill, D., Santosh, P., et al. (2006) Long-acting medications for the hyperkinetic disorders. A systematic review and European treatment guideline. *European Child & Adolescent Psychiatry* 15 (8): 476–495.

Banaschewski, T., Roessner, V., Dittmann, R.W., et al. (2004) Non-stimulant medications in the treatment of ADHD. *European Child & Adolescent Psychiatry* 13 (Supplement 1): 102–116.

Barer, M.L., Getzen, T.E., Stoddart, G.L. [eds.] (1998) *Health, health care, and health economics: perspectives on distribution.* New York, NY: Wiley.

Barkley, R.A. (2004) Driving impairments in teens and adults with attention-deficit/hyperactivity disorder. *Psychiatric Clinics of North America* 27 (2): 233–260.

Barkley, R.A. (2002) Major life activity and health outcomes associated with attention-deficit/hyperactivity disorder. *Journal of Clinical Psychiatry* 63 (Supplement 12): 10–15.

Barkley, R.A., Connor, D.F., Kwasnik, D. (2000) Challenges to determining adolescent medication response in an outpatient clinical setting: comparing Adderall and methylphenidate for ADHD. *Journal of Attention Disorders* 4: 102–113.

Barkley, R.A., Fischer, M., Edelbrock, C.S., Smallish, L. (1991) The adolescent outcome of hyperactive children diagnosed by research criteria. III. Mother-child interactions, family conflicts and maternal psychopathology. *Journal of Child Psychology and Psychiatry* 32: 233–255.

Barkley, R.A., McMurray, B., Edelbrock, C.S., Robbins, K. (1990) Side effects of methylphenidate in children with attention deficit hyperactivity disorder: a systematic, placebo-controlled evaluation. *Pediatrics* 86: 184–192.

Beneke, M., Rasmus, W. (1992) "Clinical Global Impressions" (ECDEU): some critical comments. *Pharmacopsychiatry* 25: 171–176.

Berg, M., Meurlen, R.T., van den Burg, M. (2001) Guidelines for appropriate care: the importance of empirical normative analysis. *Health Care Analysis* 9 (1): 77–99.

Berger, M.L., Teutsch, S. (2005) Cost-effectiveness analysis: from science to application. *Medical Care* 43 (7 Supplement): 49–53.

Biederman, J., Spencer, T.J., Wilens, T.E., et al. (2006a) Treatment of ADHD with stimulant medications: response to Nissen perspective in The New England Journal of Medicine. *Journal of the American Academy of Child & Adolescent Psychiatry* 45 (10): 1147–1150.

Biederman, J., Amsten, A.F., Faraone, S.V., et al. (2006b) New developments in the treatment of ADHD. *Journal of Clinical Psychiatry* 67: 148–159.

Biederman, J., Kwon, A., Aleardi, M., et al. (2005) Absence of gender effects on attention deficit hyperactivity disorder: findings in nonreferred subjects. *American Journal of Psychiatry* 162 (6): 1083–1089.

Biederman, J., Quinn, D., Weiss, M., et al. (2003) Efficacy and safety of Ritalin LA, a new, once daily, extended-release dosage form of methylphenidate, in children with attention deficit hyperactivity disorder. *Paediatric Drugs* 5: 833–841.

Biederman, J., Lopez, F.A., Boellner, S.W., Chandler, M.C. (2002) A randomized, double-blind, placebo-controlled, parallel group study of SLI381 (Adderall XR) in children with attention-deficit/hyperactivity disorder. *Pediatrics* 110 (2): 258–266.

Birch, S., Donaldson, C. (2003) Valuing the benefits and costs of health care programmes: where's the 'extra' in extra-welfarism? *Social Science & Medicine* 56 (5): 1121–1133.

Birch, S., Gafni, A. (2006a) Information created to evade reality (ICER): things we should not look to for answers. *Pharmacoeconomics* 24 (11): 1121–1131.

Birch, S., Gafni, A. (2006b) Decision rules in economic evaluation. In: Jones, A.M. (editor) *The Elgar Companion to Health Economics*. Cheltenham: Edward Elgar, 492–502.

Birch, S., Gafni, A. (1993) Changing the problem to fit the solution: Johannesson and Weinstein's (mis)application of economics to real world problems. *Journal of Health Economics* 12: 469–476.

Bird, H.R. (2000) Columbia Impairment Scale (CIS). In: American Psychiatric Association, *Handbook of Psychiatric Measures*. Washington, DC: APA, 367–369.

Bird, H.R., Andrews, H., Schwab Stone, M., et al. (1996) Global measures of impairment for epidemiological and clinical use with children and adolescents. *International Journal of Methods in Psychiatric Research* 6 (4): 295–307.

Bird, H., Shaffer, D., Fisher, P., Gould, M. (1993) The Columbia Impairment Scale (CIS): pilot findings on a measure of global impairment for children and adolescents. *International Journal of Methods in Psychiatric Research* 3: 167–176.

Blades, C.A., Culyer, A.J., Walker, A.M. (1987) Health service efficiency: appraising the appraisers: a critical review of economic appraisal in practice. *Social Science & Medicine* 25 (5): 461–472.

Blaug, M. (1998) Where are we now in British health economics? *Health Economics* 7 (Suppl. 1): S63–S78.

Bleichrodt, H., Pinto, J.L. (2006) Conceptual foundations for health utility measurement. In: Jones, A.M. (ed.) *The Elgar Companion to Health Economics*. Cheltenham, London: Edward Elgar.

Boadway, R.W., Bruce, N. (1984) *Welfare Economics*. Oxford: Basil Blackwell.

Borzak, S., Ridker, P.M. (1995) Discordance between meta-analyses and large-scale randomized, controlled trials. *Annals of Internal Medicine* 123: 873–877.

Boyd, N.F., Sutherland, H.J., Heasman, Z.K., et al. (1990) Whose utilities for decision analysis? *Medical Decision-Making* 10: 58–67.

Breggin, P. (2002) *The Ritalin Fact Book*. Cambridge, MA: Perseus.

Brennan, A., Akehurst, R. (2000) Modelling in health economic evaluation: What is its place? What is its value? *Pharmacoeconomics* 17 (5): 445–459.

Breyer, F., Zweifel, P.S., Kifmann, M. (2003) *Gesundheitsökonomie*. Berlin, Heidelberg, New York, NY: Springer (4th edition).

Bridges, J.F.P. (2005) Future challenges for the economic evaluation of healthcare. *Pharmacoeconomics* 23 (4): 317–321.

Briggs, A. (2001) Handling uncertainty in economic evaluation and presenting the results. In: Drummond, M., McGuire, A.J. (eds.) *Economic evaluation in health care: merging theory with practice*. Oxford: Oxford University Press, 172–214.

Briggs, A.H. (2000) Handling uncertainty in cost-effectiveness models. *Pharmacoeconomics* 17 (5): 479–500.

Briggs, A., Gray, A. (2000) Using cost effectiveness information. *British Medical Journal* 320: 246.

Briggs, A.H., Gray, A.M. (1999) Handling uncertainty when performing economic evaluations of healthcare interventions. *Health Technology Assessment* 3 (2): 1–134.

Briggs, A.H., O'Brien, B.J., Blackhouse, G. (2002) Thinking outside the box: recent advances in the analysis and presentation of uncertainty in cost-effectiveness studies. *Annual Review of Public Health* 23: 377–401.

Briggs, A., Sculpher, M., Buxton, M. (1994) Uncertainty in the economic evaluation of health care technologies: the role of sensitivity analysis. *Health Economics* 3 (2): 95–104.

Brown, R.T., Sexten, S.B. (1988) A controlled trial of methylphenidate in black adolescents. Attentional, behavioural, and psychological effects. *Clinical Pediatrics* 27: 74–81.

Brown, R.T., Borden, K.A., Wynne, M.E., et al. (1987) Compliance with pharmacologic and cognitive treatment for attention deficit disorder. *Journal of Child and Adolescent Psychopharmacology* 26 (4): 521–526.

Brown, R.T., Borden, K.A., Clingerman, S.R. (1985) Adherence to methylphenidate therapy in a population: a preliminary investigation. *Psychopharmacology Bulletin* 21 (1): 28–36.

Brühl B, Döpfner M, Lehmkuhl G (2000) Der Fremdbeurteilungsbogen fuer hyperkinetische Störungen (FBB-HKS) – Prävalenz hyperkinetischer Störungen im Elternurteil und psychometrische Kriterien. *Kindheit und Entwicklung* 9: 115–125.

Bryan, S., Barton, P., Burls, A. (2001) *The clinical effectiveness and cost-effectiveness of riluzole for motor neurone disease – an update*. Birmingham, January 22, 2001. Available online at: http://www.nice.org.uk/page.aspx?o=14483. Last Accessed February 01, 2004.

Bucher, H.C., Guyatt, G.H., Griffith, L.E., Walter, S.D. (1997) The results of direct and indirect comparisons in meta-analysis of randomized controlled trials. *Journal of Clinical Epidemiology* 50 (6): 683–691.

Buitelaar, J.K., Rothenberger, A. (2004) Foreword – ADHD in the scientific and political context. *European Child & Adolescent Psychiatry* 13 (Suppl. 1): 1–6.

Bundesministerium für Gesundheit (2006a) *Eckpunkte zu einer Gesundheitsreform 2006*. Berlin, July 4, 2006. Available online at www.die-gesundheitsreform.de/gesundheitspolitik/pdf/eckpunkte_gesundheitsreform_2006.pdf. Last accessed July 22, 2006.

Bundesministerium für Gesundheit (2006b) *Entwurf eines Gesetzes zur Stärkung des Wettbewerbs in der Gesetzlichen Krankenversicherung (GKV-Wettbewerbsstärkungsgesetz – GKV-WSG)*. Available online at http://www.die-gesundheitsreform.de/gesundheitspolitik/pdf/gesetzentwurf_wettbewerbsstärkungsgesetz.pdf?param=reform2006. Last accessed January 02, 2007.

Bundesministerium für Gesundheit und Soziales (2005) *Statistik über Versicherte, gegliedert nach Status, Alter, Wohnort, Kassenart: GKV Statistik KM6*. Available online at http://www.bmg.bund.de/ downloads/2004_KM6.pdf.

Burke, K. (2002) No cash to implement NICE, health authorities tell MPs. *British Medical Journal* 324: 258.

Busse, R., Orvain, J., Velasco, M., et al. (2002) Best practice in undertaking and reporting health technology assessments. Working group 4 report. *International Journal of Technology Assessment in Health Care* 18 (2): 361–422.

Buxton, M.J. (2006) Economic evaluation and decision making in the UK. *Pharmacoeconomics* 24 (11): 1133–1142.

Buxton, M. (2001) Implications of the appraisal function of the National Institute for Clinical Excellence (NICE). *Value in Health* 4 (3): 212–216.

Buxton, M.J. (1987) Economic forces and hospital technology. *International Journal of Technology Assessment in Health Care* 3: 241–251.

Buxton, M.J., Akehurst R. (2006) How NICE is the UK's fast-track system? *Scrip Magazine*, March 2006: 24–25.

Buxton, M., Drummond, M.F., Van Hout, B.A., et al. (1997) Modelling in economic evaluation: an unavoidable fact of life. *Health Economics* 6: 217–227.

Cambridge Pharma Consultancy (2002) *Delays in market access.* Cambridge, December 2002.

Caro, J.J., Salas, M., Speckman, J.L., et al. (1999a) Persistence with treatment for hypertension in actual practice. *Canadian Medical Association Journal (CMAJ)* 160 (1): 31–37.

Caro, J.J., Speckman, J.L., Salas, M., et al. (1999b) Effect of initial drug choice on persistence with antihypertensive therapy: the importance of actual practice data. *Canadian Medical Association Journal (CMAJ)* 160 (1): 41–46.

Castellanos, F.X., Giedd, J.N., Elia, J., et al. (1997) Controlled stimulant treatment of ADHD and comorbid Tourette's syndrome: effects of stimulant and dose. *Journal of the American Academy of Child & Adolescent Psychiatry* 36: 589–596.

Centre for Reviews and Dissemination [CRD] (2001) *CRD Report No. 4: Undertaking systematic reviews of research on effectiveness: CRD's guidance for those carrying out systematic reviews.* York: NHS Centre for Reviews and Dissemination, University of York (2nd edition, March 2001).

Chalmers, T.C., Levin, H., Sacks, H.S., et al. (1987a) Meta-analysis of clinical trials as a scientific discipline: I. Control of bias and comparison with large cooperative trials. *Statistics in Medicine* 6: 315–325.

Chalmers, T.C., Berrier, J., Sacks, H.S., et al. (1987b) Meta-analysis of clinical trials as a scientific discipline: II. Replicate variability and comparison of studies that agree and disagree. *Statistics in Medicine* 6: 733–744.

Chernew, M.E., Hirth, R.A., Cutler, D.M. (2003) Increased spending on health care: how much can the United States afford? *Health Affairs* 22 (4): 15–25.

Childs, M. *Eisai and Pfizer sue NICE.* Available online at: http://lists.essential.org/pipermail/ip-health/2006-November/010207.html. Last accessed December 09, 2006.

Chong, C.A.K.Y. (2003) QALYs: the best option so far. *Journal of the Canadian Medical Association (CMAJ)* 168 (11): 1394–1395.

Claxton, K., Sculpher, M., Culyer, A., et al. (2006) Discounting and cost-effectiveness in NICE – stepping back to sort out a confusion. *Health Economics* 15 (1): 1–4.

Claxton, K., Sculpher, M., McCabe, C., et al. (2005) Probabilistic sensitivity analysis for NICE technology assessment: not an optional extra. *Health Economics* 14 (4): 339–347.

Claxton, A., Cramer, J., Pierce, C. (2001) A systematic review of the associations between dose regimens and medication compliance. *Clinical Therapeutics* 23 (8): 1296–1310.

Coghill, D. (2003) Current issues in child and adolescent psychopharmacology. Part 1: Attention-deficit hyperactivity and affective disorders. *Advances in Psychiatric Treatment* 9: 86–94.

Coghill, D., Spender, Q., Barton, J., et al. (2004) Measuring quality of life in children with attention-deficit/hyperactivity disorder in the UK. *16th World Congress of the International Association for Child and Adolescent Psychiatry and Allied Professions (IACAPAP).* Book of Abstracts. Darmstadt: Steinkopff-Verlag 327.

Cohen, J. (1988) *Statistical power analysis for the behavioral sciences.* London: Academic Press (2nd edition).

Collett, B.R., Ohan, J.L., Myers, K.M. (2003) Ten-year review of rating scales. V. Scales assessing attention-deficit/hyperactivity disorder. *Journal of the American Academy for Child and Adolescent Psychiatry* 42 (9): 1015–1037.

Commission of the European Communities (2003) *Communication from the Commission to the Council, the European Parliament, the Economic and Social Committee and the Committee of the Regions: A Stronger European Based Pharmaceutical Industry for the Benefit of the Patient – A Call for Action.* Brussels, July 01, 2003: COM (2003) 383 final.

Commonwealth of Australia (1992) *Guidelines for the pharmaceutical industry on the preparation of submissions to the Pharmaceutical Benefits Advisory Committee.* Canberra, ACD: Department of Health and Family Services.

Conners, C.K. (2000) Conners' Rating Scales – Revised (CRS-R). In: American Psychiatric Association, *Handbook of Psychiatric Measures.* Washington, DC: APA, 329–332.

Conners, C. (1997) *Conners' Rating Scales-Revised Technical Manual.* North Tonawanda, NY: Multi-Health Systems.

Conners, C.K., Epstein, J.N., March, J.S., et al. (2001) Multimodal treatment of ADHD in the MTA: an alternative outcomes analysis. *Journal of the American Academy of Child and Adolescent Psychiatry* 40 (2): 159–167.

Connock, M., Juarez-Garcia, A., Frew, E. et al. (2006) A systematic review of the clinical effectiveness and cost-effectiveness of enzyme replacement therapies for Fabry's disease and mucopolysaccharidosis type 1. *Health Technology Assessment* 10 (20): 1–113.

Cook, T.D., Campbell, D.T. (1979) *Quasi-experimentation: design and analysis issues for field settings.* Boston, MA: Houghton Mifflin.

Cookson, R., McCaid, D., Maynard, A. (2001) Wrong SIGN, NICE mess: is national guidance distorting allocation of resources? *British Medical Journal* 323: 743–745.

Cox, B.M. (1990) Drug tolerance and physical dependence. In: Pratt, W.B., Taylor, P. (eds.) *Principles of Drug Action: The Basis of Pharmacology.* New York, NY: Churchill Livingstone, 639–690.

Cox, E.R., Motheral, B.R., Henderson, R.R., Mager, D. (2003) Geographic variation in the prevalence of stimulant medication use among children 5 to 14 years old: results from a commercially insured US sample. *Pediatrics* 111 (2): 237–243.

Cramer, J.A., Scheyer, R.D., Mattson, R.H. (1990) Compliance declines between clinic visits. *Archives of Internal Medicine* 150, 1509–1510.

Criado Álvarez, J.J., Romo Barrientos, C. (2003) Variabilidad y tendencias en el consumo de metilfenidato en España. Estimación de la prevalencia del trastorno por déficit de atención con hiperactividad. *Revista de Neurología* 37 (9): 806–810.

Culyer, A.J. (2006) NICE's use of cost effectiveness as an exemplar of a deliberative process. *Health Economics, Policy and Law* 1 (3): 299–318.

Culyer, A.J. (1997) The rationing debate: maximising the health of the whole community – the case for. *British Medical Journal* 314: 667–669.

Culyer, A.J. (1989) The normative economics of health care finance and provision. *Oxford Review of Economic Policy* 5: 34–58.

Culyer, A.J. (1971) The nature of the commodity "health care" and its efficient allocation. *Oxford Economic Papers* 23: 189–211.

Dahlke, F., Lohaus A., Gutzmann H. (1992) Reliability and clinical concepts underlying global judgments in dementia: implications for clinical research. *Psychopharmacology Bulletin* 28: 425–432.

Dakin, H.A., Devlin, N.J., Odeyemi, I.A.O. (2006) "Yes", "no" or "yes, but"? Multinomial modelling of NICE decision-making. *Health Policy* 77: 352–367.

Danckaerts, M., Heptinstall, E., Chadwick, O., Taylor, E. (1999) Self-report of attention deficit hyperactivity disorder in adolescents. *Psychopathology* 32 (2): 81–92.

Daniels, N. (2004) CEA and fair process: specifying the Medicare benefit package. Presentation at the Workshop "*Healing with dollars and sense: the ethics of cost-effectiveness analysis in health care decision making*". Toronto, ON: University of Toronto, Faculty of Law, December 9–10, 2004.

Daniels, N. (2001) Justice, health, and healthcare. *American Journal of Bioethics* 1 (2): 2–16.

Daniels, N. (2000) Accountability for reasonableness. Establishing a fair process for priority setting is easier than agreeing on principles. *British Medical Journal* 321: 1300–1301.

Daniels, N. (1985) *Just health care*. Cambridge, New York, NY: Cambridge University Press.

Daniels, N. (1979) Wide reflective equilibrium and theory acceptance in ethics. *Journal of Philosophy* 76: 256–282.

Daniels, N., Sabin, J.E. (2002) *Setting limits fairly – can we learn to share medical resources?* Oxford: Oxford University Press.

Daniels, N., Sabin, J. (1998) The ethics of accountability in managed care reform. *Health Affairs* 17: 50–64.

Daniels, N., Sabin, J. (1997) Limits to health care: fair procedures, democratic deliberation, and the legitimacy problem for insurers. *Philosophy and Public Affairs* 26 (4): 303–350.

Davies, C., Wetherell, M., Barnett, E., Seymour-Smith, S. (2005) *Opening the box. Evaluating the Citizens Council of NICE*. Report prepared for the National Coordinating Centre for Research Methodology, NHS Research and Development Programme. Milton Keynes: The Open University, March 2005.

De Civita, M., Regier, D., Alamgir, A.H., et al. (2005) Evaluating health-related quality-of-life studies in paediatric populations: some conceptual, methodological and developmental considerations and recent applications. *Pharmacoeconomics* 23 (7): 659–685.

DeGrandpre, R. (2000) *Ritalin nation: rapid-fire-culture and the transformation of human consciousness*. New York, NY: Norton.

Dent, T.H.S., Sadler, M. (2002) From guidance to practice: why NICE is not enough. *British Medical Journal* 324: 842–845.

Department of Health (2006) *Prescription Cost Analysis England 2005*. London: National Health Service (NHS), Health and Social Information Centre, Health Care Statistics.

Department of Health (2001) *Prescription Cost Analysis England 2000*. London: National Health Service (NHS), Health and Social Information Centre, Health Care Statistics.

Department of Health (1999) *Prescription Cost Analysis England 1998*. London: National Health Service (NHS), Health and Social Information Centre, Health Care Statistics.

De Ridder, A., De Graeve, D. (2002) Estimating willingness-to-pay for druhs to treat ADHD – a contingent valuation study in students. *Value in Health* 5 (6): 462.

Devlin, N., Parkin, D. (2004) Does NICE have cost-effectiveness threshold and what other factors influence its decisions? A binary choice analysis. *Health Economics* 13: 437–452.

Devlin, N., Parkin, D., Gold, M. (2003) WHO evaluates NICE: The report card is good, but incomplete. *British Medical Journal* 327: 1061–1062.

DiMatteo, M.R., Lepper, H.S., Croghan, T.W. (2000) Depression is a risk factor for noncompliance with medical treatment. Meta-analysis of the effects of anxiety and depression on patient adherence. *Archives of Internal Medicine* 160: 2101–2107.

Dolan, P. (2001) Utilitarianism and the measurement and aggregation of quality-adjusted life-years. *Health Care Analysis* 9 (1): 65–76.

Dolan, P. (2000) The measurement of health-related quality of life for use in resource allocation decisions in health care. In: Culyer, A.J., Newhouse, J.P. (eds.) *Handbook of Health Economics*, Vol. 1B. Amsterdam: Elsevier, 1723–1760.

Dolan, P., Shaw, R., Tsuchiya, A., Williams, A. (2005) QALY maximisation and people's preferences: a methodological review of the literature. *Health Economics* 14 (2): 197–208.

Dolan, P., Olsen, J.A., Menzel, P, Richardson, J. (2003) An inquiry into the different perspectives that can be used when eliciting preferences in health. *Health Economics* 12 (7): 545–551.

Donaldson, C., Currie, W., Mitton, C. (2002) Cost-effectiveness analysis in health care: contraindications. *British Medical Journal* 325: 891–894.

Donnelly, M., Haby, M.M., Carter, R., et al. (2004) Cost-effectiveness of dexamphetamine and methylphenidate for the treatment of childhood attention deficit hyperactivity disorder. *Australian and New Zealand Journal of Psychiatry* 38 (8): 592–601.

Drummond, M. (2006) International guidelines for pharmacoeconomic analyses: vive la différance? *ISPOR Connections* 12 (6): 6.

Drummond, M. (2005) Taking clinical trials to task. *Value in Health* 8 (5): 517–518.

Drummond, M. (2004) Economic evaluation in health care: is it really useful or are we just kidding ourselves? *Australian Economic Review* 37 (1): 3–11.

Drummond, M.F. (2003) The use of health economic information by reimbursement authorities. *Rheumatology* 42 (Supplement 3): iii60–iii63.

Drummond, M., Pang, F. (2001) Transferability of economic evaluation results. In: Drummond, M., McGuire, A., (eds.) *Economic evaluation in health care – merging theory with practice*. Oxford: Oxford University Press, 256–276.

Drummond, M., Sculpher, M. (2005) Common methodological flaws in economic evaluations. *Medical Care* 43 (7 Supplement): 5–14.

Drummond, M.F., Sculpher, M.J., Torrance, G.W., et al. (2005) *Methods for the economic evaluation of health care programmes*. Oxford: Oxford University Press, 3rd edn.

Drummond, M.F., Knapp, M.R.J., Burns, T.P., Miller, K.D., Shadwell, P. (1998) Issues in the design of studies for the economic evaluation of new atypical antipsychotics: the ESTO study. *Journal of Mental Health Policy and Economics* 1 (1): 15–22.

Drummond, M.F., O'Brien, B., Stoddart, G.L., Torrance, G.W. (1997) *Methods for the economic evaluation of health care programmes*. Oxford: Oxford University Press, 2nd edn.

Drummond, M., Brandt, A., Luce, B., Rovira, J. (1993a) Standardizing methodologies for economic evaluation in health care. Practice, problems, and potential. *International Journal of Technology Assessment in Health Care* 9 (1): 26–36.

Drummond, M., Torrance, G., Mason, J. (1993b) Cost-effectiveness league tables: more harm than good? *Social Science & Medicine* 37 (1): 33–40.

Dundar, Y., Dodd, S., Dickson, R., et al. (2006) Comparison of conference abstracts and presentations with full-text articles in the health technology assessments of rapidly evolving technologies. *Health Technology Assessment* 10 (5).

DuPaul, G.J. (1991) Parent and teacher ratings of ADHD symptoms: psychometric properties in a community-based sample. *Journal of Clinical Child Psychology* 20: 245–253.

DuPaul, G.J., Rapport, M.D. (1993) Does methylphenidate normalize the classroom performance of children with attention deficit disorder? *Journal of the American Academy of Child & Adolescent Psychiatry* 32: 190–191.

DuPaul, G.J., Power, T.J., Anastopoulos, A.D., Reid, R. (1998) *ADHD Rating Scale-IV: Checklist, Norms, and Clinical Interpretation*. New York, NY: Guilford.

Eccles, M. (2004) NICE clinical guidelines: health economics must engage with complexity of issues. (Letter) *British Medical Journal* 329: 572.

Efron, D., Jarman, F., Barker, M. (1997a) Methylphenidate versus dexamphetamine in children with attention deficit disorder: A double-blind, crossover trial. *Pediatrics* 100: e6/1–7.

Efron, D., Jarman, F., Barker, M. (1997b) Side effects of methylphenidate and dexamphetamine in children with attention deficit hyperactivity disorder. *Pediatrics* 100: 662–666.

Egger, M., Smith, G.D. (1995) Misleading meta-analysis. *British Medical Journal* 310: 752–752.

Eichler, H.G., Kong, S.X., Gerth, W.C., et al. (2004) Use of cost-effectiveness analysis in health-care resource allocation decision-making: how are cost-effectiveness thresholds expected to emerge? *Value in Health* 7 (5): 518–528.

Ekman, J.T., Gustafsson, P.A. (2000) Stimulants in AD/HD, a controversial treatment only in Sweden? *European Child & Adolescent Psychiatry* 9: 312–313.

Elia, J., Borcherding, B.G., Rapoport, J.L., Keysor, C.S. (1991) Methylphenidate and dextroamphetamine treatments of hyperactivity: Are there true nonresponders? *Psychiatry Research* 36: 141–155.

Ellis, S.J. (2001) Doctors treating patients with multiple sclerosis will lose confidence in NICE. *British Medical Journal* 322: 491.

European Commission (2002) *High level group on innovation and provision of medicines – recommendations for action*. G10 Medicines-Report, Brussels: European Communities, May 07, 2002.

Eysenck, H.J. (1978) An exercise in mega-silliness. *American Psychologist* 33: 517.

Faraone, S.V. (2003) Understanding the effect size of ADHD medications: implications for clinical care. *Medscape Psychiatry & Mental Health* 8: 1–7.

Faraone, S.V., Biederman, J., Spencer, T.J., Aleardi, M. (2006) Comparing the efficacy of medications for ADHD using meta-analysis. *Medscape General Medicine* 8 (4): 4.

Faraone, S.V., Sergeant, J., Gillberg C., Biederman J. (2003a) The worldwide prevalence of ADHD: is it an American condition? *World Psychiatry* 2 (2): 104–113.

Faraone, S.V., Spender, T., Aleardi, M., et al. (2003b) Comparing the efficacy of medications used for ADHD using meta-analysis. Program and abstracts of the 156th Annual Meeting of the American Psychiatric Association; San Francisco, CA: May 17–22, 2003.

Faraone, S.V., Pliszka, S.R., Olvera, R.L., et al. (2001) Efficacy of Adderall and methylphenidate in attention deficit hyperactivity disorder: a reanalysis using drug-placebo and drug-drug response curve methodology. *Journal of Child and Adolescent Psychopharmacology* 11: 171–180.

Fehlings, D.L., Roberts, W., Humphries, T., Dawe, G. (1991) Attention deficit hyperactivity disorder: does cognitive behavioral therapy improve home behavior? *Developmental and Behavioral Pediatrics* 12 (4): 223–228.

Feinstein, A.R. (1990) On white-coat effects and the electronic monitoring of compliance. *Archives of Internal Medicine* 150: 1377–1378.

Fendrick, A.M. (2006) The future of health economic modeling: have we gone too far or not far enough? *Value in Health* 9 (3): 179–180.

Fenwick, E., O'Brien, B.J., Brigss, A. (2004) Cost-effectiveness acceptability curves – facts, fallacies and frequently asked questions. *Health Economics* 13 (5): 405–415.

Ferner, R.E., McDowell, S.E. (2006) How NICE may be outflanked. *British Medical Journal* 332: 1268–1271.

Firestone, P. (1982) Factors associated with children's adherence to stimulant medication. *American Journal of Orthopsychiatry* 252 (3): 447-457.

Fischer, M., Barkley, R.A., Fletcher, K.E., Smallish, L. (1993) The stability of dimensions of behaviour in ADHD and normal children over an 8-year follow-up. *Journal of Abnormal Child Psychology* 21: 315–337.

Fischer, M., Newby, R.F. (1991) Assessment of stimulant response in ADHD children using a refined multimethod clinical protocol. *Journal of Clinical Child Psychology* 20: 232–244.

Fitzpatrick, P.A., Klorman, R., Brumaghim, J.T., Borgstedt, A.D. (1992) Effects of sustained-release and standard preparations of methylphenidate on attention deficit disorder. *Journal of the American Academy of Child & Adolescent Psychiatry* 31: 226–234.

Fletcher, P. (2000) Do NICE and CHI have no interest in safety? Opinion on the book NICE, CHI and the NHS reforms. Enabling excellence or imposing control? *Adverse Drug Reactions and Toxicological Reviews* 19 (3): 167–176.

Flood, C.M., Tuohy, C., Stabile, M. (2004) What is in and out of Medicare? Who decides? Draft Working Paper No. 5 – Defining the Medicare Basket. March 03, 2004.

Foster, E.M., Jensen, P.S., Schlander, M., et al. (2007) Treatment for ADHD: Is more complex treatment cost-effective for more complex cases? *Health Services Research*, 42 (1), 2007: 165–182.

Foster, E.M., Jensen, P.S., Schlander, M. (2005) *Treatment for ADD: is more complex treatment cost-effective for more complex cases?* Pennsylvania State University, The Methodology Center, University Park, PA, 2005: Technical Report No. 05–65.

Freemantle, N. (2004) Is NICE delivering the goods? *British Medical Journal* 329: 1003–1004.

Freemantle, N., Blonde, L., Bolinder, B., et al. (2005) Real-world trials to answer real-world questions. *Pharmacoeconomics* 23 (8): 747–754.

Freemantle, N., Bloor, K., Eastaugh, J. (2002) A fair innings for NICE? *Pharmacoeconomics* 20 (6): 389–391.

French, J.A., Kanner, A.M., Bautista, J., et al. (2004) Efficacy and tolerability of the new antiepileptic drugs, I: Treatment of new-onset epilepsy: report of the TTA and QSS Subcommittees of the American Academy of Neurology and the American Epilepsy Society. *Epilepsia* 45: 401–409.

Gafni, A., Birch, S. (2006) Incremental cost-effectiveness ratios (ICERS): the silence of the lambda. *Social Science & Medicine* 62: 2091–2100.

Gafni, A., Birch, S. (2003a) NICE methodological guidelines and decision making in the National Health Service in England and Wales. *Pharmacoeconomics* 21 (3): 149–157.

Gafni, A., Birch, S. (2003b) Inclusion of drugs in provincial drug benefit programs: should "reasonable decisions" lead to uncontrolled growth in expenditures? *Canadian Medical Association Journal (CMAJ)* 168 (7): 849–851.

Gafni, A., Birch, S. (1993) Guidelines for the adoption of new technologies: a prescription for uncontrolled growth in expenditures and how to avoid the problem. *Canadian Medical Association Journal (CMAJ)* 148 (6): 913–917.

Garber, A.M. (2000) Advances in cost-effectiveness analysis of health interventions. In: Culyer, A.J., Newhouse, J.P. (eds.) *Handbook of Health Economics*, Vol. 1A. Amsterdam: Elsevier, 181–221.

García-Altés, A., Ondategui-Parra, S., Neumann, P.J. (2004) Cross-national comparison of technology assessment processes. *International Journal of Technology Assessment in Health Care* 20 (3): 300–310.

Gerard, K., Smoker, L., Seymour, J. (1999) Raising the quality of cost-utility analyses: lessons learnt and still to learn. *Health Policy* 46 (3): 219–238.

Giacomini, M., Hurley, J., Gold, I., et al. (2004) The policy analysis of 'values talk': lessons from Canadian health reform. *Health Policy* 67 (1): 15–24.

Gibson, A.P., Bettinger, T.L., Patel, N.C. (2006) Atomoxetine versus stimulants for treatment of attention deficit/hyperactivity disorder. *Annals of Pharmacotherapy* 40 (6): 1134–1142.

Gibson, J.L., Martin, D.K., Singer, P.A. (2002) Priority setting for new technologies in medicine: a transdisciplinary study. *BioMed Central (BMC) Health Services Research* 2: 14 (1–5).

Gilbody, S.M., Petticrew, M. (1999) Rational decision-making in mental health: the role of systematic reviews. *Journal of Mental Health Policy and Economics* 2 (3): 99–106.

Gilbody, S.M., House, A.O., Sheldon, T.A. (2003) *Outcomes Measurement in Psychiatry. A critical review of outcomes measurement in psychiatric research and practice.* York: NHS Centre for Reviews and Dissemination (CRD), University of York, Report No. 24.

Gillberg, C., Harrington, R, Steinhausen, H.-C. (2006) *A Clinician's Handbook of Child and Adolescent Psychiatry.* Cambridge: Cambridge University Press.

Gillberg, C., Gillberg, I.C., Rasmussen, P., et al. (2004) Co-existing disorders in ADHD – implications for diagnosis and intervention. *European Child & Adolescent Psychiatry* 13 (Suppl 1): 80–92.

Gilmore, A., Milne, R. (2001) Methylphenidate in children with hyperactivity: review and cost-utility analysis. *Pharmacoepidemiology and Drug Safety* 10: 85–94.

Gilmore, A., Best, L., Milne, R. (1998) *Methylphenidate in children with hyperactivity. DEC Report No 78.* Southampton: Wessex Institute for Health Research and Development.

Ginnelly, L. (2005) *Characterising structural uncertainty in decision analytic models: review and application of currently available methods.* Oxford: Health Economists' Study Group.

Ginsberg, G., Lowe, S. (2002) Cost-effectiveness of treatments for amyotrophic lateral sclerosis: a review of the literature. *Pharmacoeconomics* 20 (6): 367–387.

Gold, M.R., Siegel, J.E., Russell, L.B., Weinstein, M.C. (1996) *Cost-Effectiveness in Health and Medicine.* New York, NY, Oxford: Oxford University Press.

Goodwin, P., Wright, G. (2004) *Decision Analysis for Management Judgment.* Chichester, England (3rd. ed): John Wiley & Sons.

Graff Low, K., Gendaszek, A.E. (2002) Illicit use of psychostimulants among college students: a preliminary study. *Health & Medicine* 7: 283–287.

Green, M., Wong, M., Atkins, D., et al. (1999) *Diagnosis and treatment of attention-deficit/hyperactivity disorder in children and adolescents.* Technical Review No 3. Rockville, MD: Agency for Health Care Policy and Research, AHCPR Publication No 99–0050.

Greenhill, L.L. (1992) Pharmacologic treatment of attention deficit hyperactivity disorder. *Psychiatric Clinics of North America* 15: 1–27.

Greenhill, L.L., Findling, R.L., Swanson, J.M. (2002) A double-blind, placebo-controlled study of modified-release methylphenidate in children with attention-deficit/hyperactivity disorder. *Pediatrics* 109: e39/1–7.

Greenhill, L.L., Swanson, J.M., Vitiello, B., et al. (2001a) Impairment and deportment responses to different methylphenidate doses in children with ADHD: the MTA titration trial. *Journal of the American Academy of Child & Adolescent Psychiatry* 40 (2): 180–187.

Greenhill, L.L., Perel, J.M., Rudolf, G., et al. (2001b) Correlations between motor persistence and plasma levels of methylphenidate-treated boys with ADHD. *International Journal of Neuropsychopharmacology* 4: 207–215.

Greenhill, L.L., Abikoff, H., Arnold, L.E., et al. (1999) Medication treatment strategies in the MTA Study: relevance to clinicians and researchers. *Journal of the American Academy of Child & Adolescent Psychiatry* 34 (10): 1304–1313.

Griebsch, I., Coast, J., Brown, J. (2005) Quality-adjusted life-years lack quality in pediatric care: a critical review of published cost-utility studies in child health. *Pediatrics* 115 : e600–e614.

Griffin, S., Claxton, K., Hawkins, N., Sculpher, M. (2006) Probabilistic analysis and computationally expensive models: necessary and required? *Value in Health* 9 (4): 244–252.

Guy, W. (2000) Clinical Global Impressions (CGI) Scale. In: American Psychiatric Association, *Handbook of Psychiatric Measures*. Washington, DC: APA, 100–102.

Guy, W. (1976) *ECDEU Assessment Manual for Psychopharmacology – Revised (DHEW Publ No ADM 76-338)*. Rockville, MD: Department of Health, Education, and Welfare, Public Health Service, Alcohol, Drug Abuse, and Mental Health Administration, 218–222.

Gyrd-Hansen, D. (2005) Willingness to pay for a QALY: theoretical and methodological issues. *Pharmacoeconomics* 23 (5): 423–432.

Hack, S., Chow, B. (2001) Pediatric psychotropic medication compliance: a literature review and research-based suggestions for improving treatment compliance. *Journal of Child and Adolescent Psychopharmacology* 11 (19): 59–67.

Handen, B., Feldman, HM., Lurier, A., Murray, P.J. (1999) Efficacy of methylphenidate among preschool children with developmental disabilities and ADHD. *Journal of the American Academy of Child & Adolescent Psychiatry* 38: 805–812.

Harris, J. (2005a) It's not NICE to discriminate. *Journal of Medical Ethics* 31: 373–375.

Harris, J. (2005b) Nice and not so nice. *Journal of Medical Ethics* 31: 685–688.

Harris, J. (1997) The rationing debate: Maximising the health of the whole community. The case against: what the principal objective of the NHS should really be. *British Medical Journal* 314: 669.

Harris, J. (1995) Double jeopardy and the veil of ignorance. *Journal of Medical Ethics* 21: 151–157.

Harris, J. (1987) QALYfying the value of life. *Journal of Medical Ethics* 13 (3): 117–123.

Hasman, A., Holm, S. (2005) Accountability for reasonableness: opening the black box of process. *Health Care Analysis* 14 (4): 261–273.

Hays, R.D., Woolley, J.M. (2000) The concept of clinically meaningful differences in health-related quality-of-life research: how meaningful is it? *Pharmacoeconomics* 18 (5): 419–423.

Hechtman, L., Abikoff, H., Klein, R.G., et al. (2004a) Academic achievement and emotional status of children with ADHD treated with long-term methylphenidate and multimodal psychosocial treatment. *Journal of the American Academy of Child & Adolescent Psychiatry* 43 (7): 812–819.

Hechtman, L., Abikoff, H., Klein, R.G., et al. (2004b) Children with ADHD treated with long-term methylphenidate and multimodal psychosocial treatment: impact on parental practices. *Journal of the American Academy of Child & Adolescent Psychiatry* 43 (7): 830–838.

Heffler, S., Smith, S., Keehan, S., et al. (2003) Health spending projections for 2002–2012. *Health Affairs* Web Exclusive, February 07, 2003: W3-54–W3-65.

Henry, D.A., Hill, S.R., Harris, A. (2005) Drug prices and value for money: the Australian Pharmaceutical Benefits Scheme. *Journal of the American Medical Association (JAMA)* 204 (20): 2630–2632.

Higgins, J.P.T., Whitehead, J. (1996) Borrowing strength from external trials in a meta-analysis. *Statistics in Medicine* 15: 1733–2749.

Hill, S.R., Mitchell, A.S., Henry, D.A. (2000) Problems with the interpretation of pharmacoeconomic analyses: a review of submissions to the Australian Pharmaceutical Benefits Scheme. *Journal of the American Medical Association (JAMA)* 283 (16): 2116–2121.

Himpel, S., Banaschewski, T., Heise, C.A., Rothenberger, A. (2005) The safety of non-stimulant agents for the treatment of attention-deficit hyperactivity disorder. *Expert Opinion on Drug Safety* 4 (2): 311–321.

Hjelmgren, J., Berggren, F., Andersson, F. (2001) Health economic guidelines – similarities, differences and some implications. *Value in Health* 4 (3): 225–250.

Hoare, P., Beattie, T. (2003) Children with attention deficit hyperactivity disorder and attendance at hospital. *European Journal of Emergency Medicine* 10 (2): 98–100.

Hoeppner, J.A., Hale, J.B., Bradley, A.M., et al. (1997) A clinical protocol for determining methylphenidate dosage levels in ADHD. *Journal of Attention Disorders* 1997, 2: 19–30.

Hollander, E., Quinn, D., Hunt, R.D., Perry, P.J. (1996) The ADHD debate: stimulants or alternative agents. *Primary Psychiatry* 3: 52–55.

Howard, S., Harrison, L. (2004) *NICE guidance implementation tracking: data sources, methodology and results. A report commissioned by NICE.* Bicester: Abacus International.

Hughes, D. (2006) Rationing of drugs for rare diseases (Editorial). *Pharmacoeconomics* 24 (4): 315–316.

Hughes, D.A., Tunnage, B., Yeo, S.T. (2005) Drugs for exceptionally rare diseases: do they deserve special status for funding? *QJM – Monthly Journal of the Association of Physicians* 98 (11): 829–836.

Hughes, D.A., Bagust, A., Haycox, A., Walley, T. (2001) Accounting for noncompliance in pharmacoeconomic evaluations. *Pharmacoeconomics* 19 (12): 1185–1197.

Hunter J.E., Schmidt, F.L. (1990) Dichotomization of continuous variables: the implications for meta-analysis. *Journal of Applied Psychology* 75 (3): 334–349.

Hurley, J. (2000) An overview of the normative economics of the health sector. In: Culyer, A.J., Newhouse, J.P. (eds.) *Handbook of Health Economics*, Volume 1A. Amsterdam: Elsevier, 55–118.

Hutton, J., McGrath, C., Frybourg, J.M., et al. (2006) Framework for describing and classifying decision-making systems using technology assessment to determine the reimbursement of health technologies (fourth hurdle systems). *International Journal of Technology Assessment in Health Care* 22 (1): 10–18.

Hwang, P., Cosby, A., Laberge, M.E. (2003) Compliance with three-times daily methylphenidate in children with attention-deficit/hyperactivity disorder. *Value in Health* 6 (3): 273.

Iliffe, S. (2005) NICE dementia proposal threatens future of evidence-based medicine. *Pulse* April 23, 2005: 54–57.

Institut für Qualität und Wirtschaftlichkeit im Gesundheitswesen [IQWiG] (2006) *Methoden. Version 2.0 vom 19.12.2006.* Available online at: http://www.iqwig.de/download/ 2006_12_19_IQWiG_Methoden_V-2-0.pdf. Last accessed December 27, 2006.

Institut für Qualität und Wirtschaftlichkeit im Gesundheitswesen [IQWiG] (2005) *Methoden. Version 1 vom 1. März 2005.* IQWiG, Cologne. Available online at www.iqwig.de/ index.download.a356e36e87a021176d 2305a0c513dc52a.pdf. Last accessed July 1, 2006.

Ioannidis, J.P.A., Cappelleri, J.C., Lau, J. (1998) Issues in comparisons between meta-analyses and large trials. *Journal of the American Medical Association* 279: 1089–1093.

Iskedjian, M., Maturi, B., Walker, J.H., et al. (2003) Cost-effectiveness of atomoxetine in the treatment of attention deficit hyperactivity disorder in children and adolescents. *Value in Health* 6 (3): 275.

Jadad, A.R., Boyle, M., Cunningham, C., et al. (1999) *Treatment of Attention-Deficit/Hyperactivity Disorder. Evidence Report / Technology Assessment No 11 (prepared by McMaster University under contract no 290-97-0017).* AHRQ Publication No 00-E005. Rockville, MD: Agency for Healthcare Research and Quality (AHRQ), November 1999.

James, R.S., Sharp, W.S., Bastain, T.M., et al. (2001) Double-blind, placebo-controlled study of single-dose amphetamine formulations in ADHD. *Journal of the American Academy of Child & Adolescent Psychiatry* 40: 1268–1276.

Jefferson, T., Demicheli, V., Vale, M. (2002) Quality of systematic reviews of economic evaluations in health care. *Journal of the American Medical Association* 287 (21): 2809–2812.

Jensen, P.S. (1999) Fact versus fancy concerning the Multimodal Treatment Study for attention-deficit hyperactivity disorder. *Canadian Journal of Psychiatry* 44: 975–980.

Jensen, P.S., Garcia, J.A., Glied, S., et al. (2005) Cost-effectiveness of ADHD treatments: findings from the multimodal treatment study of children with ADHD. *American Journal of Psychiatry* 162 (9): 1628–1636.

Jensen, P.S., Garcia, J.A., Glied, S., et al. (2004) Cost-effectiveness of attention-deficit/hyperactivity disorder (ADHD) treatments: estimates based upon the MTA study. *16th World Congress of the International Association for Child and Adolescent Psychiatry and Allied Professions (IACAPAP)*. Book of Abstracts. Darmstadt: Steinkopff-Verlag, 219.

Jensen, P.S., Hinshaw, S.P., Kraemer, H.C., et al. (2001a) ADHD comorbidity findings from the MTA Study: comparing comorbid subgroups. *Journal of the American Academy of Child & Adolescent Psychiatry* 40 (2): 147–158.

Jensen, P.S., Hinshaw, S.P., Swanson, J.M., et al. (2001b) Findings from the NIMH Multimodal treatment study of ADHD (MTA): implications and applications for primary care providers. *Journal of Developmental and Behavioral Pediatrics* 22: 1–14.

Jensen, P.S., Kettle, L., Roper, M.T., et al. (1999) Are stimulants overprescribed? Treatment of ADHD in four U.S. communities. *Journal of the American Academy of Child & Adolescent Psychiatry* 38 (7): 797–804.

Johannesson, M., Jönsson, B. (1991) Economic evaluation in health care: is there a role for cost-benefit analysis? *Health Policy* 17 (1): 1–23.

Johansson, P., Kerr, M., Andershed, H. (2005) Linking adult psychopathy with childhood hyperactivity-impulsivity-attention problems and conduct problems through retrospective self-reports. *Journal of Personality Disorders* 19 (1): 94–101.

Johnston, C., Fine S. (1993) Methods of evaluating methylphenidate in children with attention deficit hyperactivity disorder: acceptability, satisfaction, and compliance. *Journal of Pediatric Psychology* 18 (6): 717–730.

Joint Formulary Committee (2006) *British National Formulary (BNF)*. London: British Medical Association / Royal Pharmaceutical Society of Great Britain, 51st ed., March 2006.

Joint Formulary Committee (2005) *British National Formulary (BNF)*. London: British Medical Association / Royal Pharmaceutical Society of Great Britain, 50th ed., September 2005.

Joint Formulary Committee (2003) *British National Formulary (BNF)*. London: British Medical Association / Royal Pharmaceutical Society of Great Britain, 46th ed., September 2003.

Jonsen, A.R. (1986) Bentham in a box: technology assessment and health care allocation. *Law, Medicine and Health Care* 14: 172–174.

Kahneman, D., Wakker, P.P., Sarin, R. (1997) Back to Bentham? Explorations of experienced utility. *The Quarterly Journal of Economics* 112: 375–405.

Kanavos, P., Trueman, P., Bosilevic, A. (2000) Can economic evaluation guidelines improve efficiency in resource allocation? The cases of Portugal, The Netherlands, Finland, and the United Kingdom. *International Journal of Technology Assessment in Health Care* 16 (4): 1179–1192.

Kashani, J.H., Orvaschel, H., Burk, J.P., Reid, J.C. (1985) Informant variance: The issue of parent-child disagreement. *Journal of the American Academy of Child & Adolescent Psychiatry* 24: 437–441.

Kass, M.A., Gordon, M., Meltzer, D.W. (1986) Can ophthalmologists correctly identify patients defaulting from pilocarpine therapy? *American Journal of Ophthalmology* 101: 524–530.

Kauffman, R.E., Smith-Right, D., Reese, C.A., et al. (1981) Medication compliance in hyperactive children. *Pediatric Pharmacology* 1: 231–237.

Keeler, E.B., Cretin, S. (1983) Discounting of life-saving and other nonmonetary effects. *Management Science* 29: 300–306.

Keeney, R. (1992) *Value-Focused Thinking*. Cambridge, MA, Harvard University Press.

Keeney, R.L., Raiffa, H. (1993) *Decisions with multiple objectives: preferences and value trade-offs*. Cambridge: Cambridge University Press.

Kelleher, K.J., McInerny, T.K., Gardner, W.P., et al. (2001) Increasing identification of psychosocial problems: 1979–1996. *Pediatrics* 105 (6): 1313–1321.

Kelsey, D.K., Sumner, C.R., Casat, C.D., et al. (2004) Once-daily atomoxetine treatment for children with attention-deficit/hyperactivity disorder, including an assessment of evening and morning behavior: a double-blind, placebo-controlled trial. *Pediatrics* 114 (1): e1–e8.

Kemner, J.E., Lage, M.J. (2006a) Effect of methylphenidate formulation on treatment patterns and use of emergency room services. *American Journal of Health System Pharmacy* 63 (4): 317–322.

Kemner, J.E., Lage, M.J. (2006b) Impact of methylphenidate formulation on treatment patterns and hospitalizations: a retrospective analysis. *Annals of General Psychiatry* 5 (5): 1–8.

Kemner, J.E., Starr, H.L., Ciccone, P.E., et al. (2005) Outcomes of OROS methylphenidate compared with atomoxetine in children with ADHD: a multicenter, randomized prospective study. *Advances in Therapy* 22 (5): 498–512.

Kemner, J.E., Starr, H.L., Brown, D.L., et al. (2004) *Greater improvement and response rates with OROS MPH vs atomoxetine in children with ADHD.* Presentation at the XXIVth Congress of the Collegium Internationale Neuro-Psychopharmacologicum, Paris, France, June 20–24, 2004.

Keynes J.M. *The Collected Works of John Maynard Keynes.* London 1971–1989, Macmillan: Vol. IX, p. 332.

Kimko, H.C., Cross, J.T., Abernethy D.R. (1999) Pharmacokinetics and clinical effectiveness of methylphenidate. *Clinical Pharmacokinetics* 37 (6): 457–470.

King, S., Griffin, S., Hodges, Z., et al. (2006) A systematic review and economic model of the effectiveness and cost-effectiveness of methylphenidate, dexamfetamine and atomoxetine for the treatment of attention deficit hyperactivity disorder in children and adolescents. *Health Technology Assessment* 10 (23).

King, S., Riemsma, R., Hodges, Z., et al. (2004a) *Technology Assessment Report for the HTA Programme: Methylphenidate, dexamfetamine and atomoxetine for the treatment of attention deficit hyperactivity disorder. Final version.* London: NICE, June 2004.

King, S., Riemsma, R., Drummond, M., et al. (2004b) *A systematic review of the clinical and cost-effectiveness of methylphenidate hydrochloride, dexamfetamine sulphate and atomoxetine for attention deficit hyperactivity disorder (ADHD) in children and adolescents.* York: December 2004.

Klassen, A., Miller, A., Fine, S. (2004) Health-related quality of life in children and adolescents who have a diagnosis of attention-deficit/hyperactivity disorder. *Pediatrics* 114 (5): 541–547.

Klassen, A., Miller, A., Raina, P., et al. (1999) Attention-deficit hyperactivity disorder in children and youth: a quantitative systematic review of the efficacy of different management strategies. *Canadian Journal of Psychiatry* 44: 1007–1016.

Klein, R.G., Abikoff, H. (1997) Behavior therapy and methylphenidate in the treatment of children with ADHD. *Journal of Attention Disorders* 2: 89–114.

Klein, R.G., Abikoff, H.G., Hechtman, L., Weiss, G. (2004) Design and rationale of controlled study of long-term methylphenidate and multimodal psychosocial treatment in children with ADHD. *Journal of the American Academy of Child and Adolescent Psychiatry* 43 (7): 792–801.

Koch, T. (2000) Life quality vs the 'quality of life': assumptions underlying prospective quality of life instruments in health care planning. *Social Science & Medicine* 51: 419–427.

Köster, I., Schubert, I., Döpfner, M., et al. (2004) Hyperkinetische Störungen bei Kindern und Jugendlichen: Zur Häufigkeit des Behandlungsanlasses in der ambulanten Versorgung nach den Daten der Versichertenstichprobe AOK Hessen/KV Hessen (1998-2001). *Zeitschrift für Kinder – und Jugendpsychiatrie* 32 (3): 157–166.

Kolko, D.J., Bukstein, O.G., Barron, J. (1999) Methylphenidate and behavior modification in children with ADHD and comorbid ODD or CD: main and incremental effects across settings. *Journal of the American Academy of Child & Adolescent Psychiatry* 38: 578–586.

Kratochvil, C.J., Heiligenstein, F.H., Dittmann, R., et al. (2002) Atomoxetine and methylphenidate treatment in children with ADHD: a prospective, randomised, open-label trial. *Journal of the American Academy of Child & Adolescent Psychiatry* 41: 776–784.

Lam, L.T. (2002) Attention deficit disorder and hospitalization due to injury among older adolescents in New South Wales, Australia. *Journal of Attention Disorders* 6 (2): 77–82.

Lage, M., Hwang, P. (2004) Effects of methylphenidate formulation for attention deficit hyperactivity disorder on patterns and outcomes of treatment. *Journal of Child and Adolescent Psychopharmacology* 14 (4): 575–581.

Lage, M., Hwang, P. (2003) Methylphenidate formulation is associated with accident / injury rate in children with ADHD. *Value in Health* 6 (6): 688.

Laing, A., Cottrell, S., Robinson, P., et al. (2005) A modelled economic evaluation comparing atomoxetine with current therapies for the treatment of children with attention deficit/hyperactivity disorder (ADHD) in the Netherlands. *Value in Health* 8 (6): A198.

Lau, J., Ioannidis, J.P.A., Schmid, C.H. (1997) Quantitative synthesis in systematic reviews. *Annals of Internal Medicine* 127 (9): 820–826.

Laupacis, A. (2006) Economic evaluations in the Canadian Common Drug Review. *Pharmacoeconomics* 24 (11): 1157–1162.

Leaf, P., Alegria, M., Cohen, P., et al. (1996) Mental health service use in the community and schools: Results from the four-community MECA study *Journal of the American Academy of Child & Adolescent Psychiatry* 35: 889–897.

Leibson, C.L., Long, K.H. (2003) Economic implications of attention-deficit/hyperactivity disorder for healthcare systems. *Pharmacoeconomics* 21 (17): 1239–1262.

LeLorier, J., Grégoire, G., Benhaddad, A., et al. (1997) Discrepancies between meta-analyses and subsequent large, randomized trials. *New England Journal of Medicine* 337: 536–542.

Lipman, T. (2001) NICE and evidence based medicine are not really compatible. *British Medical Journal* 322: 489–490.

Littlejohns, P., Leng, G., Culyer, T., Drummond, M. (2004) NICE clinical guidelines: maybe health economists should participate in guideline development. (Letter) *British Medical Journal* 329: 571.

Llana, M.E., Crismon, M.L. (1999) Methylphenidate: increased abuse or appropriate use? *Journal of the American Pharmaceutical Association* 39 (4): 526–530.

Loeber, R., Green, S.M., Lahey, B.B., Stouthamer-Loeber, M. (1991) Differences and similarities between children, mothers, and teachers as informants on disruptive child behavior. *Journal of Abnormal Child Psychology* 19: 75–95.

Lohse, M.J., Lorenzen, A., Mueller-Oerlinghausen, B. (2004) Psychopharmaka. In: Schwabe, U., Paffrath, D. (eds.) *Arzneiverordnungs-Report 2004. Aktuelle Daten, Kosten, Trends und Kommentare.* Berlin, Heidelberg: Springer, pp. 769–810.

Loney, J., Milich, R. (1982) Hyperactivity, inattention, and aggression in clinical practice. In: Wolraich, M., Routh, D.K. (eds.) *Advances in Development and Behavioral Pediatrics, Vol. 3.* Greenwich, CT: AJI, pp. 113–147.

Lord, J., Paisley, S. (2000) *The clinical effectiveness and cost-effectiveness of methylphenidate for hyperactivity in childhood.* London: National Institute for Clinical Excellence (NICE), Version 2, August 2000.

Lu, G., Ades, A.E. (2004) Combination of direct and indirect evidence in mixed treatment comparisons. *Statistics in Medicine* 23: 3105–3124.

Macdonald, S. (2003) Increased drug spending is creating funding crisis, report says. *British Medical Journal* 326: 677.

Makridakis, S., Wheelwright, S.C., Hyndman, R.J. (1998) *Forecasting – Methods and Applications.* New York, NY: Wiley (3rd edition).

Mannuza, S., Gittelman, R. (1986) Informant variance in the diagnostic assessment of hyperactive children as young adults. In: Barrett, J.E., Rose, R.M. (eds.) *Proceedings of the 75th Annual Meeting of the American Psychopathological Association.* New York, Guilford, pp. 243–254.

Mannuzza, S., Klein, R.G. (2000) Long-term prognosis in attention-deficit/hyperactivity disorder. *Child and Adolescent Psychiatry Clinics of North America* 9 (3): 711–726.

Mannuzza, S., Klein, R.G., Abikoff, H., Moulton, J.L. 3rd (2004) Significance of childhood conduct problems to later development of conduct disorder among children with ADHD: a prospective follow-up study. *Journal of Abnormal Child Psychology* 32 (5): 565–573.

Mannuzza, S., Klein, R.G., Moulton, J.L. 3rd. (2003) Persistence of attention-deficit/hyperactivity disorder into adulthood: what have we learnt from the prospective follow-up studies? *Journal of Attention Disorders* 2003; 7 (2): 93–100.

Mannuzza, S., Klein, R.G., Bessler, A., et al. (1997) Educational and occupational outcome of hyperactive boys grown up. *Journal of the American Academy of Child & Adolescent Psychiatry* 36 (9): 1222–1227.

Manos, M.J., Short, E.J., Findling, R.L. (1999) Differential effectiveness of methylphenidate and Adderall® in school-age youths with attention deficit-hyperactivity disorder. *Journal of the American Academy of Child & Adolescent Psychiatry* 38: 813–819.

March, J.S., Silva, S.G., Compton, S., et al. (2005) The case for practical clinical trials in psychiatry. *American Journal of Psychiatry* 162 (5): 836–846.

March, J., Silva, S., Petrycki, S., et al. (2004) Fluoxetine, cognitive-behavioral therapy, and their combination for adolescents with depression: Treatment for Adolescents With Depression Study (TADS) randomized controlled trial. *Journal of the American Medical Association (JAMA)* 292: 807–820.

Marchetti, A., Magar, R., Lau, H., et al. (2001) Pharmacotherapies for attention-deficit/hyperactivity disorder: expected cost analysis. *Clinical Therapeutics* 23 (11): 1904–1921.

Marcus, S.C., Wan, G.J., Kemner, J.E., Olfson, M. (2005) Continuity of methylphenidate treatment for attention-deficit/hyperactivity disorder. *Archives of Pediatrics & Adolescent Medicine* 159: 572–578.

Marshall, T. (2005) Orphan drugs and the NHS: consider whom drug regulation is designed to protect (letter). *British Medical Journal* 331: 1144.

Mason, A. (2005) Does the English NHS have a 'health benefit basket'? *European Journal of Health Economics* 6 (Suppl. 1): S18–S23.

Matza, L.S., Paramore, C., Prasad, M. (2005a) A review of the economic burden of ADHD. *Cost Effectiveness and Resource Allocation* 3: 5.

Matza, L.S., Secnik, K., Rentz, A.M., et al. (2005b) Assessment of health state utilities for attention-deficit/hyperactivity disorder in children using parent proxy report. *Quality of Life Research* 14: 735–747.

Matza, L.S., Secnik, K., Mannix, S., Sallee, F.R. (2005c) Parent-Proxy EQ-5D Ratings of Children with Attention-Deficit Hyperactivity Disorder in the US and the UK. *Pharmacoeconomics* 23 (8): 777–790.

Matza, L.S., Rentz, A.M., Secnik, K., et al. (2004) The Link Between Health-Related Quality of Life and Clinical Symptoms Among Children with Attention-Deficit Hyperactivity Disorder. *Developmental and Behavioral Pediatrics* 25 (3): 166–174.

Mauskopf, J., Drummond, M. (2004) Publication of pharmacoeconomic data submitted to reimbursement or clinical guidelines agencies. *Value in Health* 7 (5): 515–516.

Mauskopf, J., Rutten, F., Schonfeld, W. (2003) Cost-effectiveness league tables: valuable guidance for decision makers? *Pharmacoeconomics* 21 (14): 991–1000.

Maynard, A. (2001) Ethics and health care 'underfunding'. *Journal of Medical Ethics* 27: 223–227.

Maynard, A. (2001) Towards a Euro-NICE? *Eurohealth* 7 (2): 26.

Maynard, A., Bloor, K. (1995) Help or hindrance? The role of economics in rationing in health care. *British Medical Bulletin* 51 (4): 854–868.

Maynard, A., Bloor, K., Freemantle, N. (2004) Challenges for the National Institute for Clinical Excellence. *British Medical Journal* 329: 227–229.

McCabe, C., Tsuchiya, A., Claxton, K., Raftery, J. (2006) Orphans drugs revisited. *QJM – Monthly Journal of the Association of Physicians* 99 (5): 341–345.

McCabe, C., Claxton, K., Tsuchiya, A. (2005) Orphan drugs and the NHS: should we value rarity? *British Medical Journal* 331: 1016–1019.

McCracken, J.T., McGough, J., Shah, B., et al. (2002) Risperidone in children with autism and serious behavioral problems. *New England Journal of Medicine* 347: 314–21.

McGregor, M. (2006) What decision-makers want and what they have been getting. *Value in Health* 9 (3): 181–185.

McGregor, M. (2003) Cost-utility analysis: use QALYs only with great caution. *Canadian Medical Association Journal (CMAJ)* 168 (4): 433–434.

McKie, J., Richardson, J. (2003) The rule of rescue. *Social Science & Medicine* 56 (12): 2407–2419.

McMahon, M., Morgan, S., Mitton, C. (2006) The Common Drug Review: a NICE start for Canada? *Health Policy* 77 (3): 339–351.

Menzel, P. (1990) *Strong medicine: the ethical rationing of health care*. New York, NY: Oxford University Press.

Menzel, P., Dolan, P., Richardson, J., Olsen, J.A. (2002) The role of adaptation to disability and disease in health state valuation: a preliminary normative analysis. *Social Science & Medicine* 55: 2149–2158.

Meier, A. (2003) *Der rechtliche Schutz patientenbezogener Gesundheitsdaten*. Karlsruhe, Germany: Verlag Versicherungswirtschaft, 263–311.

Menzel, P., Gold, M.R., Nord, E., et al. (1999) Toward a broader view of values in cost-effectiveness analysis of health. *Hastings Center Report* 29 (3): 7–15.

Meredith, P.A. (1999) Achieving and assessing therapeutic coverage. In: Métry, J.-M., Meyer, U.A. (eds.) *Drug Regimen Compliance: Issues in Clinical Trials and Patient Management*. Chichester: John Wiley & Sons, pp. 41–60.

Métry, J.-M. (1999) Measuring Compliance in Clinical Trials and Ambulatory Care. In: Métry, J.-M., Meyer, U.A. (eds.) *Drug Regimen Compliance: Issues in Clinical Trials and Patient Management*. Chichester: John Wiley & Sons, pp. 1–21.

Michelson, D., Allen, A.J., Busner, J., et al. (2002) Once-daily atomoxetine treatment for children and adolescents with attention deficit hyperactivity disorder: a randomized, placebo-controlled study. *American Journal of Psychiatry* 159 (11): 1896–1901.

Michelson, D., Faries, D., Wernicke, J., et al. (2001) Atomoxetine in the treatment of children and adolescents with attention-deficit/ hyperactivity disorder: a randomized, placebo-controlled, dose response study. *Pediatrics* 1008 (5): e83/1–9.

Miller, A.R., Lalonde, C.E., McGrail, K.M. (2004) Children's persistence with methylphenidate therapy: a population-based study. *Canadian Journal of Psychiatry* 49 (11): 761–768.

Miller, A.R., Lalonde, C.E., McGrail, K.M., Armstrong, R.W. (2001) Prescription of methylphenidate to children and youth, 1990–1996. *Journal of the Canadian Medical Association (CMAJ)* 165 (11): 489–494.

Miller, A., Lee, S.K., Raina, P., et al. (1998) *A review of therapies for attention-deficit/hyperactivity disorder*. Ottawa, ON: Canadian Coordinating Office for Health Technology Assessment (CCOHTA).

Mishan, E.J. (1971) Evaluation of Life and limb: a theoretical approach. *Journal of Political Economy* 79 (4): 687–705.

Mitchell, A.S. (2002) Antipodean assessment: activities, actions, and achievements. *International Journal for Technology Assessment in Health Care* 18 (2): 203–212.

Mitton, C., Donaldson, C. (2004) *Priority setting toolkit. A guide to the use of economics in healthcare decision making*. London: BMJ Books.

Morgan, S.G., McMahon, M., Mitton, C., et al. (2006) Centralized drug review processes in Australia, Canada, New Zealand, and the United Kingdom. *Health Affairs* 25 (2): 337–347.

Mortimer, D. (2006) The value of thinly spread QALYs. *Pharmacoeconomics* 24 (9): 845–853.

Motheral, B., Brooks, J., Clark, M.A., et al. (2003) A checklist for retrospective database studies – report of the ISPOR Task Force on retrospective databases. *Value in Health* 6: 90–97.

MTA Cooperative Group (2004) National Institute of Mental Health Multimodal Treatment Study of ADHD follow-up: 24-month outcomes of treatment strategies for attention-deficit/hyperactivity disorder. *Pediatrics* 113 (4): 754–761.

MTA Cooperative Group (1999a) A 14-month randomized clinical trial of treatment strategies for attention-deficit/hyperactivity disorder. *Archives of General Psychiatry* 56: 1073–1086.

MTA Cooperative Group (1999b) Moderators and mediators of treatment response for children with attention-deficit/hyperactivity disorder: the multimodal treatment study of children with attention-deficit/hyperactivity disorder. *Archives of General Psychiatry* 56: 1088–1096.

Murphy, K.R., Barkley, R.A., Bush, T. (2002) Young adults with attention deficit hyperactivity disorder: subtype differences in comorbidity, educational, and clinical history. *Journal of Nervous and Mental Disorders* 190 (3): 147–157.

Narayan, S., Hay, J. (2004) Cost effectiveness of methylphenidate versus AMP/DEX mixed salts for the first-line treatment of ADHD. *Expert Review of Pharmacoeconomics & Outcomes Research* 4 (6): 625–634.

National Health Service (NHS) Lothian (2003) *Shared care protocol and information for gps, methylphenidate for attention deficit hyperactivity disorder. Version 4.* Edinburgh, October 2003.

National Health Service (NHS) North Yorkshire Health Authority (2001) *Methylphenidate tablets (Ritalin, Equasym) shared care guidelines.*

National Health Service (NHS) Berkshire Priorities Committee (2001) *Minimum shared care arrangements for methylphenidate.* Berkshire, August 2001.

National Institute for Health and Clinical Excellence [NICE] (2007). *About the citizens council.* Available online at: www.nice.org.uk/page.aspx?o=113692. Last accessed January 7, 2007.

National Institute for Health and Clinical Excellence [NICE] (2006a) *Draft Scope: Attention deficit hyperactivity disorder: identification and management of ADHD in children, young people and adults.* London: NICE, January 31, 2006. Source: www.nice.org.uk/page.aspx?o=290880. Accessed February 12, 2006.

National Institute for Health and Clinical Excellence [NICE] (2006b) *Methylphenidate, atomoxetine and dexamfetamine for attention deficit hyperactivity disorder (ADHD) in children and adolescents. Review of Technology Appraisal 13.* London: NICE, March 2006.

National Institute for Health and Clinical Excellence [NICE] (2006c) *NICE Citizens Council to examine the "Rule of Rescue".* London: Press Release 2006/004, January 25, 2006.

National Institute for Health and Clinical Excellence [NICE] (2006d) *NICE Citizens Council to examine health inequalities.* London: Press Release 2006/025, June 02, 2006.

National Institute for Health and Clinical Excellence [NICE] (2006e) *NICE Citizens Council Report – Rule of Rescue, January 2006.* London: NICE, July 17, 2006. Available online at: www.nice.org.uk/page.aspx?o=343455. Last accessed August 1, 2006.

National Institute for Health and Clinical Excellence [NICE] (2006f) *About technology appraisals.* Available online at www.nice.org.uk/page.aspx?o=202425. Last accessed December 30, 2006.

National Institute for Health and Clinical Excellence [NICE] (2006g) *The guidelines manual 2006.* London: April 2006.

National Institute for Health and Clinical Excellence [NICE] (2006h) *The guideline development process: an overview for stakeholders, the public and the NHS.* London: NICE, September 2006 (2nd edition).

National Institute for Health and Clinical Excellence [NICE] (2006i) *Guide to the single technology appraisal (STA) process.* London: NICE, September 2006.

National Institute for Health and Clinical Excellence [NICE] (2006j) *Scope: Attention deficit hyperactivity disorder: diagnosis and management of ADHD in children, young people and adults.* London: NICE, January 31, 2006. Available online at www.nice.org.uk/page.aspx?o=351276. Last accessed October 16, 2006.

National Institute for Health and Clinical Excellence [NICE] (2006k) *Donepezil, rivastigmine, galantamine, and Memantine for the treatment of Alzheimer's disease. Appeal by Eisai Limited. Decision of the Appeal Panel.* London: October 11, 2006. Available online at: http://www.nice.org.uk/page.aspx?o=371762. Last accessed December 30, 2006.

National Institute for Health and Clinical Excellence [NICE] (2006l) *Putting NICE guidance into practice.* London: NICE, August 04, 2006. Available online at: http://www.nice.org.uk/page.aspx?o=280304. Last accessed December 02, 2006.

National Institute for Clinical Excellence [NICE] (2005a) *Appraisal Consultation Document: Methylphenidate, atomoxetine and dexamfetamine for attention-deficit/hyperactivity disorder (ADHD) in children and adolescents.* London: NICE, March 2005.

National Institute for Clinical Excellence [NICE] (2005b) *Appraisals Committee. Meeting February 15, 2005. Confirmed Meeting Minutes,* published March 17, 2005, at www.nice.org.uk/page.aspx?o=243323. Last accessed February 15, 2006.

National Institute for Health and Clinical Excellence [NICE] (2005c) *Final Appraisal Determination: Methylphenidate, atomoxetine and dexamfetamine for attention deficit hyperactivity disorder (ADHD) in children and adolescents.* London: NICE, May 2005.

National Institute for Health and Clinical Excellence [NICE] (2005d) *Appraisals Committee. Meeting April 21, 2005. Confirmed Meeting Minutes,* published May 27, 2005, at www.nice.org.uk/pdf/TAC_210405_confirmed.pdf. Last accessed February 15, 2006.

National Institute for Health and Clinical Excellence [NICE] (2005e) *Appeal details: Methylphenidate, atomoxetine and dexamfetamine for attention deficit hyperactivity disorder (ADHD) in children and adolescents.* London: NICE, July 22, 2005; updated August 25, 2005. Published at: www.nice.org.uk/page.aspx?o=adhdappeal. Last accessed December 20, 2005.

National Institute of Health and Clinical Excellence [NICE] (2005f) *Social Value Judgements. Principles for the development of NICE's guidance. Post-consultation draft.* London: NICE, September 21, 2005.

National Institute for Health and Clinical Excellence [NICE] (2005g) *NICE plans faster drugs guidance for the NHS.* London: National Institute for Health and Clinical Excellence Press Release, Friday, September 23, 2005.

National Institute for Health and Clinical Excellence [NICE] (2005h) *Appraisal of methylphenidate, atomoxetine and dexamfetamine for attention deficit hyperactivity disorder in children and adolescents: Decision of the Panel.* London: NICE, December 08, 2005. Published at: www.nice.org.uk/page. aspx?o=283566. Last accessed December 20, 2005.

National Institute for Health and Clinical Excellence [NICE] (2005i) *Appraisals in development: Attention deficit hyperactivity disorder – methylphenidate, atomoxetine and dexamfetamine (review). Project History.* Available from NICE website at www.nice.org.uk/page.aspx?o=72340 (last accessed September 28, 2005).

National Institute for Health and Clinical Excellence [NICE] (2005j) *A guide to NICE.* London: NICE, April 2005. Available online at: www.nice.org.uk/page.aspx?o=guidetonice.

National Institute of Health and Clinical Excellence [NICE] (2005k) *Social Value Judgements. Principles for the development of NICE's guidance.* London: NICE, December 08, 2005.

National Institute for Clinical Excellence [NICE] (2004a) *Guideline Development Methods: Information for National Collaborating Centres and Guideline Developers.* London: NICE, February 2004 (updated February 2005).

National Institute for Clinical Excellence [NICE] (2004b) *Guide to the Technology Appraisal Process (reference N0514).* London: NICE, April 2004.

National Institute for Clinical Excellence [NICE] (2004c) *Guide to the Methods of Technology Appraisal (reference N0515).* London: NICE, April 2004.

National Institute for Clinical Excellence [NICE] (2004d) *Technology Appraisal Process: Guidance for Appellants (reference N0520).* London: NICE, April 2004.

National Institute for Clinical Excellence [NICE] (2004e) *Special Health Authority Tenth Wave Work Programme: Attention Deficit Hyperactivity Disorder. Remit.* London: NICE, June 2004.

National Institute for Clinical Excellence [NICE] (2004f) *Press Release: NICE asked to develop guidance on the care of drug misuse, medicines for prostate cancer, and management of attention deficit hyperactivity disorder.* London: NICE, June 16, 2004.

National Institute of Clinical Excellence [NICE] (2004g) *Agreement between the Association of the British Pharmaceutical Industry (ABPI) and the National Institute for Clinical Excellence (NICE) on guidelines for the release of company data into the public domain during a health technology appraisal.* London: NICE, October 27, 2004.

National Institute for Clinical Excellence [NICE] (2004h) *Contributing to a Technology Appraisal: A Guide for Healthcare Professional Groups (reference N0517).* London: NICE, November 2004.

National Institute for Clinical Excellence [NICE] (2004i) *Contributing to a Technology Appraisal: A Guide for Manufacturers and Sponsors (reference N0518).* London: NICE, November 2004.

National Institute for Clinical Excellence [NICE] (2004j) *Contributing to a Technology Appraisal: A Guide for NHS Organisations (reference N0519).* London: NICE, November 2004.

National Institute for Clinical Excellence [NICE] (2004k) *Contributing to a Technology Appraisal: A Guide for Patient/Carer Groups (reference N0516).* London: NICE, November 2004.

National Institute for Clinical Excellence [NICE] (2004l). *Newer drugs for epilepsy in adults. Technology Appraisal Guidance 76.* London: NICE, March 2004. Available online at: http://www.nice.org.uk/page.aspx?o=ta076guidance. Last accessed December 30, 2006.

National Institute for Clinical Excellence [NICE] (2004m) *Supporting the implementation of NICE guidance.* London, NICE.

National Institute for Clinical Excellence [NICE] (2004n) *NICE Citizens Council report: ultra orphan drugs.* London: NICE, November 2004. Available online at: www.nice.org.uk/page.aspx?o=240951. Last accessed January 2, 2007.

National Institute for Clinical Excellence [NICE] (2003) *Health Technology Appraisal: Methylphenidate, atomoxetine and dexamfetamine for attention deficit hyperactivity disorder (ADHD) in children and adolescents including review of existing guidance number 13 (Guidance on the Use of Methylphenidate [Ritalin, Equasym] for Attention Deficit/Hyperactivity Disorder [ADHD] in childhood) – Scope.* London: NICE, August 2003.

National Institute for Clinical Excellence [NICE] (2002). *Technology Appraisal Guidance No. 32: Multiple sclerosis – beta-interferon and glatiramer acetate.* London: NICE, January 2002.

National Institute for Clinical Excellence [NICE] (2001). *Technology Appraisal Guidance No. 20: Guidance on the use of riluzole (Rilutek) for the treatment of motor neuron disease.* London: NICE, January 2001.

National Institute for Clinical Excellence [NICE] (2000). *Technology Appraisal Guidance No. 13: Guidance on the use of methylphenidate (Ritalin, Equasym) for attention deficit/hyperactivity disorder (ADHD) in childhood.* London: NICE, October 2000.

Netten, A. (2003) New developments and changes in guidance on the discount rate. In: Netten, A., Curtis, L. (eds.) *Unit costs of health and social care 2003.* Canterbury: University of Kent, Personal Social Services Research Unit (PSSRU), 7–12.

Netten, A., Curtis, L. (2004) *Unit costs of health and social care 2004.* Canterbury: University of Kent, Personal Social Services Research Unit (PSSRU).

Netten, A, Curtis, L. (2003) *Unit costs of health and social care 2003.* Canterbury: University of Kent, Personal Social Services Research Unit (PSSRU).

Neumann, P.J. (2004) Why don't Americans use cost-effectiveness analysis? *American Journal of Managed Care* 10: 308–312.

Neumann, P.J., Rosen, A.B., Weinstein, M.C. (2005a) Medicare and cost-effectiveness analysis. *New England Journal of Medicine* 353 (14): 1516–1522.

Neumann, P.J., Greenberg, D., Olchanski, N.V., et al. (2005b) Growth and quality of the cost-utility literature, 1976-2001. *Value in Health* 8 (1): 3–9.

Neumann, P.J., Stone, P.W., Chapman, R.H., et al. (2000) The quality of reporting in published cost-utility analyses, 1976-1997. *Annals of Internal Medicine* 132: 964–972.

Newcorn, J., Kratochvil, C.J., Allen, A.J., et al. (2005) *Atomoxetine and OROS methylphenidate for the treatment of ADHD: acute results and methodological issues.* Poster presentation at 45th Annual Meeting of the New Clinical Drug Evaluation Unit (NCDEU) of the National Institute of Mental Health (NIMH), Boca Raton, FL, June 6-9, 2005, Book of Abstracts, p. 188.

Newcorn, J.H., Owens, J.A., Jasinski, D.R., et al. (2004) *Results from recently completed comparator studies with atomoxetine and methylphenidate.* 51st Annual Meeting of the American Academy of Child & Adolescent Psychiatry (AACAP), Washington, DC: Symposium 20, October 21, 2004.

Ng, Y.-K. (2004) *Welfare economics – towards a more complete analysis.* Houndsmill, New York, NY: Palgrave Macmillan.

NICE Citizens Council (2003) *Report on age.* London: NICE, 2003. Available online: www.nice.org.uk/pdf/Citizenscouncil_report_age.pdf.

Nissen, S.E. (2006) ADHD drugs and cardiovascular risk. *New England Journal of Medicine* 354: 1445–1448.

Nord, E. (1999) *Cost-value analysis in health care: making sense out of QALYs.* Cambridge: Cambridge University Press.

Nord, E. (1995) The person-trade-off approach to valuing health care programs. *Medical Decision-Making* 15 (3): 201–208.

Nord, E. (1993) The trade-off between severity of illness and treatment effect in cost-value analysis of health care. *Health Policy* 24 (3): 227–238.

Nord, E. (1992) Methods for quality adjustment of life years. *Social Science & Medicine* 34: 559–569.

Nord, E., Pinto, J.L., Richardson, J., et al. (1999) Incorporating societal concern for fairness in numerical valuations of health programs. *Health Economics* 8 (1): 25-39.

Nord, E., Richardson, J., Street, A., et al. (1995) Who cares about cost: does economic analysis impose or reflect ethical values? *Health Policy* 34: 79–94.

Nuijten, M.J.C., Rutten, F. (2002) Combining a budgetary-impact analysis and a cost-effectiveness analysis using decision-analytic modelling techniques. *Pharmacoeconomics* 20 (12): 855–867.

O'Brien, B.J., Briggs, A.H. (2002) Analysis of uncertainty in health care cost-effectiveness studies: an introduction to statistical issues and methods. *Statistical Methods in Medical Research* 11 (6): 455–468.

O'Brien, J.T. (2006) NICE and anti-dementia drugs: a triumph of health economics over clinical wisdom? *Lancet Neurology* 5 (12): 994–996.

Office of Fair Trading [OFT] (2007) *The Pharmaceutical Price Regulation Scheme – An OFT market study*. London: OFT, February 2007.

Olfson, M. (2004) New options in the pharmacological management of attention-deficit/hyperactivity disorder. *American Journal of Managed Care* 10 (4; Supplement): S117–S124.

Ontario Ministery of Health (1994) *Ontario guidelines for economic analysis of pharmaceutical products*. Toronto, ON: Ministry of Health.

Osterdal, L.P. (2003) A note on cost-value analysis. *Health Economics* 12 (3): 247–250.

Owens, E.B., Hinshaw, S.P., Kraemer, H.C., et al. (2003) Which treatment for whom for ADHD? Moderators of treatment response in the MTA. *Journal of Consulting and Clinical Psychology* 71 (3): 540–552.

Paltiel, A.D., Neumann, P.J. (1997) Why training is the key to successful guideline implementation. *Pharmacoeconomics* 12 (2): 297–302.

Parfit, D. (2000) Equality or priority? In: Clayton M, Williams A, Editors. *The Ideal of Equality*. Basingstoke: Palgrave, 81–125.

Patakis, C.S., Feinberg, D.T., McGough, J.J. (2004) New drugs for the treatment of attention-deficit/hyperactivity disorder. *Expert Opinion on Emerging Drugs* 9 (2): 293–302.

Patrick, K.S., Mueller, R.A., Gualtieri, C.T., Breese, G.R. (1987) Pharmacokinetics and actions of methylphenidate. In: Meltzer, H.Y. (ed.) *Psychopharmacology: A Third Generation of Progress*. New York, NY: Raven Press, 1387–1395.

Pauly, M.V. (2003a) Foreword. In: Hammer, P.J., Haas-Wilson, D., Peterson, M.A., Sage, W.M. (eds.) *Uncertain times: Kenneth Arrow and the changing economics of health care*. Durham and London, Duke University Press.

Pauly, M.V. (2003b) Should we be worried about high real medical spending growth in the United States? *Health Affairs*, Web Exclusives January 2003, W3-15-W3-27

Pauly, M.V. (1995) Valuing health care benefits in money terms. In: Sloan, F.A. (editor) *Valuing Health Care*. Cambridge: Cambridge University Press, 99–124.

Pearson, S.D., Rawlins, M.D. (2005) Quality, innovation, and value for money. NICE and the British National Health Service. *Journal of the American Medical Association (JAMA)* 294 (20): 2618–2622.

Peck, C. (1999) Non-compliance and clinical trials: regulatory perspectives. In: Métry, J.-M., Meyer, U.A. (eds.) *Drug Regimen Compliance: Issues in Clinical Trials and Patient Management*. Chichester: John Wiley & Sons, pp. 97–102.

Pelham, W.E. (1999) The NIMH Multimodal Treatment Study for attention-deficit hyperactivity disorder: just say yes to drugs alone? *Canadian Journal of Psychiatry* 44: 981–990.

Pelham, W.E., Gnagy, E.M., Borroughs-Maclean, L., et al. (2001) Once-a-day Concerta methylphenidate versus three-times-daily methylphenidate in laboratory and natural settings. *Pediatrics* 107 (6): e105/1–15.

Pelham, W.E., Burrows-MacLean, L., Gnagy, E.M., et al. (2000) Once-a-day Concerta methylphenidate versus t.i.d. methylphenidate in natural settings. *Pediatrics* 121: 126–137.

Pelham, W.E., Aronoff, H.R., Midlam, J.K., et al. (1999a) A comparison of Ritalin and Adderall: efficacy and time-course in children with attention-deficit/hyperactivity disorder. *Pediatrics* 103 (4): e43/1–14.

Pelham, W.E., Gnagy, E.M., Chronis, A.M., et al. (1999b) A comparison of morning-only and morning/late afternoon Adderall to morning-only, twice-daily, and three times-daily methylphenidate in children with attention-deficit/hyperactivity disorder. *Pediatrics* 104 (6): 1300–1311.

Pelham, W.E., Carlson, C., Sams, S.E., et al. (1993) Separate and combined effects of methylphenidate and behavior modification on boys with attention deficit-hyperactivity disorder in the classroom. *Journal of Consulting and Clinical Psychology* 61: 506–515.

Pelham, W.E., Greenslade, K.E., Vodde-Hamilton, M., et al. (1990) Relative efficacy of long-acting stimulants on children with attention deficit-hyperactivity disorder: a comparison of standard methylphenidate, sustained-release methylphenidate, sustained-release dextroamphetamine, and pemoline. *Pediatrics* 86 (2): 226–237.

Pelham, W.E., Sturges, J., Hoza, J., et al. (1987) Sustained release and standard methylphenidate effects on cognitive and social behavior in children with attention deficit disorder. *Pediatrics* 80 (4): 491–501.

Petitti, D.B. (2000) *Meta-Analysis, Decision Analysis, and Cost-Effectiveness Analysis. Methods for Quantitative synthesis in Medicine.* New York, Oxford. Oxford University Press, 2nd edition.

Peto, R., Collins, R., Gray, R. (1995) Large-scale randomized evidence: large, simple trials and overviews of trials. *Journal of Clinical Epidemiology* 48: 23–40.

Philips, Z., Bojke, L., Sculpher, M., et al. (2006) Good practice guidelines for decision-analytic modelling in health technology assessment: a review and consolidation of quality assessment. *Pharmacoeconomics* 24 (4): 355–371.

Philips, Z., Ginnelly, L., Sculpher, M., et al. (2004) Review of guidelines for good practice in decision-analytic modelling in health technology assessment. *Health Technology Assessment* 2004; 8 (36): 1–174.

Pinto-Prades, J.L., Abellan-Perpinan, J.M. (2005) Measuring the health of populations: the veil of ignorance approach. *Health Economics* 14 (1): 69–82.

Pliszka, S.R. (2007) Pharmacologic treatment of attention-deficit/hyperactivity disorder: efficacy, safety, and mechanisms of action. *Neuropsychology Review*, epub ahead of print, January 23, 2007.

Pliszka, S.R., Browne, R.G., Olvera, R.L., Wynne, S.K. (2000) A double-blind, placebo-controlled study of Adderall and methylphenidate in the treatment of attention-deficit/hyperactivity disorder. *Journal of the American Academy of Child & Adolescent Psychiatry* 39 (5): 619–626.

Pollitt, C., Harrison, S., Hunter, D.J., Marnoch, G. (1990) No hiding place: on the discomforts of researching the contemporary policy process. *Journal of Social Policy* 19: 169–190.

Pope, C., Mays, N. (1995) Qualitative research: reaching the parts other methods cannot reach: an introduction to qualitative methods in health and health services research. *British Medical Journal* 311: 42–45.

Popper, K. (1935) *Logik der Forschung.* Vienna, Austria: Springer.

Porzsolt, F., Kajnar, H., Awa, A., et al. (2005) Validity of original studies in health technology assessment reports: significance of standardized reporting. *International Journal of Health Technology Assessment in Health Care* 21: 410–413.

Powell, M. (2001) Latest decision on zanamivir will not end postcode prescribing. *British Medical Journal* 322: 490.

Preuss, U., Ralston, S.J., Baldursson, G., et al. (2006) Study design, baseline patient characteristics and intervention in a cross-cultural framework: results from the ADORE study. *European Child & Adolescent Psychiatry* 15 (Suppl. 1): 4–14.

Price, M., Lloyd, A., Yuen, C., et al. (2004) The perceived benefits of dosing schedules for children with ADHD. *Value in Health* 7 (6): 782.

Quam, L., Smith, R. (2005) What can the UK and US health systems learn from each other? *British Medical Journal* 330: 530–533

Raftery, J. (2006) Review of NICE's recommendations, 1999–2005. *British Medical Journal* 332: 1266–1268.

Raftery, J. (2001) NICE: faster access to modern treatments? Analysis of guidance on health technologies. *British Medical Journal* 323: 1300–1303.

Ramsey, S., Willke, R., Briggs, A., et al. (2005) Good research practices for cost-effectiveness analysis alongside clinical trials: the ISPOR RCT-CEA Task Force report. *Value in Health* 8 (5) 521–533.

Rappley, M.D. (2005) Attention deficit-hyperactivity disorder. *New England Journal of Medicine* 352 (2): 165–173.

Rappley, M.D., Moore, J.W., Dokken, D. (2006) ADHD drugs and cardiovascular risk (letter). *New England Journal of Medicine* 354: 2296.

Rapport, M.D., DuPaul, G.J., Kelly, K.L. (1989) Attention deficit hyperactivity disorder and methylphenidate: the relationship between gross body weight and drug response in children. *Psychopharmacology Bulletin* 25: 285–290.

Rasmussen, P., Gillberg, C. (2000) Natural outcome of ADHD with developmental coordination disorder at age 22 years: a controlled, longitudinal, community-based study. *Journal of the American Academy of Child & Adolescent Psychiatry* 39 (11): 1424–1431.

Rawlins, M.D., Culyer, A.J. (2004) National Institute of Clinical Excellence and its value judgments. *British Medical Journal* 329: 224–227.

Rawlins, M., Dillon, A. (2005a) What's the evidence that NICE guidance has been implemented? More recent data on NICE implementation sho different picture. *British Medical Journal* 330: 1086.

Rawlins, M., Dillon, A. (2005b) NICE discrimination. *Journal of Medical Ethics* 31: 683–684.

Rawls, J. (1971) *A theory of justice*. Cambridge: Harvard University Press.

Redwood, H. (2006) *The use of cost-effectiveness analysis of medicines in the British National Health Service: Lessons for the United States*. (Expertise supported by the Pharmaceutical Research and Manufacturers of America, PhRMA.) Felixstowe, Suffolk: April 2006.

Reinhardt, U.E. (2004) An information infrastructure for the pharmaceutical market. *Health Affairs* 23 (1): 107–112.

Reinhardt, U.E. (2001) Perspectives on the pharmaceutical industry. *Health Affairs* 20 (5): 136–149.

Reinhardt, U.E. (1998) Abstracting from distributional effects, this policy is efficient. In: Barer, M.L., Getzen, T.E., Stoddard, G.L. (eds.) *Health, Health Care and Health Economics: Perspectives on Distribution*. Chichester: John Wiley & Sons: 1–52.

Reinhardt, U.E. (1997) Making economic evaluations respectable. *Social Science & Medicine* 45 (4): 555–562.

Reinhardt, U.E. (1992) Reflections on the meaning of efficiency. *Yale Law & Policy Review* 10 (2): 302–315.

Reinhardt, U.E., Hussey, P.S., Anderson, G.F. (2004) U.S. health care spending in an international context. *Health Affairs* 23 (3): 10–26.

Reinhardt, U.E., Hussey, P.S., Anderson, G.F. (2002) Cross-national comparisons of health systems using OECD data, 1999. *Health Affairs* 21 (3): 169–181.

Remak, E., Hutton, J., Jones, M., Zagari, M. (2003) Changes in cost-effectiveness over time. The case of Epoetin Alfa for renal replacement therapy patients in the UK. *European Journal of Health Economics* 4 (2): 115–121.

Rennie D. (2001) Cost-effectiveness analysis: making a pseudoscience legitimate. *Journal of Health Politics, Policy, and Law* 26: 2.

Rennie, D., Luft, H.S. (2000) Pharmacoeconomic analyses: making them transparent, making them credible. *Journal of the American Medical Association (JAMA)* 283 (16): 2158–2160.

Revicki, D.A., Frank, L. (1999) Pharmacoeconomic evaluations in the real world: effectiveness versus efficacy studies. *Pharmacoeconomics* 15 (5): 423–434.

Rey, J.M., Sawyer, M.G. (2003) Are psychostimulant drugs being used appropriately to treat child and adolescent disorders? *British Journal of Psychiatry* 182: 284–286.

Richardson, J. (1994) Cost utility analysis: what should be measured? *Social Science & Medicine* 39: 7–21.

Richardson, J., McKie, J. (2006) *Should economic costs be of interest in a national health scheme: or costs, fairness and reverse order analysis*. Paper presented at a seminar at the Forschungsinstitut zur Zukunft der Arbeit (IZA), Bonn, Germany, February 23, 2006, available online at: http://www.iza.org/en/papers/2526_23022006.pdf. Last accessed January 10, 2007.

Richardson, J., McKie, J. (2005) Empiricism, ethics and orthodox economic theory: what is the appropriate basis for decision-making in the health sector? *Social Science & Medicine* 60: 265–275.

Rittenhouse, B. (1996) *Uses of models in economic evaluations of medicines and other health technologies.* London: Office of Health Economics (OHE).

Robison, L.M., Skaer, T.L., Sclar, D.A., Galin, R.S. (2002) Is attention deficit hyperactivity disorder increasing among girls in the US? Trends in diagnosis and the prescribing of stimulants. *CNS Drugs* 16 (2): 129–137.

Robison, L.M., Sclar, D.A., Skaer, T.L., Galin, R.S. (1999) National trends in the prevalence of attention-deficit/hyperactivity disorder and the prescribing of methylphenidate among school-age children: 1990-1995. *Clinical Pediatrics* 38 (4): 209–217.

Romeo, R., Byford, S., Knapp, M. (2005) Annotation: economic evaluations of child and adolescent mental health interventions: a systematic review. *Journal of Child Psychology and Psychiatry* 46 (9): 919–930.

Rösler, M., Retz, W., Retz-Junginger, P., et al. (2004) Prevalence of attention-deficit/hyperactivity disorder (ADHD) and comorbid disorders in young male prison inmates. *European Archives of Psychiatry & Clinical Neuroscience* 254 (6): 365–371.

Rovira, J. (1994) Standardizing economic appraisal of health technology in the European Community. *Social Science & Medicine* 38 (12): 1675–1678.

Rothenberger, A., Coghill, D., Döpfner, M., et al. (2006) Naturalistic observational studies in the framework of ADHD health care. *European Child & Adolescent Psychiatry* 15 (Suppl. 1): I/1–I/3.

Sackett, D.L., Haynes, R.B., Guyatt, G.H., Tugwell, P. (1991) *Clinical Epidemiology: A Basic Science for Clinical Medicine.* Toronto: Little, Brown and Company, 2nd edition.

Salomon, J.A., Murray, C.J.L. (2004) A multi-method approach to measuring health-state valuations. *Health Economics* 13: 281–290.

Sanchez, R.J., Crismon, M.L., Barner, J.C., et al. (2005) Assessment of adherence measures with different stimulants among children and adolescents. *Pharmacotherapy* 25 (7): 909–917.

Sandberg, E.A. (2005) A threshold analysis: what QALY gains are needed for treatments for attention deficit hyperactivity disorder (ADHD) to be considered cost-effective? San Francisco, CA: *27th Annual Meeting of the Society for Medical Decision Making*, October 22, 2005. http://sdm.confex.com/smdm/2005ca/techprogram/P2427.htm. Last accessed February 23, 2006.

Santosh, P. (2002) *Multimodal treatment study of ADHD (MTA): impact of classificatory systems on pharmacological interventions.* Presentation at the 49th Annual Meeting of the American Academy of Child and Adolescent Psychiatry, San Francisco, CA: October 22–27, 2002.

Santosh, P.J., Taylor, E., Swanson, J., et al. (2005) Refining the diagnoses of inattention and overactivity syndromes: a reanalysis of the Multimodal Treatment study of attention deficit hyperactivity disorder (ADHD) based on ICD-10 criteria for hyperkinetic disorder. *Clinical Neuroscience Research* 5: 307–314.

Savulescu, J. (1999) Consequentialism, reasons, value and justice. *Bioethics* 12 (3): 212–235.

Sawyer, M.G., Whaites, L., Rey, J.M., et al. (2002) Health-related quality of life of children and adolescents with mental disorders. *Journal of the American Academy of Child & Adolescent Psychiatry* 41: 530–537.

Scahill, L., Schwab-Stone, M. (2000) Epidemiology of ADHD in school-age children. *Child and Adolescent Psychiatric Clinics of North America* 9 (3): 541–555.

Schachar, R., Tannock, R. (2002) Syndromes of hyperactivity and attention deficit. In : Rutter, M., Taylor, E. (eds.) *Child and Adolescent Psychiatry.* Oxford: Blackwell, 4th edition, 399–418.

Schachar, R., Jadad, A.R., Gauld, M., et al. (2002) Attention-deficit hyperactivity disorder: critical appraisal of extended treatment studies. *Canadian Journal of Psychiatry* 47 (4): 337–348.

Schirm, E., Tobi, H., Zito, J.M., de Jong-van den Berg, L.T.W. (2001) Psychotropic medication in children: a study from the Netherlands. *Pediatrics* 108 (2): e25.

Schlander, M. (2007a) NICE accountability for reasonableness. A qualitative case study of its appraisal of treatments for attention-deficit/hyperactivity disorder (ADHD). *Current Medical Research & Opinion* 23 (1): 207–222.

Schlander, M. (2007b) Is NICE infallible? A qualitative case study of its assessment of treatments for attention-deficit/hyperactivity disorder (ADHD). *Current Medical Research & Opinion*; in press.

Schlander, M. (2007c) Has NICE got it right? An international perspective considering the case of Technology Appraisal No. 98 by the National Institute for Health and Clinical Excellence (NICE). *Current Medical Research & Opinion*, submitted.

Schlander, M. (2007d) Long-acting medications for the hyperkinetic disorders: a note on cost-effectiveness. *European Child & Adolescent Psychiatry*, published online first February 6, 2007; DOI:10.1007/s00787-007-0615-2.

Schlander, M. (2007e) *Lost in translation? Over-reliance on QALYs may lead to neglect of relevant evidence.* Paper presented at the 6th World Congress of the International Health Economics Association (iHEA), Copenhagen, Denmark, July 9, 2007.

Schlander, M. (2006a) Learning from NICE technology assessments: a case study of its recent appraisal of attention-deficit/hyperactivity disorder (ADHD) treatment strategies. *Value in Health* 9 (3): A71–72.

Schlander, M. (2006b) Impact of attention-deficit/hyperactivity disorder (ADHD) on prescription drug spending for children and adolescents: increasing relevance of health economic evidence. *Technical Paper No. 02/2006.* Aschaffenburg and Eschborn, Institute for Innovation & Valuation in Health Care, July 2006.

Schlander, M. (2005a) Kosteneffektivität und Ressourcenallokation: Gibt es einen normativen Anspruch der Gesundheitsökonomie? In: Kick, H.A., Taupitz, J. (eds.) *Gesundheitswesen zwischen Wirtschaftlichkeit und Menschlichkeit.* Münster: LIT-Verlag, 37–112.

Schlander, M. (2005b) *Economic evaluation of medical interventions: answering questions people are unwilling to ask?* Presentation at the 5th World Congress of the International Health Economics Association (iHEA), Barcelona, July 12, 2005: Book of Abstracts, 194–195.

Schlander, M. (2004a) *Budgetary impact of treatments for attention-deficit/hyperactivity disorder (ADHD) in Germany: increasing relevance of health economic evidence.* In: Book of Abstracts, 16th World Congress of the International Association for Child and Adolescent Psychiatry and Allied Professions (IACAPAP). Berlin, Darmstadt: Steinkopff, August 2004: S-111-516, p. 187.

Schlander, M. (2004b) Cost-effectiveness of methylphenidate OROS for attention-deficit/hyperactivity disorder (ADHD): an evaluation from the perspective of the UK National Health Service (NHS). *Value in Health* 7 (3): 236.

Schlander, M. (2004c) Steigende Arzneimittelausgaben in Deutschland: Gesundheitsökonomische Aspekte aus einer internationalen Perspektive. *Die pharmazeutische Industrie* 66: 513–515 and 705–709.

Schlander (2003) Une Simplification Terrible? Anmerkungen zur geplanten Nutzenbewertung von Arzneimitteln aus gesundheitsökonomischer Perspektive. *Brennpunkt Gesundheitswesen* 11/03: 22–26.

Schlander, M., Schwarz, O. (2005a) The Nordbaden project for health care utilization research in Germany: database characteristics and first application. *Value in Health* 8 (6): 199.

Schlander, M., Schwarz, O. (2005b) Finanzierbarkeit steigender Gesundheitsausgaben in Deutschland: eine makroökonomische Betrachtung. *Gesundheitsökonomie & Qualitätsmanagement* 10 (6): 178–187.

Schlander M., Schwarz, O., Trott, G.-E. et al. (2007) Who cares for patients with attention-deficit/hyperactivity disorder? Insights from Nordbaden (Germany). *European Child & Adolescent Psychiatry*, published online first April 28, 2007; DOI:10.1007/s00787-007-0616-1.

Schlander, M., Schwarz, O., Hakkaart-van Roijen, L., et al. (2006a) Cost-Effectiveness of Clinically Proven Treatment Strategies for Attention-Deficit/ Hyperactivity Disorder (ADHD) in the United States, Germany, The Netherlands, Sweden, and United Kingdom. *Value in Health* 9 (6): A312.

Schlander, M., Schwarz, O., Hakkaart-van Roijen, L., et al. (2006b) Functional Impairment of Patients with Attention-Deficit/ Hyperactivity Disorder (ADHD): An Alternative Cost-Effectiveness Analysis of Clinically Proven Treatment Strategies based upon the NIMH MTA Study. *Value in Health* 9 (6): A312.

Schlander, M., Schwarz, O., Foster, E.M., et al. (2006c) Cost-Effectiveness of Clinically Proven Treatment Strategies for Attention-Deficit/ Hyperactivity Disorder (ADHD): Impact of Coexisting Conditions. *Value in Health* 9 (6): A309.

Schlander, M., Schwarz, O., Viapiano, M., Bonauer, N. (2006d) Methylphenidate Prescriptions for Children and Adolescents with Attention-Deficit/Hyperactivity Disorder (ADHD): New Data from Nordbaden / Germany. *Value in Health* 9 (6): A191–A192.

Schlander, M., Jensen, P.S., Foster, E.M., et al. (2005a) Incremental cost-effectiveness ratios of clinically proven treatments for attention-deficit/hyperactivity disorder (ADHD): impact of diagnostic criteria and comorbidity. *5th World Congress, International Health Economics Association (iHEA)*. Book of Abstracts. Barcelona: pp. 194–195.

Schlander, M., Schwarz, O., Trott, G.E., et al. (2005b) Attention-deficit/hyperactivity disorder (ADHD) in children and adolescents: mental health and physical co-morbidity in Nordbaden / Germany. *Value in Health* 8 (6): 196–197.

Schlander, M., Jensen, P.S., Foster, E.M., et al. (2004a) Kosteneffektivität alternativer Behandlungsstrategien der Aufmerksamkeitsdefizit/ Hyperaktivitätsstörung (ADHS): Erste Daten aus der amerikanischen MTA-Studie. *Monatsschrift für Kinderheilkunde* 152: Suppl. 1.

Schlander, M., Migliaccio-Walle, K., Caro, J. (2004b) *Treatment of attention-deficit/hyperactivity disorder (ADHD): modelling the cost-effectiveness of a modified-release preparation of methylphenidate from the perspective of the National Health Service (NHS) in the United Kingdom (UK).* 16th World Congress of the International Association for Child and Adolescent Psychiatry and Allied Professions (IACAPAP), Berlin, August 22–26, 2004. Book of Abstracts, Darmstadt: Steinkopff-Verlag: S-112-522, 189.

Schlander, M., Thielscher, C., Schwarz, O. (2004c) Affordability sensitive to economic growth rates. *Health Affairs* 23 (1): 276–277.

Schlander, M., Schwarz, O., Thielscher, C. (2004d) Estimating the ability to pay for health care expenditures rising faster than GDP: an international perspective comparing the USA and Germany. *Value in Health* 7 (3): 37.

Schreyögg, J., Stargardt, T., Velasco-Garrido, M., Busse, R. (2005) Defining the "health benefit basket" in nine European countries – evidence from the European Union health basket project. *European Journal of Health Economics* 6 (Suppl. 1): S2–S10.

Schubert, I., Selke, G.W., Oÿwald-Huang, P.-H., et al. (2002) *Methylphenidat-Verordnungsanalyse auf der Basis von GKV-Daten – Bericht für die Arbeitsgruppe Methylphenidat im Bundesministerium für Gesundheit.* Bonn, Germany: Wissenschaftliches Institut der AOK (WIdO).

Schubert, I., Lehmkuhl, G., Spengler, A., et al. (2001) Methylphenidat bei hyperkinetischen Störungen. *Deutsches Ärzteblatt* 98 (9): A541–A544.

Schwabe, U., Paffrath, D. (2006) *Arzneiverordnungs-Report 2006.* Heidelberg: Springer.

Schwartz, D., Lellouch, J. (1967) Explanatory and pragmatic attitudes in therapeutic trials. *Journal of Chronic Diseases* 20: 637–648.

Scottish Intercollegiate Guidelines Network [SIGN] (2003). *Diagnosis and management of epilepsy in adults. A national clinical guideline.* Edinburgh: SIGN, April 2003.

Scottish Medicines Consortium (2005a) *Atomoxetine capsules 10mg to 60mg (Strattera). No. 153/05.* February 04, 2005, published online March 07, 2005, at: http://www.scottishmedicines.org.uk/medicines/default.asp. Last accessed February 15, 2006.

Scottish Medicines Consortium (2005b) *Atomoxetine capsules 10mg to 60mg (Strattera). No. 153/05.* June 10, 2005, published online July 11, 2005, at: http://www.scottishmedicines.org.uk/medicines/default.asp. Last accessed February 15, 2006.

Scrip (2007) Eisai goes ahead with court challenge over NICE assessment. *Scrip World Pharmaceutical News* 3223: 3.

Scrip (2006) Eisai refers NICE's refusal to disclose costing models to UK Parliamentary Ombudsman. *Scrip World Pharmaceutical News* 3175: 2.

Sculpher, M.J., Drummond, M.F. (2006) Analysis sans frontiers: can we ever make economic evaluations generalisable across jurisdictions? *Pharmacoeconomics* 24 (11): 1087–1099.

Sculpher, M., Fenwick, E., Claxton, K. (2000) Assessing quality in decision analytic cost-effectiveness models. *Pharmacoeconomics* 17 (5): 461–477.

Secnik, K., Matza, L.S., Cottrell, S., et al. (2005) Health state utilities for childhood attention-deficit/hyperactivity disorder based on parent preferences in the United Kingdom. *Medical Decision Making* 25: 56–70.

Secnik, K., Cottrell, S., Matza, L.S., et al. (2004) Assessment of health state utilities for Attention-Deficit/Hyperactivity Disorder in children using parent-based standard gamble scores. *Value in Health* 7 (3): 236.

Sen, A. (2002) Why health equity? *Health Economics* 11: 659–666.

Sen, A.K. (1985) *Capabilities and commodities*. Amsterdam: Elsevier.

Sendi, P.P., Briggs, A.M. (2001) Affordability and cost-effectiveness: decision-making on the cost-effectiveness plane. *Health Economics* 10 (7): 675–680.

Sergeant, J. (2004) EUNETHYDIS – searching for valid aetiological candidates for attention-deficit hyperactivity disorder. *European Child & Adolescent Psychiatry* 13 (Suppl. 1): 43–49.

Sharp, W.S., Alter, J.M., Marsh, W.L., et al. (1999) ADHD in girls: clinical comparability of a research sample. *Journal of the American Academy of Child & Adolescent Psychiatry* 38: 40–47.

Shatin, D., Drinkard, C.R. (2002) Ambulatory use of psychotropics by employer-insured children and adolescents in a national managed care organization. *Ambulatory Pediatrics* 2 (2): 111-119.

Sheehan, M. (2005) Orphan drugs and the NHS: fairness in health care entails more than cost effectiveness. *British Medical Journal* 331: 1144–1146.

Sheldon, T.A., Cullum, N., Dawson, D., et al. (2004) What's the evidence that NICE guidance has been implemented? Results from a national evaluation using time series analysis, audit of patients' notes, and interviews. *British Medical Journal* 329: 999–1006.

Shukla, V.P., Otten, N. (1999) *Assessment of attention deficit/hyperactivity disorder therapy: a Canadian perspective*. Ottawa, ON: Canadian Coordinating Office for Health Technology Assessment (CCOHTA).

Siegel, J.E. (2005) Cost-effectiveness analysis in US healthcare decision-making: where is it going? *Medical Care* 43 (7 Supplement): 1–4.

Siegel, J.E., Torrance, G.W., Russell, L.B., et al. (1997) Guidelines for pharmacoeconomic studies. Recommendations from the panel on cost effectiveness in health and medicine. *Pharmacoeconomics* 11 (2): 159–168.

Singer, P., McKie, J., Kuhse, H., Richardson, J. (1995) Double jeopardy and the use of QALYs in health care allocation. *Journal of Medical Ethics* 21 (3): 144–150.

Siponmaa, L., Kristiansson, M., Jonson, C., et al. (2001) Juvenile and young adult mentally disordered offenders: the role of child neuropsychiatric disorders. *Journal of the American Academy of Psychiatry & Law* 29 (4): 420–426.

Sleator, E.K., Ullmann, R.K., von Neumann, A. (1982) How do hyperactive children feel about taking stimulants and will they tell the doctor? *Clinical Pediatrics* 21 (8): 474–479.

Smith, R. (2004) The triumph of NICE. *British Medical Journal* 329: 0.

Smith, R. (2000) The failings of NICE. Time to start work on version 2. *British Medical Journal* 321: 1363–1364.

Smith, B.H., Pelham, W.E. Jr., Gnagy, E. et al. (2000) The reliability, validity, and unique contributions of self-report by adolescents receiving treatment for attention-deficit/hyperactivity disorder. *Journal of Consulting and Clinical Psychology* 68 (3): 489–499.

Song, F., Altman, D.G., Glenny, A-M., Deeks, J.J. (2003) Validity of indirect comparison for estimating efficacy of competing interventions: empirical evidence from published meta-analyses. *British Medical Journal* 326: 472–476.

Sourander, A., Elonheimo, H., Niemela, S., et al. (2006) Childhood predictors of male criminality: a prospective population-based follow-up study from age 8 to late adolescence. *Journal of the American Academy of Child & Adolescent Psychiatry* 45 (5): 578–586.

Spencer, T., Heiligenstein, J.H., Biederman, J., et al. (2002) Results from 2 proof-of-concept, placebo-controlled studies of atomoxetine in children with attention-deficit/hyperactivity disorder. *Journal of Clinical Psychiatry* 63 (12): 1140–1147.

Spilker, B. (1991) *Guide to clinical trials*. New York, NY: Raven Press.

Statistical Office of the European Communites (2005) *Population by age in Germany*. Available online at http://epp.eurostat.cec.eu.int.

Statistisches Landesamt Baden-Württemberg (2005) *Bevölkerung am 31.12.2004 nach Altersjahren, Nationalität und Geschlecht; Regierungsbezirk Karlsruhe*. Available online at http://www.statistik.baden-wuerttemberg.de/SRDB/.

Steele, M., Weiss, M., Swanson, J., et al. (2006) A randomized, controlled, effectiveness trial of OROS-methylphenidate compared to usual care with immediate-release-methylphenidate in Attention-Deficit-Hyperactivity-Disorder. *Canadian Journal of Clinical Pharmacology* 13 (1): e50–e62.

Steele, M., Riccardelli, R., Binder, C. (2004) *Effectiveness of OROS-methylphenidate vs. usual care with immediate release methylphenidate in ADHD children*. Presentation at the American Psychiatric Association (APA) annual meeting, New York, NY, May 1–6th.

Stewart, A., Sandercock, J., Bryan, S., et al. (2000) *The clinical effectiveness of riluzole for motor neurone disease*. Birmingham, August 1, 2000. Available online at: http://www.nice.org.uk/page.aspx?o=14479. Last Accessed February 01, 2004.

Stein, M.A. (2004) Innovations in attention-deficit/hyperactivity disorder pharmacotherapy: long-acting stimulant and nonstimulant treatments. *American Journal of Managed Care* 10 (4, Supplement): S89–S98.

Stein, M.A., Sarampote, C.S., Waldman, I.D., et al. (2003) A dose-response study of OROS methylphenidate in children with attention-deficit/hyperactivity disorder. *Pediatrics* 112: e404–e413.

Stein, M.A., Blondis, T.A., Schnitzler, E.R., et al. (1996) Methylphenidate dosing: twice daily versus three times daily. *Pediatrics* 98 (4): 748–756.

Steinhausen, H.-C., Nøvik, T.S., Baldursson, G., et al. (2006) Co-existing psychiatric problems in ADHD in the ADORE cohort. *European Child & Adolescent Psychiatry* 15 (Suppl. 1): 4–14.

Steinhoff, K. (2004) Attention-deficit/hyperactivity disorder: medication treatment-dosing and duration of action. *American Journal of Managed Care* 10 (4): S99–S106.

Steinhoff, K., Wigal, T., Swanson, J. (2003) Single daily dose ADHD medication effect size evaluation. Poster presentation, *50th Annual Meeting of the American Academy for Child and Adolescent Psychiatry*, Miami, FL, October 22–27, 2003.

Stevens, A., Milne, R. (2004) Health technology assessment in England and Wales. *International Journal of Technology Assessment in Health Care* 20 (1): 11–24.

Stewart, M., Mendelson, W., Johnson, M. (1973) Hyperactive children as adolescents: how they describe themselves. *Child Psychiatry & Human Development* 4: 3–11.

Stolk, E.A., Busschbach, J.J., Caffa, M., et al. (2000) Cost utility analysis of sildenafil compared with papaverine-phentolamine injections. *British Medical Journal* 320: 1165–1168.

Swanson, J. (2003) Compliance with stimulants for attention-deficit / hyperactivity disorder. Issues and approaches for improvement. *CNS Drugs* 17 (2): 117–131.

Swanson, J. (1992) *School-based assessments and interventions for ADD students*. Irvine, CA: K.C. Publishing.

Swanson, J.M., Wigal, S.B., Wigal, T., et al. (2004) A comparison of once-daily extended-release methylphenidate formulations in children with attention-deficit/hyperactivity disorder in the laboratory school (the Comacs study). *Pediatrics* 113: e206–e216.

Swanson, J.M., Gupta, S., Lam, A., et al. (2003) Development of a new once-a-day formulation of methylphenidate for the treatment of attention-deficit/hyperactivity disorder: proof-of-concept and proof-of-product studies. *Archives of General Psychiatry* 60 (2): 204–211.

Swanson, J.M., Kraemer, H.C., Hinshaw, S.P., et al. (2001) Clinical relevance of the primary findings of the MTA: success rates based on severity of ADHD and ODD symptoms at the end of treatment. *Journal of the American Academy of Child & Adolescent Psychiatry* 40 (2): 168–179.

Swanson, J.M., Kinsbourne, M., Roberts, W., Zucker, K. (1978) A time-response analysis of the effect of stimulant medication on the learning ability of children referred for hyperactivity. *Pediatrics* 61: 21–29.

Swensen, A., Birnbaum, H.G., Ben Hamadi, R., et al. (2004) Incidence and costs of accidents among attention-deficit/hyperactivity disorder patients. *Journal of Adolescent Health* 35 (4): 346.e1–9

Swensen, A.R., Birnbaum, H.G., Secnik, K., et al. (2003) Attention-deficit/hyperactivity disorder: increased costs for patients and their families. *Journal of the American Academy of Child & Adolescent Psychiatry* 42 (12): 1415–1423.

Taylor, E. (2006) Hyperkinetic disorders. In: Gillberg, C., Harrington, R., Steinhausen, H.-C. (eds.) *A Clinician's Handbook of Child and Adolescent Psychiatry*. Cambridge: Cambridge University Press, 489–521.

Taylor, E. (2004) ADHD is best understood as a cultural construct – against. *British Journal of Psychiatry* 184: 9.

Taylor, E. (1999) Development of clinical services for attention-deficit/ hyperactivity disorder. *Archives of General Psychiatry* 56: 1097–1099.

Taylor, E., Doepfner, M., Sergeant, J., et al. (2004) European guidelines for hyperkinetic disorder – first upgrade. *European Child & Adolescent Psychiatry* 13 (Suppl 1): 7–30.

Taylor, E., Sergeant, J., Doepfner, M., et al. (1998) Clinical guidelines for hyperkinetic disorder. *European Child & Adolescent Psychiatry* 7: 184–200.

Taylor, E., Chadwick, O., Heptinstall, E., et al. (1996) Hyperactivity and conduct problems as risk factors for adolescent development. *Journal of the American Academy of Child and Adolescent Psychiatry* 35: 1213–1226.

Taylor, E., Sandberg, S., Thorley, C., et al. (1991) *The epidemiology of childhood hyperactivity*. New York, NY: Oxford University Press.

Taylor, R. (2002) Generating national guidance: a NICE model? Presentation at the *5th International Conference on Strategic Issues in Health Care Policy, Finance, and Performance in Health Care*. St. Andrews, Scotland, April 11–13, 2002.

Technical Review Panel on the Medicare Trustees Reports (2000) *Review of the assumptions and methods of the Medicare Trustees' financial projections*. Baltimore, MD: Centers for Medicare & Medicaid Services (CMS).

Tervo, R.C., Azuma, S., Fogas, B., Fiechtner, H. (2002) Children with ADHD and motor dysfunction compared with children with ADHD only. *Developmental Medicine and Child Neurology* 44: 383–390.

Thapar, A., van den Bree, M., Fowler, T., et al. (2006) Predictors of antisocial behaviour in children with attention deficit hyperactivity disorder. *European Child & Adolescent Psychiatry* 15 (2): 118–125.

Tilden, D., Richardson, R, Nyhus, K., et al. (2005) A modelled economic evaluation of atomoxetine (Strattera) for the treatment of three patient groups with attention deficit hyperactivity disorder. *Value in Health* 8 (6): A197.

Timimi, S. (2004) ADHD is best understood as a cultural construct – for. *British Journal of Psychiatry* 184: 8–9.

Timimi, S. (2003) Inappropriate use of psychostimulants. *British Journal of Psychiatry* 183: 173.

Timimi, S. (2002) *Pathological Child Psychiatry and the Medicalization of Childhood*. Hove: Brunner-Routledge.

Torrance, G.W. (2006) Utility measurement in healthcare: the things I never got to. *Pharmacoeconomics* 24 (11): 1069–1078.

Towse, A., Pritchard, C. (2002) National Institute of Clinical Excellence (NICE): is economic appraisal working? *Pharmacoeconomics* 20 (Suppl 3): 95–105.

Towse, A., Pritchard, C., Devlin, N. (2002) *Cost-Effectiveness Thresholds: Economic and Ethical Issues*. London: King's Fund and Office of Health Economics.

Tripp, G., Luk, S.L., Schaughency, E.A., Singh, R. (1999) DSM-IV and ICD-10: a comparison of the correlates of ADHD and hyperkinetic disorder. *Journal of the American Academy of Child & Adolescent Psychiatry* 38 (2): 156–164.

Trueman, P., Drummond, M, Hutton, J. (2001) Developing guidance for budget impact analysis. *Pharmacoeconomics* 19 (6): 609–621.

Tunis, S.R. (2004) Economic analysis in healthcare decisions. *American Journal of Managed Care* 10 (5): 301–304.

Tversky, A., Kahneman, D. (1974) Judgment under uncertainty: Heuristics and biases. *Science* 185: 1124–1131.

Ubel, P.A. (2000) *Pricing Life: Why It's Time for Health Care Rationing*. Cambridge, MA, London: The MIT Press.

Ubel, P.A. (1999a) How stable are people's preferences for giving priority to severely ill patients? *Social Science & Medicine* 49 (7): 895-903.

Ubel, P.A. (1999b) The challenge of measuring community values in ways appropriate for setting health care priorities. *Kennedy Institute of Ethics Journal* 9 (3): 263–284.

Ubel, P.A., Nord, E., Gold, M.R., et al. (2000) Improving value measurement in cost-effectiveness analysis. *Medical Care* 38 (9): 892–890.

United Nations (1948) *Universal declaration of human rights*. United Nations, Resolution 217A III UN General Assembly.

Urquhart, J. (1999) Pharmacoeconomic Impact of Variable Compliance. In: Métry, J.-M., Meyer, U.A. (eds.) *Drug Regimen Compliance: Issues in Clinical Trials and Patient Management*. Chichester: John Wiley & Sons, 119–145.

Valentine, J. Zubrick, S., Sly, P. (1995) National trends in the use of stimulant medication for attention deficit hyperactivity disorder. *Journal of Paediatrics and Child Health* 32 (3): 223–227.

Vanness, D.J., Mullahy, J. (2006) Perspectives on the mean-based evaluation of health care. In: Jones, A.M. (editor) *The Elgar Companion to Health Economics*. Cheltenham: Edward Elgar, 526–536.

Vanoverbeke, N., Annemans, L., Ingham, M., Adriaenssen, I. (2003) A cost analysis of the management of attention-deficit/hyperactivity disorder (ADHD) in children in the UK. *Journal of Medical Economics* 6: 79–94.

Vitiello, B., Burke, L. (1998) Generic methylphenidate versus brand Ritalin: which should be used. In: Greenhill L, Osman B, Editors. *Ritalin: Theory and Practice*. Larchmont, NY: Mary Ann Liebert, 221–226.

Vitiello, B., Severe, J.B., Greenhill, L.L., et al. (2001) Methylphenidate dosage for children with ADHD over time under controlled conditions: lessons from the MTA. *Journal of the American Academy of Child & Adolescent Psychiatry* 40 (2): 188–196.

von Ferber, L., Lehmkuhl, G., Köster, I., et al. (2003) Methylphenidatgebrauch in Deutschland: Versichertenbezogene epidemiologische Studie über die Entwicklung von 1998 bis 2000. *Deutsches Ärzteblatt* 100 (1–2): C38–C43.

Wailoo, A, Roberts, J., Brazier, J., McCabe, C. (2004) Efficiency, equity, and NICE clinical guidelines. Clinical guidelines need a broader view than just the clinical. (Editorial) *British Medical Journal* 328: 536–537.

Walkup, J.T., Labellarte, M.J., Riddle, M.A., (2001) et al. Fluvoxamine for the treatment of anxiety disorders in children and adolescents. *New England Journal of Medicine* 344: 1279–85.

Wasson, J., Gausette, C., Whaley, F., et al. (1992) Telephone care as a substitute for routine clinical follow-up. *Journal of the American Medical Association (JAMA)* 267: 1788–1793.

Waxmonsky, J.G. (2005) Nonstimulant therapies for attention-deficit hyperactivity disorder (ADHD) in children and adults. *Essential Psychopharamcology* 6 (5): 262–276.

Weinstein, A.G. (1995) Clinical management strategies to maintain compliance in asthmatic children. *Annals of Allergy, Asthma & Immunology* 74 (4): 304–310.

Weinstein, M.C. (2006) Decision rules for incremental cost-effectiveness analysis. In: Jones, A.M. (editor) *The Elgar Companion to Health Economics*. Cheltenham: Edward Elgar, 469–478.

Weinstein, M. C., Stason, W.B. (1977) Foundations of cost-effectiveness analysis for health and medical practices. *New England Journal of Medicine* 296: 716–721.

Weinstein, M.C., Zeckhauser, R. (1973) Critical ratios and efficient allocation. *Journal of Public Economics* 2: 147–157.

Weinstein, M.C., O'Brien, B., Hornberger, J., et al. (2003) Principles of good practice for decision analytic modeling in health-care evaluation: report of the ISPOR Task Force on good research practices – modeling studies. *Value in Health* 6 (1): 9–17.

Weinstein, M.C., Toy, E.L., Sandberg, E.A., et al. (2001) Modeling for health care and other policy decisions: uses, roles, and validity. *Value in Health* 4 (5): 9–17.

Weiss, M., Gadow, K., Wasdell, M.B. (2006) Effectiveness outcomes in attention-deficit/hyperactivity disorder. *Journal of Clinical Psychiatry* 67 (Supplement 8): 38–45.

Weiss, M. Tannock, R., Kratochvil, C., et al. (2005) A randomized, placebo-controlled study of once-daily atomoxetine in the school setting in children with ADHD. *Journal of the American Academy of Child & Adolescent Psychiatry* 44 (7): 647–655.

Weiss et al. (2004) has been referenced in the Assessment Report (King et al., 2004b) as– "commercial-in-confidence – a submission [by . . .] Lilley Research Laboratories; 2004"; this reference could be identified in the public domain as Weiss et al., 2005.

Wells, K.C. (2001) Comprehensive versus matched psychosocial treatment in the MTA Study: conceptual and empirical issues. *Journal of Clinical Child Psychology* 30 (1): 131–135.

Wells, K.C., Pelham, W.E., Kotkin, R.A., et al. (2000) Psychosocial treatment strategies in the MTA Study: rationale, methods, and critical issues in design and implementation. *Journal of Abnormal Child Psychology* 28 (6): 483–505.

Wichmann, H.E., Raspe, H.H., Jöckel, K.H. [Deutsche Arbeitsgemeinschaft für Epidemiologie, DAE], and Hamm, R., Wellbrock, R. [Arbeitskreis Wissenschaft der Konferenz der Datenschutzbeauftragten des Bundes und der Länder] (1998) *Epidemiologie und Datenschutz.*

Wilby, J., Kainth, A., McDaid, C., et al. (2003) *A rapid and systematic review of the clinical effectiveness, tolerability and cost effectiveness of newer drugs for epilepsy in adults (commercial-in-confidence [CIC] data removed).* York, February 21, 2003.

Wilens, T. (2004) *Subtypes of ADHD at risk for substance abuse.* Presentation at the 157th Annual Meeting of the American Psychiatric Association; New York, NY: May 1–6, 2004.

Wilens, T.E., Biederman, J. (2006) Alcohol, drugs, and attention-deficit/hyperactivity disorder: a model for the study of addictions in youth. *Journal of Psychopharmacology* 20 (4): 580–588.

Wilens, T.E., Dodson, W. (2004) A clinical perspective of attention-deficit/hyperactivity disorder into adulthood. *Journal of Clinical Psychiatry* 65 (10): 1301–1313.

Wilens, T., Pelham, W., Stein, M., et al. (2003) ADHD treatment with once-daily OROS methylphenidate: interim 12-months results from a long-term open-label study. *Journal of the American Academy of Child & Adolescent Psychiatry* 42 (4): 424–433.

Wilensky, G.R. (2006) Developing a center for comparative effectiveness information. *Health Affairs* 25: w572–w585.

Williams, A. (2004) *What could be nicer than NICE? Annual Lecture 2004.* London: Office of Health Economics.

Williams, A. (1997) Intergenerational equity: an exploration of the 'fair innings' argument. *Health Economics* 6: 117–132.

Williams, A. (1996) QALYs and ethics: a health economist's perspective. *Social Science & Medicine* 43 (12): 1795–1804.

Wolraich, M.L., McGuinn, L., Doffing, M. (2007) Treatment of attention deficit hyperactivity disorder in children and adolescents: safety considerations. *Drug Safety* 30 (1): 17–26.

Wolraich, M.L., Wibbelsman, C.J., Brown, T.E., et al. (2005) Attention-deficit/hyperactivity disorder among adolescents: a review of diagnosis, treatment, and clinical implications. *Pediatrics* 115 (6): 1734–1746.

Wolraich, M.L., Greenhill, L.L., Pelham, W.L., et al. (2001) Randomized, controlled trial of OROS methylphenidate once a day in children with attention-deficit/hyperactivity disorder. *Pediatrics* 108 (4): 883–892.

Wolraich, M.L., Hannah, J.N., Baumgaertel, A., Feurer, I.D. (1998) Examination of DSM-IV criteria for attention deficit/hyperactivity disorder in a county-wide sample. *Journal of Developmental and Behavioral Pediatrics* 19: 162–168.

Wonder, M.J., Neville, A.M., Parsons, R. (2006) Are Australians able to access new medicines on the Pharmaceutical Benefits Scheme in a more or less timely manner? An analysis of Pharmaceutical Benefits Advisory Committee recommendations, 1999–2003. *Value in Health* 9 (4): 205–212.

Wong, I.C.K., Murray, M.L., Camilleri-Novak, D., Stephens, P. (2004) Increased prescribing trends of paediatric psychotropic medications. *Archives of Disease in Childhood* 89: 1131–1132.

World Health Organization [WHO] (2003) *Technology appraisal programme of the National Institute for Clinical Excellence. A review by WHO. June-July 2003.* Copenhagen: World

Health Organization (WHO). Available online at www.nice.org.uk/Docref.asp?d=85797. Last accessed June 30, 2004

World Health Organization [WHO] (1992) *International statistical classification of diseases and related health problems (ICD-10)*. Geneva, Switzerland: The World Health Organization, 10th edition.

Young, S., Chadwick, O., Heptinstall, E., et al. (2005) The adolescent outcome of hyperactive girls. Self-reported interpersonal relationships and coping mechanisms. *European Child & Adolescent Psychiatry* 14 (5): 245–253.

Zuckerbrot, R.A., Jensen, P.S. (2006) Improving recognition of adolescent depression in primary care. *Archives of Pediatrics & Adolescent Medicine* 160: 694–704.

Zupancic, J.A.F., Miller, A., Raina, P., et al. (1998) Economic evaluation of pharmaceutical and psychological/behavioural therapies for attention-deficit/hyperactivity disorder. In: Miller, A., Lee, S.K., Rain,. P., et al. (eds.) *A review of therapies for attention-deficit/hyperactivity disorder*. Ottawa, ON: Canadian Coordinating Office for Health Technology Assessment (CCO-HTA).

About the Author

Michael Schlander, born in Offenbach am Main (Germany) in 1959, studied medicine and psychology at the University of Frankfurt am Main, Germany (1978–1985), and has since been licensed as a physician in Germany. He also studied business administration and management at the City University of Bellevue, Washington (1992–1994, completing the postgraduate program with an M.B.A. degree as *valedictorian* of the class of 1994), and health economics at the Stockholm School of Economics (Diploma, 2002).

He spent five years in experimental brain research and clinical neurology, obtaining his M.D. (*summa cum laude*) in this field. From 1987 to 2002, he held management positions (in clinical development, as director of a strategic business unit, and as chairman of the board) with pharmaceutical companies in Germany, Belgium, and the United States.

As of 1996, he has been founding member of the Scientific Steering Committee for a postgraduate study program in pharmaceutical medicine at the Universities of Witten/Herdecke (1996–2005) and Duisburg-Essen (since 2005), both in Germany. A professor at the University of Applied Economic Sciences Ludwigshafen, Germany (since 2002), he is also serving as chairman and scientific director of the Institute for Innovation & Valuation in Health Care (InnoVal^{HC}), a not-for-profit research organization, founded in June 2005.

He is a member of numerous professional organizations, including the International Health Economics Association (iHEA), the International Society for Pharmacoeconomics and Outcomes Research (ISPOR), and the association of German-speaking economists (Verein für Socialpolitik).

www.innoval-hc.com
www.michaelschlander.com

Index

Printed in the United States of America